Fluids&Electrolytes

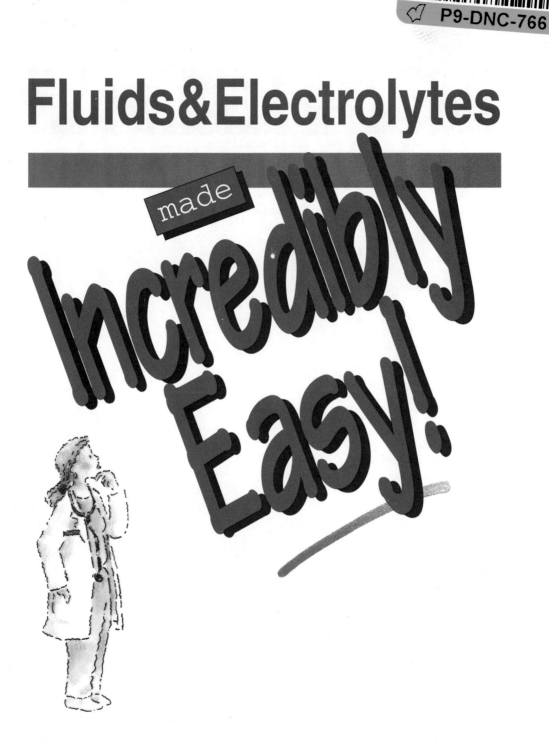

made Incredibly Easy!

Springhouse Corporation
Springhouse, Pennsylvania

Staff

Executive Director
Matthew Cahill

Editorial Director
Patricia Dwyer Schull, RN, MSN

Art Director
John Hubbard

Clinical Manager
Judith A. McCann, RN, MSN

Managing Editor
A. T. McPhee, RN, BSN

Clinical Editors
Ann M. Barrow, RN, MSN, CCRN (project manager); Joanne M. Bartelmo, RN, MSN, CCRN

Editors
Mary Lou Ambrose, Kathy E. Goldberg, Peter H. Johnson, Elizabeth Mauro, Joann Nash, Barbara L. Sabella, Michael Shaw

Copy Editors
Cynthia C. Breuninger (manager), Brenna H. Mayer, Christine Cunniffe

Designers
Arlene Putterman (associate art director), Matie Patterson (assistant art director), Lorraine Lostracco (book designer), Mary Ludwicki, Joseph Clark

Illustrators
Scott Thorn Barrows, Barbara Cousins, John Cymerman, Mark Lefkowitz, Judy Newhouse, Bot Roda, Mary Stangl, Nina Wallace, Larry Ward

Typography
Diane Paluba (manager), Joyce Rossi Biletz, Phyllis Marron, Valerie Rosenberger

Manufacturing
Deborah Meiris (director), T.A. Landis, Otto Mezei

Production Coordinator
Margaret A. Rastiello

Editorial Assistants
Carol Caputo, Beverly Lane, Mary Madden, Jeanne Napier

Indexer
Barbara Hodgson

Printed in the United States of America.

IEF&E-021197

 A member of the Reed Elsevier plc group

Library of Congress Cataloging-in Publication Date

Fluids and electrolytes made incredibly easy.
    p. cm.
    Includes index
    1. Water-electrolyte imbalances.   2. Body fluid disorders.
    I. Springhouse Corporation.
    [DNLM: 1. Water-Electrolyte Imbalance—nurses' instruction. 2. Water-Electrolyte Balance—nurses' instruction. WD 220 F6462 1997]
RC630.F596 1997
616.3'992—dc21
DNLM/DLC
ISBN 0-87434-886-2 (alk. paper)   96-47450
                                                              CIP

Contents

Contributors and consultants

Deborah Becker, RN, MSN, CCRN
Clinical Lecturer
School of Nursing
University of Pennsylvania
Philadelphia
Staff Nurse
Coronary Care Unit
The Graduate Hospital
Philadelphia

Kathleen Ellstrom, RN, MS, CS
Pulmonary Clinical Nurse Specialist
University of California, Los Angeles
Medical Center

Theresa P. Fulginiti, RN, BSN, CEN
Staff Nurse
Doylestown (Pa.) Hospital

Joyce Lyne Heise, RN, MSN
Director of Nursing
Kent State University
East Liverpool, Ohio

Luana Martindale, RN, MSN
Associate Professor
University of Arkansas at Little Rock

Karen E. Michael, RN, MSN
Manager
Concurrent Review–Case Management
QualMed Plans for
Health–Philadelphia

Barbara A. Moyer, RN, EdD
Education Nurse Specialist
Lehigh Valley Hospital
Allentown, Pa.
Assistant Professor
Allentown College of St. Francis de Sales
Center Valley, Pa.

Carol Muha-Ronneau, RN, MSN
Associate Professor
Purdue University
Westville, Ind.

Denise Netz, CRNP, MSN
Nurse Practitioner
Nazareth Hospital–St. Agnes
Medical Center
Philadelphia

Margaret R. Rateau, RN, MSN
Assistant Professor of Nursing
Kent State University
East Liverpool, Ohio

Lucille A. Rosso, RN, MSN
Independent Nurse Consultant
Columbus, N.J.

Carla Roy, RN, BSN
Staff Nurse
Medical Intensive Care Unit
The Graduate Hospital
Philadelphia

Mary Ellen Santucci, RN, MSN, CRRN
Instructor
Thomas Jefferson University
Philadelphia

Patricia P. Shoemaker, RN, MSN
Chair
Health Technology Division
Davidson County Community College
Lexington, N.C.

Dawn M. Specht, RN, MSN, CEN, CCRN, PHRN
Clinical Nurse Specialist
Cooper Health System
Camden, N.J.

Patricia D. Weiskittel, RN, MSN, CNN
Renal Clinical Nurse Specialist
University Hospital
Cincinnati

Alice Vrsan, RN, MSN, CCRN
Educational Nurse Specialist
Lehigh Valley Hospital
Allentown, Pa.

Foreword

Almost every major illness has the potential to cause fluid, electrolyte, or acid-base imbalances. Evaluating patients with those imbalances and assessing pertinent diagnostic findings can challenge even the most experienced nurse.

If you want to be able to spot fluid-and-electrolyte problems quickly and if you want to know exactly what arterial blood gas results mean, then *Fluids & Electrolytes Made Incredibly Easy* is the book for you! This reader-friendly book makes sense of the maze of lab tests, the subtle signs and symptoms of common fluid and electrolyte imbalances, and the teaching you need to do each day to help your patients prevent recurrences of the imbalances.

In a world of increasingly ill patients and increasingly difficult patient loads, you need a text that can explain complex topics clearly and easily, without making you wade through long explanations that don't directly affect bedside care. *Fluids & Electrolytes Made Incredibly Easy* is that book.

Packed with crystal-clear explanations, charts, and illustrations, the book takes you step-by-step through some of the most complex concepts in nursing today, concepts such as recognizing respiratory acidosis with metabolic compensation, understanding the clinical significance of an anion gap, and knowing why a serum calcium level should always be evaluated along with the serum albumin level.

Fluids & Electrolytes Made Incredibly Easy is organized into four sections. Part I reviews fundamental information about fluids, electrolytes, and acid-base balance. Part II covers imbalances in sodium, potassium, magnesium, calcium, phosphorus, and chloride, as well as imbalances in acids, fluids, and bases. The section explains how the body regulates fluids, electrolytes, acids, and bases; how imbalances occur; what the major causes of each imbalance are; what diagnostic tests are used to evaluate the imbalance; and what the common nursing interventions are.

Part III discusses major health problems — including congestive heart failure and respiratory failure — and the fluid, electrolyte, and acid-base imbalances associated with each. Part IV explains how to correct fluid and electrolyte imbalances. It also tells you how to recognize and treat an adverse reaction to lipid emulsions, how to identify incompatible blood types, and how to administer crystalloids through a central line, among many other topics.

The clear and easy-to-understand illustrations in each section will help you understand what really happens when a patient experiences a fluid and electrolyte imbalance. One illustration, for instance, shows step-by-step what happens during hypovolemic shock. After reviewing the illustration, you'll truly understand the complicated pathophysiology of shock. As a result, you'll be able to care more effectively for hypovolemic patients.

In addition, the book contains numerous organizational tools to help you rapidly absorb content. These tools include a summary of key chapter contents, easy-to-remember memory joggers (such as S-A-L-T, which can help you remember how to assess for signs of hypernatremia), lots of highlighted key points, and terms defined right in the text. A self-test at the end of each chapter helps you evaluate what you've learned.

Of particular interest are special logos that alert you to critical pieces of information. "Uh-oh" lists signs and symptoms to help you quickly recognize trouble. "It's not working" tells you what to do when standard interventions aren't getting results. "Chart smart" outlines all the points you'll want to document about each imbalance. "Parting points" focuses on topics you'll need to teach patients about their imbalances. And *"Now* I get it!" puts pathophysiology in a whole new, incredibly simple light.

In short, this book can help experienced and inexperienced nurses alike really understand fluid and electrolyte imbalances. Many nurses still cringe at the mere mention of a fluid or electrolyte imbalance. I remember a day when those imbalances set my own heart to jumping. Those days are gone now, thank goodness, and they can be gone for you too.

In this day of increased litigation, increased expectations of nursing knowledge, and increased complexity of patient illnesses, you need a concise, clearly written text to explain fluids and electrolytes plainly and simply. If you've been feeling the least bit insecure about caring for a patient with a fluid or electrolyte imbalance, this book is for you.

One look at *Fluids & Electrolytes Made Incredibly Easy* will make the book an important part of your clinical library and a purchase you'll never regret.

Sheri Innerarity, RN, PhD, CNS, FNP
Assistant Professor for Clinical Nursing
The University of Texas at Austin
Clinical Nurse Specialist, Adult Health and Family Nurse Practitioner
Smithville (Tex.) Internal Medicine Clinic

Part I

Balancing basics

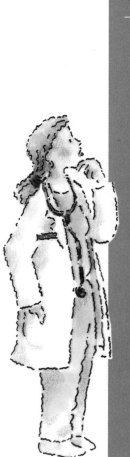

Balancing fluids

Just the facts

This chapter lays the groundwork for understanding fluids and how they're balanced by the body. Like the chapters to come, Balancing Fluids contains definitions and a list of concepts covered. In this chapter, you'll learn:

♦ how fluids are distributed throughout the body

♦ what certain fluid-related terms mean

♦ how fluid moves through the body

♦ what roles hormones and the kidneys play in fluid balance.

A look at fluids

Where would we be without body fluids? Not very far. Fluids are vital to all forms of life, help to maintain body temperature and cell shape, and are involved in transporting nutrients, gases, and wastes. Let's take a close look at fluids and how the body balances them.

Making gains = losses

The skin, the lungs, the kidneys — just about all major organs — work together to maintain the proper balance of fluid. To maintain that balance, the amount of fluid gained throughout the day must equal the amount lost. Some of those losses can be measured; others can't.

It's insensible

Fluid losses from the skin and the lungs are referred to as insensible losses because they can't be measured or seen.

Losses from the evaporation of fluid through the skin are fairly constant but depend on the person's body surface area. For example, the body surface area of an infant is greater than that of an adult relative to their respective weights. As a result, infants typically lose more water from their skin than adults.

Changes in humidity levels affect the amount of fluid lost through the skin. Likewise, respiratory rate and depth affect the amount of fluid lost through the lungs. Tachypnea, for example, causes more water to be lost; bradypnea causes less. Fever increases insensible losses of fluid from both the skin and the lungs.

Now that's sensible

Losses of fluid that can be measured are referred to as sensible losses. Sensible losses include fluids lost through urination, defecation, wounds, perspiration, and other means.

A typical adult loses 100 ml to 200 ml of fluid per day through defecation. In cases of severe diarrhea, losses may exceed 5,000 ml a day. (For more information about sensible and insensible losses, see *Sites involved in fluid loss,* page 4.)

Where has all the fluid gone?

The body holds fluid in two basic areas, or compartments — inside the cells and outside them. Fluid found inside the cells is called intracellular fluid. Fluid found outside the cells is called extracellular fluid. Capillary walls and cell membranes separate the intracellular and extracellular compartments. (See *Fluid compartments.*)

To maintain proper fluid balance, the distribution of fluid between the two compartments must remain relatively constant. In an adult, the total amount of intracellular fluid averages 40% of the person's body weight, or about 28 L. The total amount of extracellular fluid averages 20% of the person's body weight, or about 14 L.

Extracellular fluid can be broken down further into interstitial fluid, which surrounds the cells, and intravascular fluid or plasma, which is the liquid portion of blood. In an adult, interstitial fluid accounts for the majority of extracellular fluid, about 75%. Plasma accounts for the remaining 25%.

The body contains other fluids, called transcellular fluids, in the cerebrospinal column, the pleural cavity, the

Fluid compartments

This illustration shows the three primary fluid compartments in the body — intracellular, interstitial, and intravascular. Intracellular fluids are separated from interstitial and intravascular fluids (extracellular fluids) by capillary walls and cell membranes.

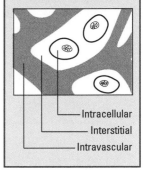

Intracellular
Interstitial
Intravascular

Memory jogger

To help you remember which fluid belongs to which compartment, keep in mind that "inter" means between (as in interval — between two events) and "intra" means within or inside (as in intravenous — inside a vein)

Sites involved in fluid loss

Each day the body gains and loses fluid through several different processes. The illustration here shows the primary sites involved and normal daily fluid losses. Gastric, intestinal, pancreatic, and biliary secretions are almost completely reabsorbed and aren't usually counted in daily fluid gains and losses.

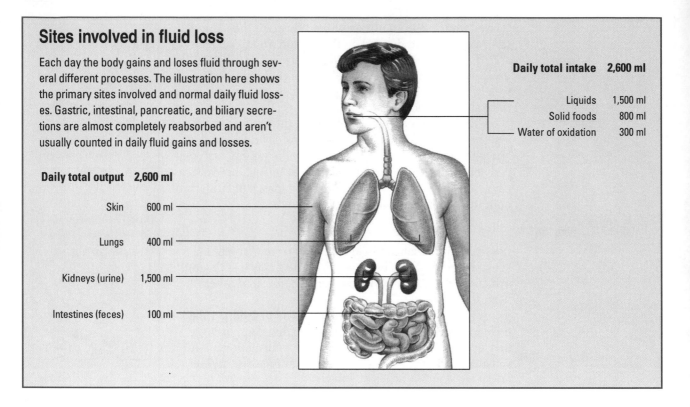

Daily total intake	2,600 ml
Liquids	1,500 ml
Solid foods	800 ml
Water of oxidation	300 ml

Daily total output	2,600 ml
Skin	600 ml
Lungs	400 ml
Kidneys (urine)	1,500 ml
Intestines (feces)	100 ml

lymph system, the joints, and the eyes. Transcellular fluids are generally not subject to significant gains and losses throughout the day, however, so they won't be covered here.

Water here, water there

The distribution of fluid within the body's compartments varies with age. Compared with adults, infants have a greater percentage of body water stored inside interstitial spaces. About 80% of the body weight of a full-term neonate consists of water. About 90% of the body weight of a premature infant is water. The amount of water as a percentage of body weight decreases with age until the person reaches puberty. In a typical 154-lb (70-kg) lean adult male, 60% or about 93 lb (42 kg) of body weight is water.

Skeletal muscle cells hold much of that water; fat cells contain little of it. Women, who normally have a higher ratio of fat to skeletal muscle than men, typically have a somewhat lower relative water content. Likewise, an obese person may have a relative water content level as low as 45%. Accumulated body fat in these individuals increases weight without boosting the body's water content. That's why, if an obese patient gains or loses a significant amount of fluid, he stands a greater-than-average risk of suffering a fluid imbalance.

Older, but drier

The risk of suffering a fluid imbalance also increases with age. As a person ages, skeletal muscle mass declines and the proportion of fat within the body increases. After age 60, water content drops to about 45%.

Likewise, the distribution of fluid within the body changes with age. For instance, about 15% of a typical young adult's total body weight is made up of interstitial fluid. That percentage progressively decreases with age.

About 5% of the body's total fluid volume is made up of plasma. Plasma volume remains stable throughout life.

Fluids and their movements

Fluids in the body generally aren't found in pure forms. They're most often found in three different types of solutions: isotonic, hypotonic, and hypertonic.

Meet Iso "the Match" Tonic

An isotonic solution has the same solute concentration as another solution. For instance, if two fluids in adjacent compartments are equally concentrated, they're already in balance so the fluid inside each compartment stays put. No imbalance means no net fluid shift. (See *Isotonic fluids.*)

For example, normal saline solution is considered isotonic because the concentration of sodium in the solution nearly equals the concentration of sodium in the blood.

Meet Hypo "Low-Low" Tonic

A hypotonic solution has a lower solute concentration than another solution. For instance, say one solution contains only a little sodium and another solution contains more. The first solution is hypotonic, compared with the second solution. As a result, fluid from the first solution — the hypotonic solution — would shift into the second solution until the two solutions had equal concentrations. (See

Isotonic fluids

No net fluid shifts occur between isotonic solutions because the solutions are equally concentrated.

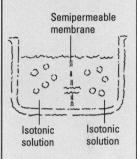

Semipermeable membrane

Isotonic solution   Isotonic solution

Hypotonic fluids

When a less concentrated, or hypotonic, solution is placed next to a more concentrated solution, fluid shifts from the hypotonic solution into the more concentrated compartment to equalize concentrations.

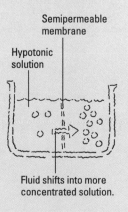

Semipermeable membrane

Hypotonic solution

Fluid shifts into more concentrated solution.

Hypotonic fluids.) Remember that the body constantly strives to maintain a state of balance, or equilibrium.

Half-normal saline solution is considered hypotonic because the concentration of sodium in the solution is lower than the concentration of sodium in the patient's blood.

Meet Hyper "Over the Top" Tonic

A hypertonic solution has a higher solute concentration than another solution. For instance, say one solution contains a large amount of sodium and a second solution contains hardly any. The first solution is hypertonic compared to the second solution.

As a result, fluid would be drawn from the second solution into the first solution — the hypertonic solution — until the two solutions had equal concentrations. (See *Hypertonic fluids.*) Again, the body constantly strives to maintain a state of equilibrium.

For instance, a solution of dextrose 5% in normal saline is considered hypertonic because the concentration of solutes in the solution is greater than the concentration of solutes in the patient's blood.

Fluid movement

Just as the heart beats constantly, fluids and solutes move constantly within the body. That movement allows the body to maintain homeostasis, the constant state of balance the body seeks. (See *Fluid tips.*)

Movement within the cells

Solutes within the various compartments of the body (intracellular, interstitial, and intravascular) move through the membranes separating those compartments in different ways. The membranes are semipermeable, meaning that they allow some solutes to pass through, but not others. Here are the different ways fluids and solutes move through membranes at the cellular level.

Diffusion goes with the flow

In diffusion, solutes move from an area of higher concentration to an area of lower concentration, which eventually results in an equal distribution of solutes within the two areas. Diffusion is a form of passive transport because no energy is required to make it happen; it just happens. It's

---

Hypertonic fluids

If one solution is more solute concentrated than an adjacent solution, it has less fluid relative to the adjacent solution. Fluid will move out of the less concentrated solution into the more concentrated, or hypertonic, solution until both solutions are equal in concentration of solutes and fluid.

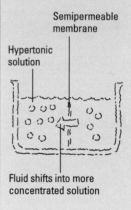

Semipermeable membrane

Hypertonic solution

Fluid shifts into more concentrated solution

Now I get it!

Fluid tips

Fluids, nutrients, and waste products constantly shift within the body's compartments—from the cells to the interstitial spaces to the blood vessels and back again. A change in one compartment can affect all of the others.

That continuous fluid shifting can have important implications for your nursing care. For instance, if you give a hypotonic fluid to a patient, it may cause too much fluid to move from the veins into the cells. As a result, the cells can swell.

Conversely, if you give a hypertonic solution to a patient, it may cause too much fluid to be pulled from cells into the bloodstream, and the cells can shrink.

For more information about I.V. solutions, see Chapter 18.

Diffusion

Solutes move from areas of higher concentration to areas of lower concentration until their concentration is equal in both areas.

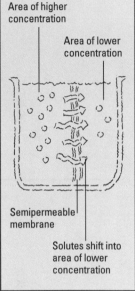

Area of higher concentration

Area of lower concentration

Semipermeable membrane

Solutes shift into area of lower concentration

kind of like fish traveling downstream. They just go with the flow. (See *Diffusion*.)

Actively transporting

In active transport, solutes move from an area of lower concentration to an area of higher concentration. Think of active transport as swimming upstream. When a fish swims upstream, it has to expend energy, which it gets from food.

The energy required for a solute to move against a concentration gradient comes from a substance called adenosine triphosphate, or ATP. Stored in all cells, ATP supplies energy for solute movement in and out of cells. (See *Active transport*, page 8.)

Some solutes, such as sodium and potassium, use ATP to move in and out of cells in a form of active transport called the sodium-potassium pump. (For more information on this physiologic pump, see Chapter 5.) Other solutes that require active transport to cross cell membranes include calcium ions, hydrogen ions, amino acids, and certain sugars.

Osmosis lets fluids through

Osmosis refers to the passive movement of fluid across a membrane from an area of lower solute concentration and comparatively more fluid into an area of higher solute concentration and comparatively less fluid. Osmosis stops when enough fluid has moved through the membrane to

Active transport

In active transport, energy from a molecule called adenosine triphosphate (ATP) moves solutes from an area of lower concentration to an area of higher concentration, an action opposite that of diffusion.

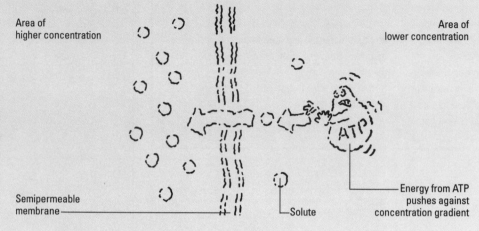

Area of higher concentration

Area of lower concentration

Energy from ATP pushes against concentration gradient

Semipermeable membrane

Solute

Osmosis

In osmosis, fluid moves passively from an area with more fluid (and fewer solutes) to one with less fluid (and *more* solutes). Remember that in osmosis fluid moves, not solutes.

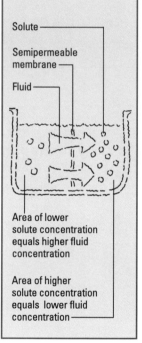

Solute

Semipermeable membrane

Fluid

Area of lower solute concentration equals higher fluid concentration

Area of higher solute concentration equals lower fluid concentration

equalize the solute concentration on both sides of the membrane. (See *Osmosis*.)

Movement within the vascular system

Within the vascular system, only capillaries have walls thin enough to let solutes pass through. The movement of fluids and solutes through the walls of the body's capillaries plays a critical role in fluid balance.

The pressure is on

The movement of fluids through capillaries — a process called capillary filtration — results from blood pushing against the walls of the capillary. That pressure, called hydrostatic (or "fluid-pushing") pressure, forces fluids and solutes through the capillary wall.

When the hydrostatic pressure inside a capillary is greater than the pressure in the surrounding interstitial space, fluids and solutes inside the capillary are forced out into the interstitial space. When the pressure inside the capillary is less than the pressure outside of it, fluids and solutes move back into the capillary. (See *Hydrostatic pressure*.)

Keeping the fluid in

A process called reabsorption prevents too much fluid from leaving the capillaries, no matter how much hydrostatic pressure exists within the capillaries. When fluid filters through a capillary, the protein albumin remains behind in the diminishing volume of water. Albumin is a large molecule that normally can't pass through capillary membranes. As the concentration of albumin inside a capillary increases, fluid begins to move back into the capillaries through osmosis.

Think of albumin as a "water magnet." The osmotic, or pulling, force of albumin in the intravascular space is referred to as the plasma colloid osmotic pressure (COP). The plasma COP in capillaries averages about 25 mm Hg. (See *Albumin*.)

As long as capillary blood pressure (the hydrostatic pressure) exceeds plasma COP, water and solutes can leave the capillaries and enter the interstitial fluid. When capillary blood pressure falls below plasma COP, water and diffusible solutes return to the capillaries.

Normally, blood pressure in a capillary exceeds plasma COP in the arteriole end and falls below it in the venule end. As a result, capillary filtration occurs along the first half of the vessel; reabsorption, along the second half. As long as capillary blood pressure and plasma albu-

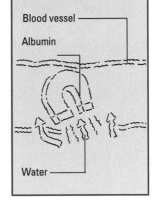

Albumin

Albumin, a large protein molecule, acts like a magnet to attract water and hold it inside the blood vessel.

Blood vessel —

Albumin

Water —

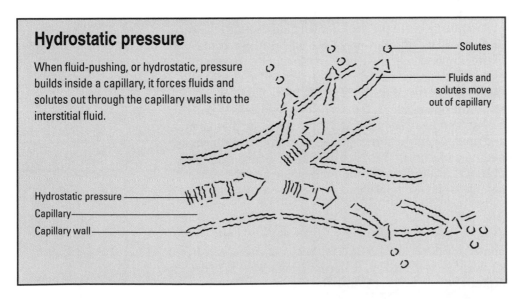

Hydrostatic pressure

When fluid-pushing, or hydrostatic, pressure builds inside a capillary, it forces fluids and solutes out through the capillary walls into the interstitial fluid.

Solutes

Fluids and solutes move out of capillary

Hydrostatic pressure ——

Capillary ——

Capillary wall ——

min levels remain normal, the amount of water that moves into the vessel equals the amount that moves out.

Occasionally, extra fluid filters out of the capillary. When that happens, the excess fluid shifts into the lymphatic vessels located just outside the capillaries and eventually returns to the heart for recirculation.

Maintaining the balance

A number of body processes work together to maintain fluid balance. A problem in any of those processes can affect the entire fluid-maintenance system. Here's a closer look at those processes.

Role of the kidneys

The kidneys play a vital role in fluid balance. If the kidneys don't work properly, the body has great difficulty controlling fluid balance. The workhorse of the kidney is the nephron, which forms urine. The body puts the nephrons through their paces every day. (See *Typical nephron*.)

A nephron consists of a glomerulus and a tubule. The tubule, sometimes convoluted, ends in a collecting duct. The glomerulus is a cluster of capillaries that filter blood. Like a vascular cradle, Bowman's capsule surrounds the glomerulus.

Capillary blood pressure forces fluid through the capillary walls and into Bowman's capsule at the proximal end of the tubule. Along the length of the tubule, water and electrolytes are either excreted or retained according to the body's needs. If the body needs more fluid, for instance, it retains more. If it needs less fluid, less is reabsorbed and more is excreted. Electrolytes, such as sodium and potassium, are either filtered or reabsorbed throughout the same area. The resulting filtrate, which eventually becomes urine, flows through the tubule into the collecting ducts and eventually into the bladder as urine.

Superabsorbent

The nephrons filter blood at a rate of about 125 ml/minute, or about 180 L/day. That rate, called the glomerular filtration rate leads to the production of 1 to 2 L/day of urine. The nephrons reabsorb the remaining 178 L or

Typical nephron

The nephron (shown here) filters blood and excretes excess solutes, electrolytes, fluids, and metabolic waste products while keeping blood composition and volume constant.

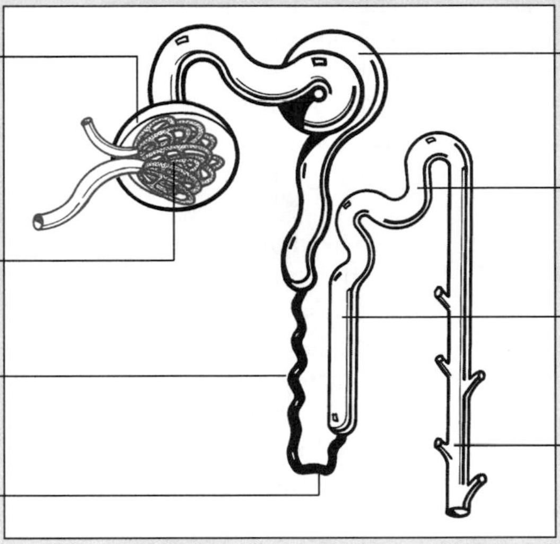

Bowman's capsule — Proximal tubule

Distal tubule

Glomerulus — Ascending limb

Descending limb — Collecting duct

Loop of Henle —

more of fluid, an amount equivalent to more than 30 oil changes for the family car!

Conserve, conserve, conserve

If the body loses even 1% or 2% of its fluid, the kidneys take steps to conserve water. Perhaps the most important step involves reabsorbing more water from the filtrate, which forms a more concentrated urine.

The kidneys must continue to excrete at least 20 ml/hour of urine (500 ml/day) to eliminate body wastes. A urinary excretion rate below 20 ml/hour usually indicates renal pathology.

The minimum excretion rate varies with age. Infants and young children excrete urine at a higher rate than adults because their higher metabolic rates produce more waste. In addition, an infant's kidneys can't concentrate urine until about age 3 months and remain less efficient than an adult's kidneys until about age 2 years.

The kidneys respond to fluid excesses by excreting a more dilute urine, which rids the body of fluid and conserves electrolytes.

Antidiuretic hormone

Several hormones affect fluid balance, among them a water retainer called antidiuretic hormone (ADH). (You may also hear the hormone called "vasopressin.") The hypothalamus produces ADH, but the posterior pituitary gland stores and releases it. If you can remember what ADH stands for, you can remember its job — to restore blood volume by reducing diuresis and increasing water retention. (See *How antidiuretic hormone works.*)

Sensitive to changes

Increased serum osmolality or decreased blood volume stimulates the release of ADH, which in turn increases the reabsorption of water by the kidneys. The increased reabsorption of water results in more concentrated urine.

Likewise, decreased serum osmolality or increased blood volume inhibits the release of ADH and causes less water to be reabsorbed, making the urine less concentrated. The amount of ADH released varies throughout the day, depending on needs.

This up-and-down cycle of ADH release keeps fluid levels in balance all day long. Like a dam on a river, the body holds water when fluid levels drop and releases it when fluid levels rise.

How antidiuretic hormone works

Antidiuretic hormone (ADH) regulates fluid balance through a series of steps, outlined here.

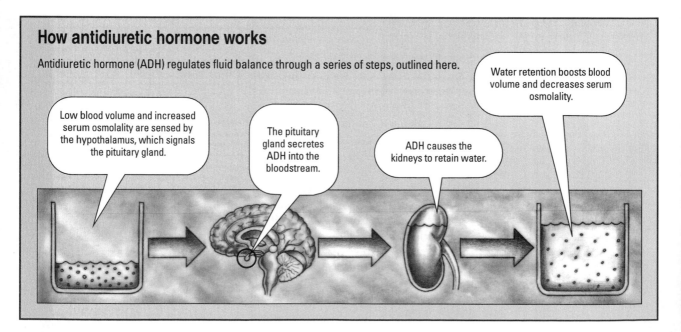

Low blood volume and increased serum osmolality are sensed by the hypothalamus, which signals the pituitary gland.

The pituitary gland secretes ADH into the bloodstream.

ADH causes the kidneys to retain water.

Water retention boosts blood volume and decreases serum osmolality.

Renin and angiotensin

To help maintain a balance of sodium and water in the body, as well as to maintain a healthy blood volume and blood pressure, special cells (called juxtaglomerular cells) near each glomerulus secrete an enzyme called renin. Through a complex series of steps, renin leads to the production of angiotensin II, a powerful vasoconstrictor. (See *Renin-angiotensin system*.)

Angiotensin II causes peripheral vasoconstriction and stimulates the production of aldosterone. Both actions raise blood pressure.

As soon as the blood pressure reaches a normal level, the body stops releasing renin and this feedback cycle of renin to angiotensin to aldosterone stops.

Renin ups and downs

The amount of renin secreted depends on blood flow and the level of sodium in the bloodstream. If blood flow to the kidneys diminishes, as happens in a patient who's hemorrhaging, or if the amount of sodium reaching the

Renin-angiotensin system

This illustration shows the steps involved in the production of aldosterone (a hormone that helps to regulate fluid balance) through the renin-angiotensin system.

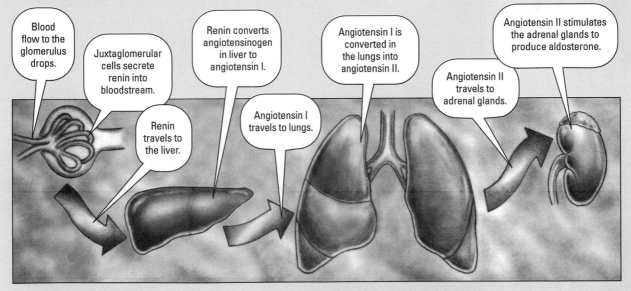

glomerulus drops, the juxtaglomerular cells secrete more renin. The renin causes vasoconstriction and a subsequent increase in blood pressure.

Conversely, if blood flow to the kidneys increases, or if the amount of sodium reaching the glomerulus increases, juxtaglomerular cells secrete less renin. A drop-off in renin secretion reduces vasoconstriction and helps to normalize blood pressure.

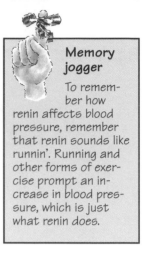

Memory jogger

To remember how renin affects blood pressure, remember that renin sounds like runnin'. Running and other forms of exercise prompt an increase in blood pressure, which is just what renin does.

Aldosterone

Like the renin-angiotensin system, a hormone called aldosterone also plays a role in maintaining blood pressure and fluid balance. Secreted by the adrenal cortex, aldosterone regulates the reabsorption of sodium and water within the nephron. (See *How aldosterone works*.)

When blood volume drops, aldosterone initiates the active transport of sodium from the distal tubules and the collecting ducts into the bloodstream. That active transport forces sodium back into the bloodstream. When sodium is forced into the bloodstream, more water is reabsorbed and blood volume expands.

How aldosterone works

Aldosterone, produced as a result of the renin-angiotensin system, acts to regulate fluid volume as described below.

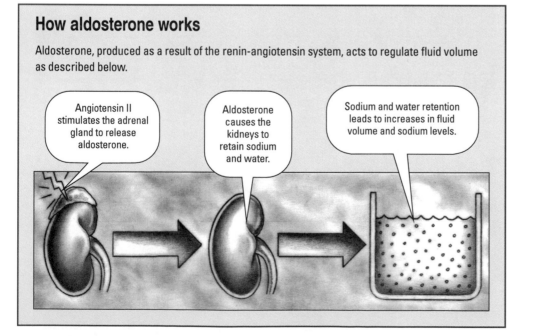

Atrial natriuretic peptide

Aldosterone and the renin-angiotensin system aren't the only processes that maintain fluid balance. A cardiac hormone called atrial natriuretic peptide (ANP) also helps keep that balance. Stored in the cells of the atria, ANP is released when atrial pressure increases. The hormone opposes the renin-angiotensin system by decreasing blood pressure and reducing intravascular blood volume. (See *How atrial natriuretic peptide works.*)

This powerful hormone:
- suppresses serum renin levels
- decreases aldosterone release by the adrenal glands
- increases glomerular filtration, which increases urinary excretion of sodium and water
- decreases ADH release by the posterior pituitary gland
- reduces vascular resistance by causing vasodilation.

Stretch that atrium

The amount of ANP released by the atria rises in response to a number of conditions, including chronic renal failure and congestive heart failure.

How atrial natriuretic peptide works

When blood volume and blood pressure rise and begin to stretch the atria, the heart's atrial natriuretic peptide (ANP) "shuts off" the renin-angiotensin system, which keeps blood volume and blood pressure stable.

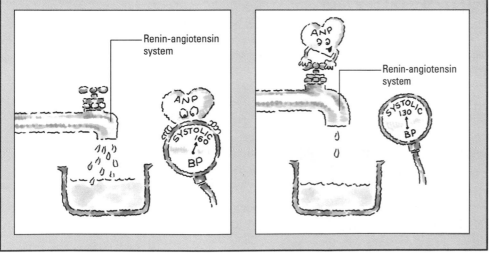

Conditions that cause atrial stretching can also lead to increases in the amount of ANP released. Those conditions include postural changes, atrial tachycardia, high sodium intake, infusions of sodium chloride, and use of drugs that cause vasoconstriction.

Thirst

Perhaps the simplest mechanism for maintaining balance is the thirst mechanism. Thirst occurs as a result of even small losses of fluid. Losing body fluids or eating highly salty foods leads to an increase in extracellular fluid osmolality. This increase leads to the drying of mucus membranes in the mouth, which in turn stimulates the thirst center in the hypothalamus.

In an elderly person, the thirst mechanism is less effective than it is in a younger person, leaving the older person more prone to dehydration.

Quenching that thirst

Normally, when a person is thirsty, he drinks fluid. The ingested fluid is absorbed from the intestine into the bloodstream, where it moves freely between fluid compartments. This movement leads to an increase in the amount of fluid in the body and a decrease in the concentration of solutes, thus balancing fluid levels throughout the body.

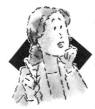

Quick quiz!

1. If you were walking across the Sahara Desert with an empty canteen, the amount of ADH secreted would most likely:

    A. increase.

    B. decrease.

    C. stay the same.

Answer: A. Since your body would most likely be dehydrated, it would try to retain as much fluid as possible. To retain fluid, the amount of ADH secreted would increase.

2. If you placed two containers next to each other, separated only by a semipermeable membrane, and the solu-

tion in one container was hypotonic relative to the other, fluid in the hypotonic container would:
- A. move out of the hypotonic container into the other.
- B. pull fluid from the other container into the hypotonic container.
- C. stay unchanged within the hypotonic container.

Answer: A. Fluid would move out of the hypotonic container into the other container to equalize the concentration of fluid within the two containers.

3. Hydrostatic pressure, which pushes fluid out of the capillaries, is opposed by colloid osmotic pressure, which involves:
- A. reduced renin secretion.
- B. the pulling power of albumin to reabsorb water.
- C. an increase in the amount of ADH released.

Answer: B. Albumin in capillaries draws water toward it, a process called reabsorption.

4. When a person's blood pressure drops, the kidneys respond by:
- A. secreting renin.
- B. producing aldosterone.
- C. slowing the release of antidiuretic hormone.

Answer: A. Juxtaglomerular cells in the kidneys secrete renin in response to low blood flow or a low sodium level. The eventual effect of renin secretion is an increase in blood pressure.

5. Giving a hypertonic I.V. solution to a patient may cause too much fluid to be:
- A. pulled from the cells into the bloodstream.
- B. pulled out of the bloodstream into the cells.
- C. pushed out of the bloodstream into the extravascular spaces.

Answer: A. Because the concentration of solutes in the I.V. solution is greater than the concentration of solutes in the patient's blood, a hypertonic solution may cause fluid to be pulled from the cells into the bloodstream.

Scoring

☆☆☆   If you answered all five questions correctly, congratulations! You're a fluid whiz.

☆☆   If you answered three or four questions correctly, take a swig of water; you're just a little dry.

☆   If you answered fewer than three questions correctly, pour yourself a glass of sports drink and and enjoy an invigorating burst of fluid refreshment!

Balancing electrolytes

Just the facts

In this chapter, you'll learn:

♦ what the difference is between cations and anions

♦ what normal and abnormal serum electrolyte results are

♦ what role nephrons play in electrolyte balance

♦ how and where diuretics affect electrolytes in the kidney

♦ what concentration of electrolytes are found in selected I.V. fluids.

A look at electrolytes

Electrolytes work with fluids to maintain health and well-being. They can be found in various concentrations, depending on whether they're inside or outside the cells. Electrolytes are crucial for nearly all cellular reactions and for controlling cell functions. Let's take a look at what electrolytes are, how they function, and what upsets their balance.

Defining electrolytes

Electrolytes are substances that, when in solution, separate (or dissociate) into electrically charged particles called ions. Some ions are positively charged; others, negatively charged. Several pairs of opposite-charged ions are so closely linked that a problem with one ion causes a problem with the other. Sodium and chloride are linked that way, as are calcium and phosphorus.

The normal balance of electrolytes in the body can be offset by a wide variety of diseases. Understanding electrolytes and recognizing their imbalances makes patient assessment more accurate.

Anions and cations

Anions are electrolytes that generate a negative charge. Cations are electrolytes that generate a positive charge. An electrical charge makes cells function normally. Chloride, phosphorus, and bicarbonate are anions; sodium, potassium, calcium, and magnesium are cations.

The anion gap reflects serum anion-cation balance. The test is useful in distinguishing types and causes of acid-base imbalances. (The anion gap is discussed in Chapter 3.)

Keeping those +'s and -'s balanced

Electrolytes operate outside the cell in extracellular fluid compartments and inside the cell in intracellular fluid compartments. Individual electrolytes differ in concentration, but electrolyte totals balance to achieve a neutral electrical charge (positives and negatives balance each other). This is called electroneutrality.

Interacting electrolytes

Most electrolytes interact with hydrogen ions to maintain acid-base balance. The major electrolytes have specialized functions that contribute to metabolism and fluid and electrolyte balance.

Major electrolytes outside the cell

Sodium and chloride, the major electrolytes in extracellular fluid, exert most of their effects outside the cell. Sodium concentration makes a major contribution to serum osmolality (solute concentration in a solution) and to extracellular fluid volume. Sodium also helps nerve and muscle cells interact. Chloride helps maintain osmotic pressure (water-pulling pressure). Gastric mucosal cells need chloride to produce hydrochloric acid, which breaks down food into absorbable components.

Calcium and bicarbonate are two other electrolytes found in extracellular fluid. Calcium is the major cation involved in the structure and function of bones and teeth and is needed to:

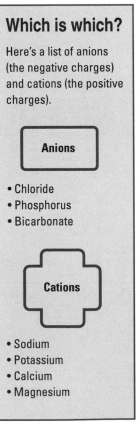

Memory jogger
To remind yourself about the difference between anions and cations, remember that the "t" in "cation" looks like the positive symbol, "+."

Which is which?

Here's a list of anions (the negative charges) and cations (the positive charges).

Anions

• Chloride
• Phosphorus
• Bicarbonate

Cations

• Sodium
• Potassium
• Calcium
• Magnesium

- stabilize the cell membrane and reduce its permeability to sodium
- transmit nerve impulses
- contract muscles
- coagulate blood
- form bone and teeth.

Major electrolytes inside the cell

Potassium, phosphate, and magnesium are among the most abundant electrolytes inside the cell.

The body contains phosphorus in the form of phosphate salts. *Sometimes the words phosphorus and phosphate are used interchangeably.*

Potassium plays an important role in:
- the regulation of cell excitability
- nerve impulse conduction
- resting membrane potential
- muscle contraction and myocardial membrane responsiveness
- control of intracellular osmolality.

Phosphate is also essential for energy metabolism. Combined with calcium, phosphate has a key role in the mineralization of bones and teeth. It also helps maintain acid-base balance.

Magnesium acts as a catalyst for enzyme reactions. It regulates neuromuscular contraction, promotes normal functioning of the nervous and cardiovascular systems, and aids in protein synthesis and sodium and potassium ion transportation.

Electrolyte movement

When cells die (for example, from trauma or chemotherapy), their contents spill into the extracellular area and upset the balance. In this case, elevated levels of intracellular electrolytes, such as phosphorus and potassium, are found in plasma.

Although electrolytes are concentrated in one compartment or another, they're not locked or frozen in these areas. Just like fluids, electrolytes move about trying to maintain balance and electroneutrality.

What affects electrolyte balance

Electrolytes function in the body both individually and in relation to other electrolytes. Imbalances in one electrolyte often affect the balance of others. (See *Understanding electrolytes.*)

Electrolyte balance is influenced by fluid intake and output, acid-base balance, hormone secretion, and normal cell functioning.

Measuring serum levels

Even though electrolytes exist inside and outside the cell, only the levels outside the cell (in the bloodstream) are measured. Serum levels stay fairly stable throughout a person's lifespan. However, you need to understand which level is normal and which is abnormal in order to react quickly and appropriately to a patient's electrolyte imbalance.

The patient's condition determines how often electrolyte levels are checked. Lab results are often reported in milliequivalents per liter (mEq/L)—a measure of the ion's chemical activity or its power. (See *Recognizing serum electrolyte results,* page 24, for a look at normal and abnormal electrolyte levels in the blood.)

See the whole picture

When you see an abnormal lab result, apply it to what you know about the patient. For instance, a potassium level of 7 mEq/L reported on a patient with previously normal potassium levels and no apparent reason for the increase may be an inaccurate result. Perhaps the patient's blood sample was hemolyzed from trauma to the cells. Look at the whole picture. Review what you know about the patient, his symptoms, and electrolyte levels before acting. (See *Documenting electrolyte imbalances.*)

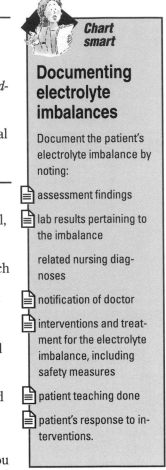

Chart smart

Documenting electrolyte imbalances

Document the patient's electrolyte imbalance by noting:

- assessment findings
- lab results pertaining to the imbalance
- related nursing diagnoses
- notification of doctor
- interventions and treatment for the electrolyte imbalance, including safety measures
- patient teaching done
- patient's response to interventions.

Fluid regulation

Many activities and factors are involved in regulating fluid and electrolyte balance. A quick review of some of the basics will help you understand this regulation better.

Understanding electrolytes

Electrolytes help regulate water distribution, govern acid-base balance, and transmit nerve impulses. They also contribute to energy generation and blood clotting. This table summarizes what the body's major electrolytes do. Check the illustration below to see how electrolytes are distributed in and around the cell.

Potassium (K)
- The dominant cation in intracellular fluid (ICF)
- Regulates cell excitability
- Permeates cell membranes, thereby affecting the cell's electrical status
- Helps to control ICF osmolality and, consequently, ICF osmotic pressure

Magnesium (Mg)
- A leading ICF cation
- Contributes to many enzymatic and metabolic processes, particularly protein synthesis
- Modifies nerve impulse transmission and skeletal muscle response. (Unbalanced Mg concentrations dramatically affect neuromuscular processes.)

Phosphorus (P)
- The major ICF anion
- Promotes energy storage and carbohydrate, protein, and fat metabolism
- Acts as a hydrogen buffer

Sodium (Na)
- The main extracellular fluid (ECF) cation

- Helps govern normal ECF osmolality (A shift in Na concentrations triggers a fluid volume change to restore normal solute and water ratios.)
- Helps maintain acid-base balance
- Activates nerve and muscle cells
- Influences water distribution (with chloride)

Chloride (Cl)
- The main ECF anion
- Helps maintain normal ECF osmolality
- Affects body pH
- Plays a vital role in maintaining acid-base balance; combines with hydrogen ions to produce hydrochloric acid

Calcium (Ca)
- A major cation in teeth and bones; found in fairly equal concentrations in ICF and ECF
- Also found in cell membranes, where it helps cells adhere to one another and maintain their shape
- Acts as an enzyme activator within cells (Muscles must have Ca to contract.)
- Aids coagulation
- Affects cell membrane permeability and firing level

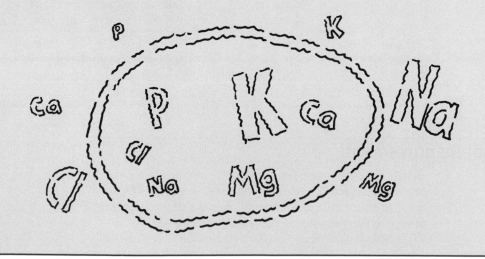

Recognizing serum electrolyte results

Use the quick-reference chart below to interpret serum electrolyte results in adult patients. This chart also lists some disorders that can cause imbalances.

Electrolyte	Results	Implications	Common causes
Serum sodium	135 to 145 mEq/L	Normal	
	<135 mEq/L	Hyponatremia	Syndrome of inappropriate antidiuretic hormone secretion
	>145 mEq/L	Hypernatremia	Diabetes inspidus
Serum potassium	3.5 to 5 mEq/L	Normal	
	< 3.5 mEq/L	Hypokalemia	Diarrhea
	> 5 mEq/L	Hyperkalemia	Burns
Total serum calcium	8.9 to 10.1 mg/dL	Normal	
	< 8.9 mg/dL	Hypocalcemia	Acute pancreatitis
	>10.1 mg/dL	Hypercalcemia	Hyperparathyroidism
Ionized calcium	4.5 to 5.1 mg/dL	Normal	
	< 4.5 mg/dL	Hypocalcemia	Massive transfusion
	> 5.1 mg/dL	Hypercalcemia	Acidosis
Serum phosphorous	2.5 to 4.5 mg/dL or 1.8 to 2.6 mEq/L	Normal	
	< 2.5 mg/dL or 1.8 mEq/L	Hypophosphatemia	Diabetic ketoacidosis
	> 4.5 mg/dL or 2.6 mEq/L	Hyperphosphatemia	Renal insufficiency
Serum magnesium	1.5 to 2.5 mEq/L	Normal	
	<1.5 mEq/L	Hypomagnesemia	Malnutrition
	>2.5 mEq/L	Hypermagnesemia	Renal failure
Serum chloride	96 to 106 mEq/L	Normal	
	< 96 mEq/L	Hypochloremia	Prolonged vomiting
	>106 mEq/L	Hyperchloremia	Hypernatremia

Fluid and solute movement

Active transport moves solutes upstream and requires physiologic (body) pumps to move the substances from areas of lesser concentration to areas of higher concentration — against a concentration gradient. Adenosine triphosphate is the energy that moves solutes upstream.

The sodium-potassium pump, an example of active transport, moves sodium ions from intracellular fluid (an area of lesser concentration) to extracellular fluid (an area of greater concentration). With potassium, the reverse happens: A large amount of potassium in intracellular fluid causes an electrical potential at the cell membrane. As ions rapidly shift in and out of the cell, electrical impulses are conducted. These impulses are essential for maintaining life.

Organ and gland involvement

Most major organs and glands in the body—the lungs, liver, adrenal glands, heart, hypothalamus, pituitary gland, skin, GI tract, and kidneys—help to regulate fluid and electrolyte balance. As part of the renin-angiotensin system, the lungs and liver help regulate sodium and water balance as well as blood pressure. The adrenal glands secrete aldosterone, which keeps sodium in the kidneys and affects potassium levels. These levels are affected because the kidneys excrete potassium, or hydrogen ions, in exchange for retained sodium.

The heart opposes the renin-angiotensin system when it secretes atrial natriuretic peptide (ANP), causing sodium excretion. The hypothalamus and posterior pituitary gland produce and secrete an antidiuretic hormone that causes the body to retain water, which, in turn, affects the solute concentration in the blood.

Where electrolytes are lost

Sodium, potassium, chloride, and water are lost in sweat. Electrolytes can also be lost from the GI tract, but a functional GI tract is vital for electrolyte absorption as well. Discussion of individual electrolytes in upcoming chapters explains how their balance is affected by GI absorption of foods and fluids.

Don't forget the parathyroid glands

The parathyroid glands also play a role in electrolyte balance, specifically calcium and phosphorus. The parathyroid glands (usually two pairs) are located behind and to the side of the thyroid gland where they secrete parathyroid hormone. This hormone draws calcium into the blood from the bones, intestines, and kidneys and helps move phosphorus from the blood to the kidneys to be excreted in urine.

The thyroid gland is also involved in electrolyte balance by secreting calcitonin. This hormone lowers an elevated calcium level by preventing calcium release from bone. Calcitonin also decreases intestinal absorption and kidney reabsorption of calcium.

Kidney involvement

Remember filtration? It's the movement of water and dissolved substances from an area of higher pressure to one of lower pressure through a semipermeable membrane. Filtration occurs in the nephron (the anatomic and functional unit of the kidney). As blood circulates through the glomerulus (a tuft of capillaries), fluids and electrolytes are filtered and collected in the nephron's tubule.

Who's at risk?

Some fluids and electrolytes are reabsorbed through capillaries at various points along the nephron; others are secreted. The immature kidneys of an infant can't concentrate urine or reabsorb electrolytes as well as the kidneys of an adult, which puts infants at a higher-than-normal risk for electrolyte imbalances. Older adults are also at risk electrolyte imbalances. Their kidneys have fewer functional nephrons, a decrease in the glomerular filtration rate, and a diminished ability to concentrate urine.

Keeping electrolyte levels in check

A vital part of the kidney's job is to regulate electrolyte levels in the body. A normally functioning kidney maintains the correct fluid level in the body. Sodium and fluid balance are closely related. When too much sodium is released, the body's fluid level drops.

The kidneys also rid the body of excess potassium. When the kidneys fail, potassium builds up in the body. High levels of potassium in the blood can be fatal. (For more information about which areas of the nephron control fluid and electrolyte balance, see *How the nephron regulates the balance.*)

How the nephron regulates the balance

Here, the nephron is stretched out to show where and how fluid and electrolyte regulation takes place.

Glomerulus
- Filters 180 L/day of fluid
- Acts as bulk filter to pass along protein-free and red blood cell–free filtrate (liquid that has been filtered)

Proximal tubule
- Has freely permeable cell membranes
- Reabsorbs most electrolytes, glucose, urea, and amino acids
- Carries large amounts of water with electrolytes back to circulation
- Reduces water content of filtrate by 70%

Loop of Henle
- Contains high concentrations of salts, mostly sodium
- Further concentrates filtrate because of water lost by osmosis
- Pulls chloride and sodium out of filtrate without water and reabsorbs them in ascending limb
- Causes filtrate to become more dilute as it moves into distal tubule

Distal tubule
- Reabsorbs water and concentrates urine due to ADH action
- Reabsorbs sodium and water; secretes potassium due to aldosterone action

Collecting duct
- ADH acts here to reabsorb water
- Reabsorbs or secretes potassium, sodium, urea, hydrogen ions, and ammonia, according to body's needs

How diuretics affect the balance

Many patients — both hospitalized and at home — receive diuretics, medications to increase urine production. Diuretics are used to treat many different disorders, such as hypertension, congestive heart failure, electrolyte imbalances, and certain kidney diseases.

Monitoring a diuretic's effects

The health care team monitors the effects of diuretics, including their effects on electrolyte balance. Diuretics can cause electrolytes to be lost, whereas I.V. fluids replace electrolyte losses.

Older adults, who are already at risk for fluid and electrolyte imbalances, need careful monitoring because diuretics can worsen their imbalances. Once you know how the nephron functions normally, you can predict a diuretic's effects on your patient by knowing where the drug acts along the nephron.

This knowledge and understanding can help you provide optimal care for patients on diuretics. (See *Where diuretics work.*)

I.V. fluids

As with diuretics, I.V. fluids affect the electrolyte balance in the body. When providing I.V. fluids, keep in mind the patient's normal electrolyte requirements. For instance, the patient requires:
• sodium: 1 to 2 mEq/kg/day
• potassium: 0.5 to 1 mEq/kg/day
• chloride: 1 to 2 mEq/kg/day.

Is the I.V. working?

To evaluate I.V. fluid treatment, ask:
• Are the I.V. solutions providing the correct amount of electrolytes?
• How long has the patient been receiving I.V. fluids?
• Is the patient receiving any oral supplementation of electrolytes?

For more about I.V. fluids, see Chapter 17. (For the electrolyte content of some commonly used I.V. fluids, see *What I.V. solutions contain,* page 30.)

Where diuretics work

Here's a look at the effects of diuretics and other drugs along the nephron.

Glomerulus

Dopamine. Not generally classified as a diuretic, dopamine is included here because it may increase urine output. Dopaminergic receptor sites exist along the afferent arterioles (tiny vessels that bring blood to the glomerulus). Dopamine in low doses (0.5 to 3 mcg/kg/min) acts here to dilate the vessels to increase blood flow to the glomerulus. This, in turn, increases the amount of filtration in the nephron.

Proximal tubule

Osmotic diuretics (mannitol, glucose). Mannitol is not reabsorbed in the tubule; it remains in high concentrations throughout its journey, increasing the osmolality of the filtrate, and hindering water, sodium, and chloride reabsorption, which increases their excretion.

High levels of blood sugar cause excess glucose to spill over into the tubules, and its osmotic effect also results in increased urine output.

Carbonic anhydrase inhibitors (acetazolamide [Diamox]). These drugs reduce hydrogen ion (think acid) concentration in the tubule, which causes increased excretion of bicarbonate, water, sodium, and potassium.

Loop of Henle

Loop diuretics (furosemide [Lasix], bumetanide [Bumex], ethacrynic acid [Edecrin]). These diuretics act on the ascending loop of Henle to prevent reabsorption of water and sodium. This increases volume in the tubules and shrinks blood volume. Potassium and chloride are also excreted here.

Distal tubule

Thiazide diuretics (hydrochlorothiazide [Hydro-DIURIL], metolazone [Zaroxolyn]). Thiazide diuretics act high up in the distal tubule to prevent sodium reabsorption, which increases the amount of tubular fluid and electrolytes farther down the nephron. Blood volume shrinks, aldosterone increases sodium reabsorption and, in exchange, potassium is lost from the body.

Potassium-sparing diuretics (spironolactone [Aldactone]). These diuretics interfere with sodium and chloride reabsorption in the tubule. Potassium is spared and sodium, chloride, and water are excreted. Urine output increases and the body retains potassium.

What I.V. solutions contain

This table lists the electrolyte content of some commonly used I.V. fluids.

I.V. solution	Electrolyte	Amount
Dextrose	None	——
Sodium chloride		
0.45%	Sodium chloride	77 mEq/L
0.9%	Sodium chloride	154 mEq/L
3%	Sodium chloride	513 mEq/L
5%	Sodium chloride	855 mEq/L
Dextrose-Sodium Chloride		
5% dextrose and 0.45% sodium chloride	Sodium chloride	77 mEq/L
5% dextrose and 0.9% sodium chloride	Sodium chloride	154 mEq/L
Ringer's Solution (plain)		
	Sodium	147 mEq/L
	Potassium	4 mEq/L
	Calcium	4.5 mEq/L
	Chloride	156 mEq/L
Lactated Ringer's Solution		
	Sodium	130 mEq/L
	Potassium	4 mEq/L
	Calcium	3 mEq/L
	Chloride	109 mEq/L
	Lactate	28 mEq/L

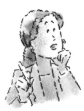

Quick quiz

1. When cells are damaged by a burn, you would expect the damaged cells to release the major electrolyte:

    A. calcium.
    B: chloride.
    C: potassium.

Answer: C. Potassium is the major electrolyte inside the cell that leaks out into the extracellular fluid after a major trauma like a burn. This puts the patient at risk for hyperkalemia.

2. Diuretics affect the kidneys by altering the reabsorption and excretion of:

    A. water only.
    B. electrolytes only.
    C. water and electrolytes.

Answer: C. Diuretics generally affect how much water and sodium is excreted by the body. As they are lost by the body, other electrolytes such as potassium can also be lost through the urine.

3. The major extracellular cation is:

    A. calcium.
    B. potassium.
    C. sodium.

Answer: C. Sodium is the major extracellular cation. Among other things, it's important in the regulation of fluid balance in the body.

4. In the nephron, most electrolytes are reabsorbed in the:

    A. proximal tubule.
    B. glomerulus.
    C. loop of Henle.

Answer: A. The proximal tubule reabsorbs most of the electrolytes from the filtrate. It also reabsorbs glucose, urea, amino acids, and water.

5. Potassium is essential for conducting electrical impulses because it causes ions to:

    A. clump together to generate a current.
    B. shift in and out of the cell to conduct a current.
    C. trap sodium inside the cell to maintain a current.

Answer: B. Potassium in the intracellular fluid causes ions to shift in and out of the cell, which allows electrical impulses to be conducted from cell to cell.

Scoring

☆☆☆ If you answered all five correctly, congratulations! You're a real juggler, able to balance lots of things at once.

☆☆ If you answered four or five correctly, great! You're a juggler's apprentice. Study hard, and you too shall one day dazzle audiences with your balancing skills!

☆ If you answered three or fewer correctly, no problem. Take a few lessons from a master juggler and you'll be juggling behind your back before you know it!

Balancing acids and bases

Just the facts

In this chapter you'll learn:

♦ what acids and bases are

♦ what pH is and what role it plays in metabolism

♦ how the body regulates its acid-base balance

♦ which diagnostic tests are used to assess acid-base balance.

A look at acids and bases

The chemical reactions that sustain life depend on a delicate balance — or homeostasis — between acids and bases in the body. Even a slight imbalance can profoundly affect metabolism and essential body functions. Acid-base balance can be affected by a number of conditions, such as infection and trauma, and by medications. To understand acid-base balance in the body, you need to understand some basic chemistry.

All about pH

Understanding acids and bases requires an understanding of pH, a calculation based on the percentage of hydrogen ions in a solution. The calculation is based on the amount of acids and bases in the solution.

Acids are substances that consist of molecules that can give up, or donate, hydrogen ions (H) to other molecules. Carbonic acid is an example of an acid that occurs naturally in the body. Bases — such as bicarbonate — are substances that consist of molecules that can accept hydrogen ions.

A solution that contains more base than it does acid has fewer hydrogen ions and so has a higher pH. A pH higher than 7 makes the solution a base.

A solution that contains more acid than it does base has more hydrogen ions and so has a lower pH. A pH lower than 7 makes the solution an acid.

Getting to know your pH

You can assess a patient's acid-base balance if you know the pH of his blood. Since arterial blood is used most often to measure pH, this discussion will focus on arterial samples.

Arterial blood is normally slightly alkaline, ranging from 7.35 to 7.45. That pH represents a balance between the percentage of hydrogen ions and the percentage of bicarbonate (HCO_3) ions.

Generally, the pH is maintained in a ratio of 20 parts bicarbonate to 1 part carbonic acid. A pH lower than 6.8 or higher than 7.8 is usually fatal. (See *Normal pH*.)

Low pH

Under certain conditions, the pH of arterial blood may deviate significantly from its narrow normal range. A de-

---

Normal pH

The illlustration shows that the blood pH normally stays slightly alkaline, in the range of 7.35 to 7.45. At that point, the amount of acid (H) is balanced with the amount of base. A pH < 7.35 is considered abnormally acidic; a pH > 7.45 is considered abnormally alkaline.

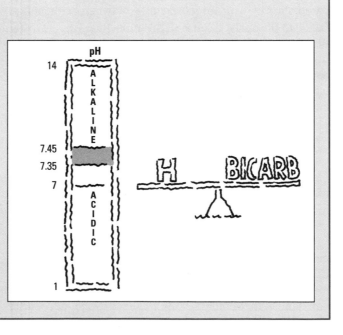

creased pH may occur if the hydrogen ion concentration (acid) of the blood increases or if the HCO_3 level decreases. In either case, a drop in pH below 7.35 signals acidosis. (See *Acidosis.*)

High pH

The pH can increase if the level of bicarbonate increases or the level of hydrogen ions decreases, the opposite effect of a low pH. In either case, an increase in pH above 7.45 signals alkalosis. (See *Alkalosis,* page 36.)

Regulating acids and bases

A person's well-being depends on maintenance of a normal pH. A deviation in the pH can compromise essential body processes including electrolyte balance, the activity of critical enzymes, muscle contraction, and basic cellular function. The body normally maintains pH within a narrow range by carefully balancing acidic and alkaline elements. When one aspect of that balancing act breaks down, the body can't maintain a healthy pH as easily and problems arise.

Acidosis

Acidosis, a condition in which the pH is < 7.35, occurs when acids (H) accumulate or bases such as bicarbonate are lost.

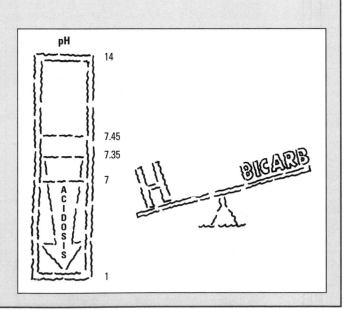

Alkalosis

Alkalosis, a condition in which the pH is >7.45, occurs when bases such as bicarbonate accumulate or acids (H) are lost.

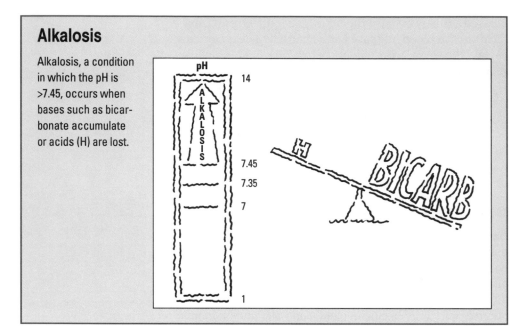

The Big Three regulators

The body regulates acids and bases to avoid those potentially serious consequences. Three regulatory systems come into play when pH rises or falls.
• Chemical buffers act immediately to protect tissues and cells. Those buffers instantly combine with the offending acid or base, neutralizing harmful effects until other regulatory systems take over.
• The respiratory system, through hypoventilation or hyperventilation, acts as a buffer to regulate the excretion of acids or the retention of them within minutes of the change in pH.
• The kidneys kick in by excreting more acids or bases, or by conserving them, according to the body's needs. Renal regulation can restore normal H concentration within hours or days.

Regulating method 1

The body maintains a healthy pH in part through buffers, substances that minimize changes in pH by combining with excess acids or bases. Chemical buffers in the blood, the intracellular fluid, and the interstitial fluid serve as the body's most efficient pH-balancing weapon. The three main chemical buffering systems include the bicarbonate-buffer system, the phosphate-buffer system, and the protein-buffer system.

Bicarb buffer

The bicarbonate-buffer system is the major buffer system in the body and is responsible mainly for buffering blood and interstitial fluid. The bicarbonate system relies on a series of chemical reactions in which pairs of weak acids and bases (such as carbonic acid and bicarbonate) combine with the stronger acids (such as hydrochloric acid) and bases to weaken them.

Decreasing the strength of potentially damaging acids and bases reduces the danger those chemicals pose to pH balance. The kidneys assist the bicarbonate-buffer system in regulating production of bicarbonate. The lungs assist by regulating the production of carbonic acid, which results from combining carbon dioxide and water.

Phosphate buffer

Like the bicarbonate-buffer system, the phosphate-buffer system also depends on a series of chemical reactions to minimize pH changes. Phosphate buffers react with either acids or bases to form compounds that slightly alter pH, which can provide extremely effective buffering. This system proves especially effective in renal tubules, where greater concentrations of phosphates exist.

Protein buffers

Protein buffers, the most plentiful buffers in the body, work inside and outside cells. They are composed of hemoglobin as well as other proteins. Behaving chemically like bicarbonate buffers, protein buffers bind with acids and bases to neutralize them. In red blood cells, for instance, hemoglobin combines with hydrogen ions to act as a buffer.

Regulating method 2

The respiratory system serves as the second line of defense against acid-base imbalances. The lungs regulate blood levels of carbon dioxide, a gas that combines with water to form carbonic acid. Increased levels of carbonic acid lead to a decrease in pH.

Chemoreceptors in the medulla of the brain sense those pH changes and vary the rate and depth of breathing to compensate (See *CO_2 and hyperventilation.*) Breath-

---

CO_2 and hyperventilation

When a patient's ventilatory rate increases, carbon dioxide is "blown off" and the CO_2 level drops.

Respiratory rate

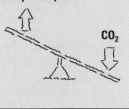

ing faster or more deeply eliminates more CO_2 from the lungs. The more CO_2 is lost, the less carbonic acid is made and, as a result, the pH rises.

The body normalizes such a pH change by slowing the rate or decreasing the depth of breathing, thus reducing CO_2 excretion.

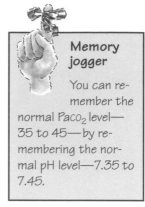

Check the $Paco_2$

The effectiveness of ventilation can be assessed by looking at the partial pressure of CO_2 in arterial blood ($Paco_2$). The normal $Paco_2$ level in the body is 35 to 45 mm Hg. $Paco_2$ levels reflect the concentration of carbon dioxide in the blood. As the concentration of the gas increases, so does its partial pressure.

Keep in mind that the respiratory system of an older adult may be compromised and less able to regulate acid-base balance.

Twice as good

As a buffer, respiratory regulation can maintain acid-base balance twice as effectively as chemical buffers because it can handle twice the amount of acids and bases. The respiratory system also responds to pH changes quickly — within minutes. However, the lungs can restore normal pH only temporarily. Long-term adjustments to pH are accomplished by the kidneys.

Regulating method 3

The kidneys serve as yet another of the body's mechanisms for maintaining acid-base balance. They can reabsorb or excrete acids and bases into the urine. They can also produce bicarbonate to replenish lost supplies. Adjustments to pH made by the kidneys can take hours to days.

Measuring bicarb

The level of bicarbonate is also regulated by the kidneys. Evaluating the bicarbonate level helps to assess the metabolic component of acid-base balance. Normally, the bicarbonate level is reported with arterial blood gas (ABG) results. The normal bicarbonate level is 22 to 26 mEq/L. Bicarbonate is also reported with serum electrolytes as total serum CO_2 content.

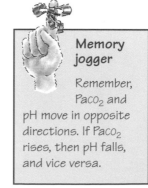

Making an adjustment

If the blood contains too much acid or not enough base, the pH drops and the kidneys reabsorb bicarbonate (in the form of sodium bicarbonate). The kidneys also excrete hydrogen (in combination with phosphate or ammonia). In those situations, the urine becomes more acidic than normal. Urine tends to be acidic because the body usually produces slightly more acids than bases.

The reabsorption of bicarbonate and the increased excretion of hydrogen causes more bicarbonate to be formed in the renal tubules and eventually retained by the body. The bicarbonate level in the blood then rises to a more normal level, increasing pH.

Remember that an infant's kidneys can't acidify urine as well as an adult's can. In addition, because ammonia production decreases with age, the kidneys of an older adult can't handle excess acid as well as kidneys of a younger adult can.

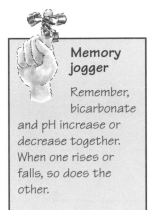

Memory jogger

Remember, bicarbonate and pH increase or decrease together. When one rises or falls, so does the other.

In, out, in, out

If the blood contains more base and less acid, the pH rises. The kidneys compensate by excreting bicarbonate and retaining more hydrogen ions. As a result, urine becomes more alkaline and the bicarbonate level in the blood drops. Conversely, if the blood contains less bicarbonate and more acid, the pH drops.

The body responds to acid-base imbalances by activating compensatory mechanisms that minimize pH changes. Returning the pH to a normal or near-normal level mainly involves changes in the component (metabolic or respiratory) not primarily affected by the imbalance.

If the body compensates only partially for an imbalance, tests will indicate that the pH is still out of the normal range. Full, or complete, compensation means that the pH will be back to normal.

Respiratory helps metabolic

If a metabolic disturbance is the primary cause of an acid-base imbalance, the lungs can compensate in one of two ways. In the case of acidosis caused by a lack of bicarbonate, the lungs increase the rate of ventilation, which "blows off" CO_2 and helps to raise the pH to normal. With alkalosis caused by an excess of bicarbonate, the lungs hypoventilate to retain CO_2 and bring down the pH.

Metabolic helps respiratory

If the respiratory system disturbs the acid-base balance, the kidneys can compensate for it by altering levels of bicarbonate and hydrogen ions. When the $Paco_2$ level is high — a state of acidosis — the kidneys retain bicarbonate and excrete more acid to raise the pH. In the case of alkalosis, when the $Paco_2$ level is low, the kidneys excrete bicarbonate and hold on to more acid, to lower the pH.

Diagnosing imbalances

A number of diagnostic tests are used to diagnose acid-base disturbances. Here's a look at the more common ones.

Arterial blood gases

An ABG analysis is a diagnostic test that uses a sample of blood obtained from an arterial puncture. The test allows for the assessment of the effectiveness of ventilation and overall acid-base balance. The information can prove useful not only for diagnosing acid-base imbalances and problems with oxygenation but also for monitoring the patient's response to treatment. (See *Taking an ABG sample*.)

Keep in mind that an ABG analysis is a tool to be used in conjunction with a full assessment of the patient. Only by assessing all information can you gain a clear picture of what's happening.

An ABG analysis involves several separate test results, only three of which relate to acid-base balance: pH, $Paco_2$, and HCO_3. Here again are normal adult values of those results:
- pH: 7.35 to 7.45
- $Paco_2$: 35 to 45 mm Hg
- HCO_3: 22 to 26 mEq/L.

An ABG overview

Recall that pH is a measure of the hydrogen ion concentration of the blood. $Paco_2$ measures the partial pressure of carbon dioxide in arterial blood, which indicates the effectiveness of ventilation. $Paco_2$ levels move in the opposite direction as pH. HCO_3, which moves in the same direction

---

Taking an ABG sample

When a needle puncture is necessary for obtaining an arterial blood gas (ABG) sample, the radial, brachial, or femoral artery may be used. The angle of penetration will vary. For the radial artery — the artery most often used — the needle should enter bevel up at a 45-degree angle, as shown. For the brachial artery, the angle should be 60 degrees, and for the femoral artery, 90 degrees.

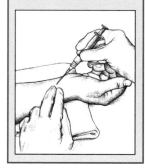

as pH, represents the metabolic component of the body's acid-base balance.

Other pieces of information are routinely reported with ABG results, including PaO_2 and SaO_2. The PaO_2 is a measurement of the partial pressure exerted by oxygen dissolved in arterial blood. The normal PaO_2 is 80 to 100 mm Hg. The PaO_2 varies with age. After age 60, the PaO_2 may drop below 80 mm Hg without signs of hypoxia.

The SaO_2 measures the percentage of hemoglobin actually carrying oxygen as opposed to the percentage that could (100%). The normal SaO_2 value is 95% to 100%.

Steps in interpreting an ABG

When interpreting results from an ABG analysis, be consistent in the sequence you use to analyze information. Here's a step-by-step process you might feel comfortable using. (See *Quick look at ABGs*.)

Step 1: Check the pH

First, check the pH. This figure will form the basis for understanding just about all of the others.

If the pH is abnormal, does it reflect acidosis (less than 7.35) or alkalosis (greater than 7.45)?

Once you determine whether the patient is acidotic or alkalotic, determine which system — respiratory or metabolic — is at fault.

Step 2: What's the CO_2?

Remember that the $PaCO_2$ level provides information about the respiratory component of acid-base balance. If the $PaCO_2$ isn't normal, determine whether it's low (less than 35 mm Hg) or high (greater than 45 mm Hg).

If the $PaCO_2$ level is either high or low, does the abnormal result correspond with the change in pH? For example, if the pH is high, you would expect the $PaCO_2$ to be low. If ABG results indicate that the $PaCO_2$ is indeed low (hypocapnia), the problem is primarily respiratory in origin. Conversely, for a low pH, you would expect a high $PaCO_2$ (hypercapnia), indicating respiratory acidosis.

Step 3: Watch the bicarb

Next, examine the bicarbonate level (HCO_3), which provides information about the metabolic aspect of acid-base

---

Quick look at ABGs

Here's a quick look at how to interpret arterial blood gas (ABG) results.

• Check the pH. Is it normal (7.35 to 7.45), acidotic (below 7.35), or alkalotic (above 7.45)?
• Check the $PaCO_2$. Is it normal (35 to 45 mm Hg), low, or high?
• Check the bicarbonate. Is it normal (22 to 26 mEq/L), low, or high?
• Check for signs of compensation. Which value ($PaCO_2$ or bicarbonate) more closely corresponds to the change in pH?
• Check the PaO_2 and the SaO_2. Is the PaO_2 normal (80 to 100 mm Hg), low, or high? Is the SaO_2 normal (95% to 100%), low, or high?

balance. If that level isn't normal, determine whether it's low (< 22 mEq/L) or high (> 26 mEq/L).

If the bicarb is either high or low, does the abnormal result correspond with the change in pH? For example, if the pH is high, you would expect the bicarb also to be high. If ABG results indicate that the bicarb is indeed high, the problem is primarily metabolic in origin. Conversely, for a low pH, you would expect a low bicarb, indicating metabolic acidosis.

Step 4: Look for compensation

Sometimes you'll see a change in both the $Paco_2$ and the bicarbonate level. One of the levels will indicate the primary source of the pH change. The other reflects the body's effort to compensate for that disturbance.

The body's ability to compensate may be so good (complete compensation) that the pH falls within the range of normal. Partial compensation occurs when the pH remains outside of the normal range.

Compensation involves opposites. For instance, if results indicate a primary metabolic acidosis, any compensation will come in the form of respiratory alkalosis. For example, here's a set of blood gases from a patient who has metabolic acidosis with compensatory respiratory alkalosis:

- pH: 7.27
- $Paco_2$: 27 mm Hg
- HCO_3: 10 mEq/L.

Note that the low pH indicates acidosis. Note also that the $Paco_2$ is low. A low $Paco_2$ normally causes alkalosis. The bicarb is also low, which normally leads to acidosis.

The bicarb level, then, more closely corresponds with the pH, making the metabolic component the primary problem. The resultant decrease in the $Paco_2$ reflects a respiratory compensation.

Normal values for pH, $Paco_2$, and HCO_3 indicate that the patient's acid-base balance is also normal.

Step 5: Last, what's the Pao_2 and Sao_2?

Last, check the Pao_2 and Sao_2, which yield information about the patient's oxygenation status. If the levels aren't normal, determine whether they are high (Pao_2 greater than 100 mm Hg) or low (Pao_2 less than 80 mm Hg; Sao_2 less than 95%).

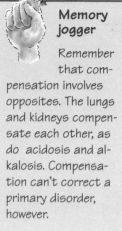

Memory jogger

Remember that compensation involves opposites. The lungs and kidneys compensate each other, as do acidosis and alkalosis. Compensation can't correct a primary disorder, however.

Remember that PaO_2 reflects the ability of the body to pick up oxygen from the lungs. A low PaO_2 represents hypoxemia and can cause hyperventilation. This level also indicates when to make adjustments in the concentration of oxygen being administered to a patient. (See *Inaccurate ABG results.*)

Anion gap

You may come across a test result called the anion gap. Earlier chapters discussed how the strength of cations (positively charged ions) and anions (negatively charged ions) must be equal in the blood to maintain a proper balance of electrical charges. The anion gap result allows clinicians to differentiate among various types of acidotic conditions. Take a look at the main cations and anions and how they affect acid-base balance.

Identifying the gap

The anion gap refers to the relationship among the body's cations and anions. (See *Crossing the great anion gap.*) Sodium accounts for more than 90% of the circulating cations. Chloride and bicarbonate (HCO_3) together account for 85% of the counterbalancing anions. (Potassium

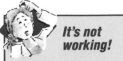

It's not working!

Inaccurate ABG results

Arterial blood gas (ABG) results can be altered by using poor technique when drawing a sample of arterial blood.

• A delay in getting the sample to the lab or drawing an ABG within 15 to 20 minutes of a procedure, such as suctioning or administering a respiratory treatment, could alter results.
• Air bubbles in the syringe could affect the oxygen level.
• Venous blood in the syringe could alter carbon dioxide, oxygen, and pH levels.

Crossing the great anion gap

The illustration below represents the normal anion gap. The gap is calculated by adding the chloride level and the bicarb level, and then subtracting that total from the sodium level. It normally ranges from 8 to 14 mEq/L and represents the level of unmeasured anions in extracellular fluid.

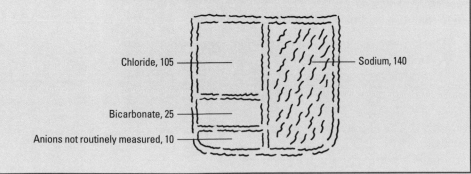

Chloride, 105

Bicarbonate, 25

Anions not routinely measured, 10

Sodium, 140

is generally omitted because it occurs in such low, stable amounts).

The gap between the two measurements represents the anions not routinely measured, including sulfates, phosphates, proteins, and organic acids, such as lactic acid and ketone acids. Since those anions aren't measured in routine laboratory tests, the anion gap is a way of determining their presence.

What do the results mean?

An increase in the anion gap (greater than 14 mEq/L) indicates an increase in the percentage of one or more unmeasured anions in the bloodstream. Increases can occur with acidotic conditions characterized by higher-than-normal amounts of organic acids. Such conditions include lactic acidosis and ketoacidosis.

The anion gap remains normal for certain other conditions, including hyperchloremic acidosis, renal tubular acidosis, and severe bicarbonate-wasting conditions, such as biliary or pancreatic fistulas and poorly functioning ileal loops.

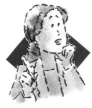

Quick quiz

1. A measurement of the partial pressure of carbon dioxide in the blood indicates the effectiveness of:
    A. kidney function.
    B. lung ventilation.
    C. phosphate buffers.

Answer: B. The $Paco_2$ reflects how well ventilation is helping to maintain acid-base balance.

2. The kidneys respond to acid-base disturbances by:
    A. adjusting $Paco_2$ levels.
    B. producing phosphate buffers.
    C. excreting or reabsorbing hydrogen or bicarbonate.

Answer: C. The kidneys respond to particular acid-base imbalances by excreting or reabsorbing hydrogen or bicarbonate, according to the body's needs.

3. If your patient is breathing rapidly, his body is attempting to:

    A. retain carbon dioxide.

    B. get rid of excess carbon dioxide.

    C. improve the buffering ability of bicarbonate.

Answer: B. High carbon dioxide levels in the blood, measured as $Paco_2$, cause a drop in pH. Chemoreceptors in the brain sense this decrease and stimulate the lungs to hyperventilate, causing more CO_2 to be exhaled.

4. If your patient has a higher-than-normal pH (alkalosis), you would expect to also see:

    A. a high $Paco_2$.

    B. a low $Paco_2$.

    C. a low HCO_3.

Answer: B. A low $Paco_2$ means less carbon dioxide (acid) is in the blood, which raises the pH.

5. The lab reports the following ABG results on your patient:

    pH: 7.33

    $Paco_2$:   40 mm Hg

    HCO_3:   20 mEq/L

You interpret these results as:

    A. respiratory acidosis.

    B. metabolic acidosis.

    C. respiratory alkalosis.

Answer: B. The pH is low, which indicates acidosis. Since the $Paco_2$ is normal and the bicarbonate is low (matching the pH), the metabolic component is the primary source of the disorder.

6. A Pao_2 level of 49 mm Hg indicates:

    A. acidosis.

    B. hypoxia.

    C. hypercapnia.

Answer: B. A Pao_2 of 49 mm Hg is below the normal range of 80 to 100 mm Hg and therefore indicates hypoxia.

7. A colleague hands you these blood gas results:

    pH: 7.52

    $Paco_2$:   47 mm Hg

    HCO_3:   36 mEq/L

You interpret the results as:
A. respiratory acidosis.
B. respiratory alkalosis with respiratory compensation.
C. metabolic alkalosis with respiratory compensation.

Answer: C. The pH is alkalotic. Although there are changes in both $Paco_2$ and HCO_3, the HCO_3 matches the pH. The elevated $Paco_2$ represents the efforts of the respiratory system to compensate for the alkalosis by retaining carbon dioxide.

Scoring

☆☆☆   If you answered all seven items correctly, congratulations! What great acid-base balance you have!

☆☆   If you answered four to six correctly, great! You can donate hydrogen ions to us anytime!

☆   If you answered fewer than four correctly, not to worry. Your base is solid with us!

Part II

Fluid and electrolyte imbalances

When fluids tip the balance

Just the facts

This chapter will help you learn how to assess patients with fluid imbalances and how to care for those patients. In this chapter, you'll learn:

♦ how to assess a patient's fluid-volume status

♦ which patients are at risk for developing fluid imbalances

♦ what to watch for in a patient with a fluid imbalance

♦ what to teach the patient about his particular fluid imbalance

♦ how to document the care given and teaching done for a patient with a fluid imbalance.

A look at fluid volume

Blood pressure is related to the amount of blood pumped by the heart and the extent of vasoconstriction present. Fluid volume affects these elements and makes blood pressure measurements key in assessing a patient's fluid status. Some pressure measurements, such as pulmonary artery pressure or central venous pressure, are obtained through specialized catheters. These measurements also contribute to the assessment of fluid volume.

Cuff measurements

A simple blood-pressure measurement, using a stethoscope and a sphygmomanometer, is still one of the best tools you can use to assess fluid volume. It's quick, easy, and carries little risk for the patient. Direct and indirect blood pressure measurements are frequently related to the amount of blood flowing through the patient's circulatory system.

To properly position a blood pressure cuff, wrap the cuff snugly around the upper arm, above the antecubital space. For adults, place the lower border of the cuff about 1" (2.5 cm) above the antecubital space. For children, place the lower border appropriately closer to the antecubital space.

Place the center of the cuff's bladder directly over the medial aspect of the arm, over the brachial artery. Most cuffs have a reference mark to help you position the bladder. After positioning the cuff, palpate the brachial artery and place the bell of the stethoscope directly over the point where you can feel the strongest pulsations. (See *Positioning a blood pressure cuff.*)

BPs automatically

You may also have access to an automated blood pressure unit. The unit is designed to take blood pressure measurements repeatedly, helpful for a patient whose blood pressure is expected to change frequently (as with a fluid imbalance). The unit automatically computes and digitally records blood pressure readings.

Using the monitor is a snap. Place the cuff on the arm and turn the unit on. The cuff automatically inflates to check the blood pressure and deflates immediately afterward. You can program the monitor to inflate the cuff

Positioning a blood pressure cuff

This illustration shows how to properly position a blood pressure cuff and stethoscope bell.

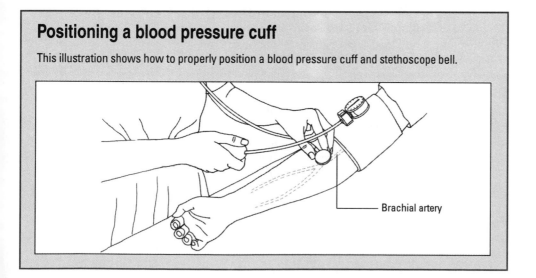

Brachial artery

as often as needed and set alarms for high, low, and mean blood pressures. The monitor displays each blood pressure reading until the next pressure is taken. Before using an automated system, obtain a baseline blood pressure reading your usual way; then compare the manual reading with the digital display.

Palpable pressures

Sometimes you can't hear blood pressure well. If you have trouble hearing the patient's blood pressure, which often happens when a patient is hypotensive, palpate the blood pressure to estimate systolic pressure.

To palpate the blood pressure, place a cuff on the upper arm and palpate the brachial pulse or the radial pulse. Inflate the cuff until you no longer feel the pulse. Then slowly deflate the cuff, noting the point at which you feel the pulse again. The point at which you can feel the pulse again is the systolic blood pressure. If you palpate a patient's blood pressure at 90 mm Hg, for example, chart it as "90/P" (the P stands for palpable).

The Doppler difference

What would you do if your patient's arm was swollen or his blood pressure was so low you couldn't feel his pulse? First, palpate his carotid artery to make sure he has a pulse. Then use a Doppler device to obtain a reading of the patient's systolic blood pressure. (See *How to take a Doppler blood pressure*.)

The Doppler probe uses ultrasound waves directed at the blood vessel to detect blood flow. Through the Doppler unit, you'll be able to hear the patient's blood flow with each pulse.

To obtain a Doppler blood pressure, place a blood pressure cuff on the arm as you normally would. Apply lubricant to the antecubital area where you would expect to find the brachial pulse. Turn the unit on, and place the probe lightly on the arm, over the brachial artery. Adjust the volume control and the placement of the probe until you hear the pulse clearly. (See *Correcting problems of blood pressure measurement*.)

Inflate the blood-pressure cuff until the pulse sound disappears. Slowly deflate the cuff, and note the point at which the pulse sound returns — the systolic pressure. If you hear the pulse at 80 mm Hg, for instance, record it as "80/D" (the D stands for Doppler).

How to take a Doppler blood pressure

When you can't hear or feel a patient's blood pressure, try using a Doppler probe, as shown below.

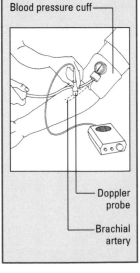

Blood pressure cuff

Doppler probe

Brachial artery

It's not working!

Correcting problems of blood pressure measurement

Use this chart to figure out what to do for each possible cause of a falsely high or low BP reading.

Problem and possible cause	What to do
False-high reading	
• Cuff too small	• Make sure the cuff bladder is 20% wider than the circumference of the arm or leg being used for measurement.
• Cuff wrapped too loosely, reducing its effective width	• Tighten the cuff.
• Slow cuff deflation causing venous congestion in the arm or leg	• Never deflate the cuff more slowly than 2 mm Hg/heartbeat.
• Tilted mercury column	• Read pressures with the mercury column vertical.
• Poorly timed measurement — after the patient has eaten, ambulated, appeared anxious, or flexed arm muscles	• Postpone blood pressure measurement, or help the patient relax before taking pressures.
• Multiple attempts at blood pressure in the same arm (causes venous congestion)	• Don't attempt to measure blood pressure more than twice in the same arm; wait several minutes between attempts.
False-low reading	
• Incorrect position of the arm or leg	• Make sure the arm or leg is level with the patient's heart.
• Mercury column below eye level	• Read mercury column at eye level.
• Failure to notice auscultatory gap (sound fades out for 10 to 15 mm Hg, then returns)	• Estimate systolic pressure by palpation before actually measuring it. Then check this pressure against the measured pressure.
• Inaudible or low-volume sounds	• Before reinflating the cuff, instruct the patient to raise his arm or leg to decrease venous pressure and amplify low-volume sounds. After inflating the cuff, tell the patient to lower his arm or leg. Then deflate the cuff and listen. If you still fail to detect low-volume sounds, chart the palpable systolic pressure.

Direct measurements

Direct measurement refers to an invasive method of obtaining blood pressure readings. Direct blood pressure monitoring is indicated when highly accurate or frequent blood pressure measurements are required, as with severe fluid imbalances.

A-lines

Arterial lines, or A-lines, are inserted into the radial or the brachial artery (or the femoral artery, if necessary). A-lines monitor blood pressure continuously and can also be used to sample arterial blood for blood gas analysis or other lab tests. Because the lines require a certain level of technology and staff training, patients who have these lines are usually placed in intermediate or critical care units.

Lines under pressure

The catheter is connected to a continuous flush system — a bag of normal saline solution (often containing heparin) inside a pressurized cuff. This system maintains the patency of the line. (See *Pulmonary artery catheter.*)

The line is connected to a transducer, and then to a bedside monitor. The transducer converts fluid-pressure waves from the catheter into an electronic signal that can be analyzed and displayed by the monitor. Since the patient's blood pressure is displayed continuously, you can instantly note changes in the measurements and respond quickly.

To maintain the accuracy of whatever blood pressure measurement system you use, periodically compare the readings of automated and direct measurement systems with manual readings.

PA caths

While an A-line directly measures blood pressure, a pulmonary artery (PA) catheter directly measures other pressures. PA catheters are usually inserted into the subclavian or internal jugular veins, though the lines are sometimes inserted into a vein in the arm or the leg.

The tip of the catheter is advanced through the vein into the right atrium, then into the right ventricle, and finally into the pulmonary artery. The hubs of the catheter are then connected to a pressurized transducer system similar to the system used for an A-line.

Getting a clearer picture

The PA catheter provides a clearer picture of the patient's fluid volume status than other measurement techniques.

Pulmonary artery catheter

The many ports on a pulmonary artery catheter, shown here, can be used for pacing, infusing solutions, or monitoring oxygen saturation, body temperature, cardiac output, or various intraluminal pressures, such as central venous pressure (through the proximal lumen) or pulmonary capillary wedge pressure (through the distal lumen).

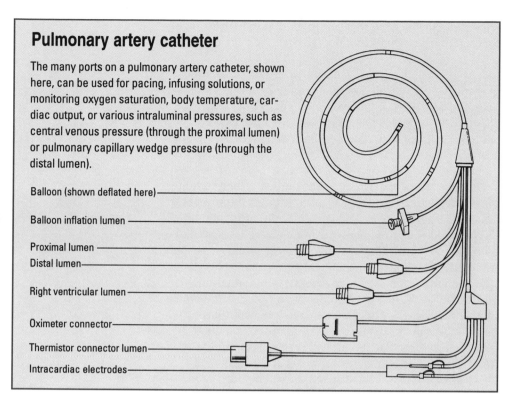

Balloon (shown deflated here)

Balloon inflation lumen

Proximal lumen

Distal lumen

Right ventricular lumen

Oximeter connector

Thermistor connector lumen

Intracardiac electrodes

The catheter allows for the evaluation of pulmonary artery pressure (PAP), pulmonary artery wedge pressure, cardiac output, and even central venous pressure (CVP). Those measurements provide information about the function of the left side of the heart, including the heart's pumping ability, its filling pressures, and its vascular volume.

The PAP is the pressure routinely displayed on the monitor. The normal systolic PAP is 15 to 25 mm Hg and reflects pressure from the contraction of the right atrium. The normal diastolic PAP is 8 to 15 mm Hg and reflects the lowest pressure in the pulmonary vessels. The mean PAP is 10 to 20 mm Hg.

Wedging the balloon

When you inflate the small balloon at the catheter tip, blood carries the catheter tip farther into the pulmonary artery. The tip floats inside the artery until it stops — or becomes wedged — in a smaller branch.

When the tip is wedged in a branch of the pulmonary artery, the catheter measures pressures coming from the left side of the heart, a measurement that may prove useful in gauging changes in blood volume. The normal pulmonary artery wedge pressure is 6 to 12 mm Hg.

In general, these two values — PAP and the wedge pressure — are elevated in cases of fluid overload and decreased in cases of fluid-volume deficit. That's why a PA catheter is useful when assessing and treating an acutely ill patient with a fluid imbalance.

Cardiac output, too

PA catheters also measure cardiac output, either continuously or after injections of I.V. fluid through the proximal lumen. Cardiac output is a measurement of the amount of blood pumped by the heart in 1 minute and is calculated by multiplying the heart rate by the stroke volume. (Don't worry, the monitor makes that calculation for you!)

The stroke volume is the amount of blood pumped out by the ventricle with each beat and is also calculated by the bedside monitor. The normal cardiac output is between 4 and 8 L/minute. If a person lacks adequate blood volume, cardiac output will be low (assuming the heart can pump normally otherwise). If the person is overloaded with fluid, cardiac output will be high.

Central pressures

A central venous catheter can measure CVP, another useful indication of a patient's fluid status. The term CVP refers to the pressure of the blood inside the central venous circulation. The tip of a CVP catheter is usually placed in one of the jugular veins in the neck or in a subclavian vein in the chest.

The normal CVP ranges from 0 to 7 mm Hg (5 to 10 cm H_2O). If the CVP is high, it usually means the patient is overloaded with fluid. If it's low, it usually means the patient is low on fluid. (To estimate CVP yourself, see *Estimating central venous pressure*.)

How the body compensates

Most of the time, the body adequately compensates for minor fluid imbalances and keeps blood pressure readings and other measurements pretty much normal. But sometimes the body can't compensate for fluid deficits or

Estimating central venous pressure

To estimate a patient's central venous pressure (CVP), follow these steps.

1. Place the patient at a 45-degree angle.

2. Use tangential lighting to observe the internal jugular vein.

3. Note the highest level of visible pulsation.

4. Locate the angle of Louis, or sternal notch, by palpating the point at which the clavicles join the sternum (the suprasternal notch).

5. Place two of your fingers on the suprasternal notch and slide them down the sternum until they reach a bony protuberance — the angle of Louis. The right atrium lies about 2" (5 cm) below this point.

6. Measure the height between the angle of Louis and the highest level of visible pulsation. Normally, this distance is less than 1.2" (3 cm).

7. Add 2" to this figure to estimate the distance between the highest level of pulsation and the right atrium. A distance greater than 4" (10 cm) may indicate elevated CVP.

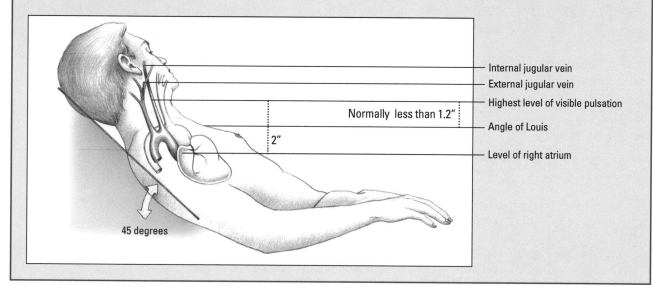

Internal jugular vein
External jugular vein
Highest level of visible pulsation
Normally less than 1.2"
Angle of Louis
2"
Level of right atrium
45 degrees

excesses. When that happens, any of several problems may result, including dehydration, hypovolemia, hypervolemia, and water intoxication. Let's look at dehydration first.

Dehydration

The body loses water all the time. A person responds to the thirst reflex by drinking fluids and eating foods that contain water. However, if water isn't replaced adequately, the body's cells can lose water, a condition called dehydration. (See *Try our Fluid Shift Game,* page 59.)

How it happens

The loss of body fluids causes an increase in the concentration of solutes in the blood (increased osmolality). Serum sodium levels rise. In an attempt to regain fluid balance between the two spaces — intracellular and extracellular — water molecules shift out of the cells into the more concentrated blood. This process, combined with water retention by the kidneys and increased water intake, usually restores the body's fluid volume.

Meanwhile, back in the cells...

Without an adequate supply of water in the extracellular space, fluid continues to shift out of the cells into the extracellular space, causing even greater fluid loss from the cells. The cells begin to shrink as that process continues. Because water is essential for obtaining nutrients, expelling wastes, and maintaining the shape of the cell, dry cells can't function properly.

Who's at risk?

Failure to respond adequately to the thirst stimulus risks dehydration. Confused, comatose, or bedridden patients are particularly vulnerable, as are infants, who can't drink fluid on their own and have immature kidneys that can't concentrate urine efficiently.

Older patients are also prone to dehydration. The body of an older person has a lower body-water content, diminished kidney function, and a reduced ability to sense thirst so it can't correct fluid-volume deficits as easily as the body of a younger adult can. A patient may also become dehydrated if he is receiving highly concentrated feedings without receiving enough supplemental water.

Dry diseases

Any situation that accelerates fluid loss can lead to dehydration. For instance, in diabetes insipidus, the brain fails to secrete antidiuretic hormone (ADH), due to injury or tumor. If the brain doesn't secrete enough ADH, the result is a greater-than-normal diuresis.

The body of a patient with diabetes insipidus produces large amounts of highly dilute urine — as much as 30 L a day. The patient is also thirsty and tends to drink large amounts of fluids, though he generally can't keep up with the diuresis.

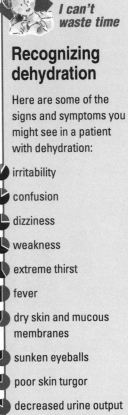

I can't waste time

Recognizing dehydration

Here are some of the signs and symptoms you might see in a patient with dehydration:

- irritability
- confusion
- dizziness
- weakness
- extreme thirst
- fever
- dry skin and mucous membranes
- sunken eyeballs
- poor skin turgor
- decreased urine output (with diabetes insipidus, urine will be pale and plentiful)
- increased heart rate with falling blood pressure.

Other causes of dehydration include prolonged fever, watery diarrhea, and certain cases of renal failure and hyperglycemia in which the person produces large amounts of dilute urine.

What to look for

As dehydration progresses, watch for changes in mental status. (See *Recognizing dehydration.*) The patient may complain of dizziness, weakness, or extreme thirst. He may have a fever (since less fluid is available for perspiration, which lowers body temperature), dry skin, or dry mucous membranes. Skin turgor may be poor. *Keep in mind that the skin of an older patient often lacks elasticity, so checking skin turgor in those patients may be unreliable.*

In addition, the urine output starts to fall because less fluid is circulating in the body. If the person has diabetes insipidus, the urine will most likely be pale and produced in large volume. The heart rate may go up, and the blood pressure may fall. In severe cases, seizures and coma may result. (See *Danger signs of dehydration.*)

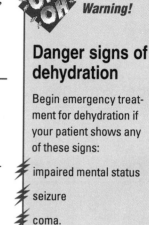

Warning!

Danger signs of dehydration

Begin emergency treatment for dehydration if your patient shows any of these signs:

- impaired mental status
- seizure
- coma.

What tests show

Diagnostic test results you may see include:
- elevated serum osmolality: more than 300 mOsm/kg
- elevated serum sodium: more than 145 mEq/L
- urine specific gravity: more than 1.030.

In patients with diabetes insipidus, because the urine is so dilute, the specific gravity is usually less than 1.005, and osmolality is 50 to 200 mOsm/kg.

How dehydration is treated

Treatment for dehydration aims to replace missing fluids. Because a dehydrated patient's blood is concentrated, avoid hypertonic solutions. If the patient can handle oral fluids, encourage them. Because the serum sodium is elevated, make sure the fluids given are salt-free.

A severely dehydrated patient will receive I.V. fluids to replace lost fluids. Most patients receive hypotonic, low-sodium fluids, such as dextrose 5% in water (D_5W).

Remember, though, if you give a hypotonic solution too quickly, the fluid will move from the veins into the cells and cause them to become edematous. Swelling of cells in the brain can create cerebral edema. *To avoid such potentially devastating problems, give fluids gradually, over a period of about 48 hours.*

How you intervene

Monitor at-risk patients closely to detect impending dehydration early. If a patient develops dehydration, here are some things you'll want to do:
• Monitor symptoms and vital signs closely.
• Accurately record the patient's intake and output.
• Maintain I.V. access as ordered. Monitor I.V. infusions. Remember to be alert for signs of cerebral edema when your patient is receiving hypotonic fluids. Those signs include headache, confusion, irritability, lethargy, nausea, vomiting, widening pulse pressure, decreased pulse rate, and seizures. (See *Teaching about dehydration.*)
• Keep in mind that vasopressin may be ordered for patients with diabetes insipidus.
• Monitor serum sodium, urine osmolality, and urine specific gravity.
• Insert a urinary catheter, as ordered.
• Provide a safe environment for the patient who is confused, dizzy, or at risk of suffering a seizure, and teach his family to do the same.
• Obtain daily weights (same scale, same time of day) to evaluate treatment progress. (See *Documenting dehydration.)*
• Provide skin and mouth care to maintain the integrity of the skin surface and oral mucous membranes.

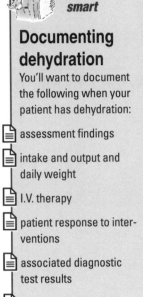

Chart smart

Documenting dehydration
You'll want to document the following when your patient has dehydration:

📄 assessment findings

📄 intake and output and daily weight

📄 I.V. therapy

📄 patient response to interventions

📄 associated diagnostic test results

📄 patient teaching done and the patient's response.

Parting points

Teaching about dehydration
Make sure to cover these topics and to evaluate your patient's learning:

🎓 explanation of condition and its treatment

🎓 warning signs and symptoms

🎓 prescribed medications

🎓 importance of complying with therapy.

Hypovolemia

Hypovolemia refers to isotonic fluid loss (which includes loss of fluids plus solutes) from the extracellular space. Children and older people are especially vulnerable to hypovolemia. Some of the initial signs and symptoms of hypovolemia can be subtle as the body tries to compensate for the loss of circulating blood volume. Subtle signs can become more serious and, if not detected early and treated properly, can progress to hypovolemic shock, a common form of shock. (See *Hypovolemic shock,* page 60.)

(Text continues on page 63.)

Try our Fluid Shift Game

When extracellular fluid accumulates and becomes trapped in the interstitial space, the body can't readily transport the fluid back into the circulation. As a result, the fluid remains in the third space, making it physiologically useless.

Several disorders can cause fluid to shift into the third space, as you can see in our Fluid Shift Game. The game is designed to show the movement of body fluid among the vascular, interstitial, and lymph compartments.

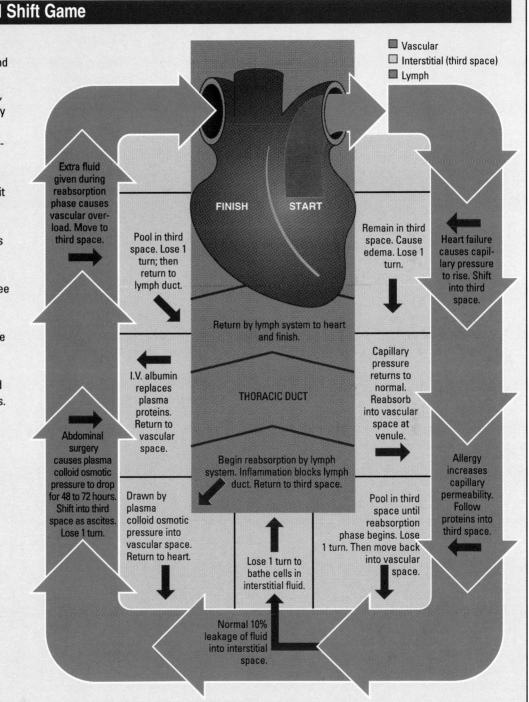

■ Vascular
□ Interstitial (third space)
■ Lymph

FINISH   START

Extra fluid given during reabsorption phase causes vascular overload. Move to third space.

Pool in third space. Lose 1 turn; then return to lymph duct.

Remain in third space. Cause edema. Lose 1 turn.

Heart failure causes capillary pressure to rise. Shift into third space.

Return by lymph system to heart and finish.

Capillary pressure returns to normal. Reabsorb into vascular space at venule.

I.V. albumin replaces plasma proteins. Return to vascular space.

THORACIC DUCT

Begin reabsorption by lymph system. Inflammation blocks lymph duct. Return to third space.

Abdominal surgery causes plasma colloid osmotic pressure to drop for 48 to 72 hours. Shift into third space as ascites. Lose 1 turn.

Drawn by plasma colloid osmotic pressure into vascular space. Return to heart.

Pool in third space until reabsorption phase begins. Lose 1 turn. Then move back into vascular space.

Allergy increases capillary permeability. Follow proteins into third space.

Lose 1 turn to bathe cells in interstitial fluid.

Normal 10% leakage of fluid into interstitial space.

Hypovolemic shock

In hypovolemic shock, fluid circulating in the blood vessels decreases, lowering cardiac output and leading to hypotension. Recognizing hypovolemic shock promptly is crucial. Untreated, this condition can lead to progressive hypoxia, tissue death and, ultimately, cardiac and respiratory arrest.

Jump start for the heart

Sensory nerves in the aortic arch respond to decreased blood pressure by stimulating the sympathetic nervous system, causing tachycardia, increased cardiac contractility, and venous constriction. This temporarily improves cardiac output. Look for a progressive drop in blood pressure accompanied by a rapid, thready pulse.

Meanwhile, in the kidneys

Blood pressure sensors in the kidney activate the renin-angiotensin system, which causes increased sodium and water retention in the kidneys. This mechanism helps the body preserve fluid.

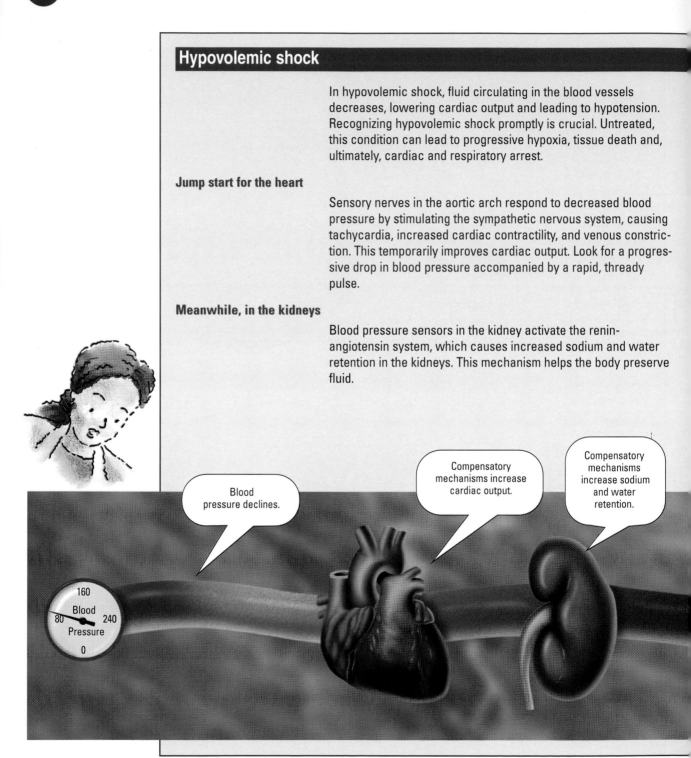

Blood pressure declines.

Compensatory mechanisms increase cardiac output.

Compensatory mechanisms increase sodium and water retention.

160
Blood
80   240
Pressure
0

One heck of a hormone

When the brain senses low blood pressure, antidiuretic hormone (ADH) stimulates thirst, a mechanism to increase volume. You may note decreased urine output.

Now, the bad news...

Without prompt treatment, compensatory mechanisms cannot maintain circulation for long and blood pressure falls dramatically. When the blood pressure falls below 80 mm Hg, tissue perfusion decreases and not enough blood reaches the coronary arteries. Be alert for arrhythmias and myocardial ischemia or infarction.

Dangerous complications

Hypoxia from poor tissue perfusion may cause dilation of the arterioles, which causes blood to become trapped in the capillaries. This can lead to disseminated intravascular coagulation. Watch for signs of this life-threatening complication: petechiae, bruising, bleeding, or oozing from the gums.

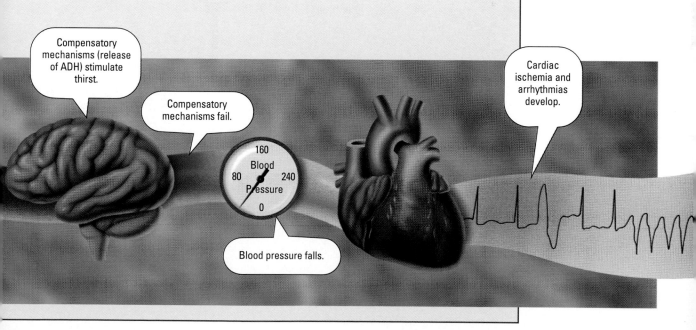

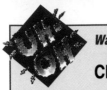

Warning!

Checking for orthostatic hypotension

If you suspect hypovolemia, check for orthostatic, or postural, hypotension, which can be a sign of impending hypovolemic shock. Orthostatic hypotension is defined as a fall in systolic blood pressure of at least 20 mm Hg or an increase in heart rate of at least 20 beats/minute when the patient changes position as shown below.

When documenting blood pressures and pulses, indicate the patient's position each time using the appropriate stick figure as shown below.

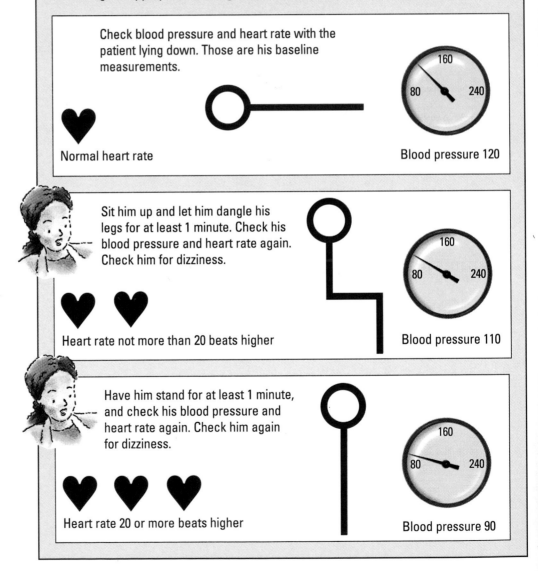

Check blood pressure and heart rate with the patient lying down. Those are his baseline measurements.

Normal heart rate

Blood pressure 120

Sit him up and let him dangle his legs for at least 1 minute. Check his blood pressure and heart rate again. Check him for dizziness.

Heart rate not more than 20 beats higher

Blood pressure 110

Have him stand for at least 1 minute, and check his blood pressure and heart rate again. Check him again for dizziness.

Heart rate 20 or more beats higher

Blood pressure 90

How hypovolemia happens

Several possible paths can lead to hypovolemia. Excessive fluid loss (bleeding, for instance) is a risk factor, especially when found in combination with reduced fluid intake. Patients who are unable or unwilling to take in adequate amounts of fluids are at an increased risk for hypovolemia. Hypovolemia can also result from a third-space fluid shift, which occurs when fluid moves out of the intravascular space but not into the intracellular space. For instance, fluid may shift into the abdominal cavity (ascites), the pleural cavity, or the pericardial sac. These third-space fluid shifts may occur as a result of increased permeability of the capillary membrane or a decrease in plasma colloid osmotic pressure.

Extracellular losses

Fluid loss from the extracellular compartment can be caused by a number of conditions, including:
• abdominal surgery
• diabetes mellitus (with increased urination)
• excessive diuretic therapy
• excessive laxative use
• excessive sweating
• fever
• fistulas
• hemorrhage (Remember, bleeding may be frank or occult.)
• nasogastric drainage
• renal failure with increased urination
• vomiting or diarrhea. (Younger patients are at higher risk for hypovolemia because of their relatively large GI tracts.)

Third-space shifting

Fluid shifts into the third space can be caused by a number of conditions, including:
• acute intestinal obstruction
• acute peritonitis
• burns (during the initial phase)
• crush injuries
• hip fracture
• hypoalbuminemia
• pleural effusion.

What to look for

If volume loss is minimal (10% to 15% of an average of about 5 L of total circulating blood volume), the body tries to compensate for its lack of circulating volume by increasing the heart rate. You may also note orthostatic hypotension, restlessness, or anxiety. The patient will most likely still produce urine at a rate of more than 30 ml/per hour but may still have delayed capillary refill time and cool, pale skin over the arms and legs. (See *Recognizing hypovolemia*.)

Weighty evidence

The hypovolemic patient may also lose weight. Acute weight loss can indicate rapid fluid changes. A drop in weight of 5% to 10% can indicate mild to moderate loss; more than 10%, severe loss. As hypovolemia progresses, the patient's symptoms worsen. Central venous and pulmonary pressures may fall as well. Be alert for such subtle signs in your patient, including the presence of orthostatic hypotension. (See *Checking for orthostatic hypotension,* page 62.)

Dazed and confused

With moderate intravascular volume loss (approximately 25%), the patient may become more confused and irritable and complain of extreme thirst. The pulse usually becomes rapid and thready, and the blood pressure drops. The patient may become cool and clammy, and the urine output can drop to 10 to 30 ml/hour.

Shock!

Severe hypovolemia (40% or more of intravascular volume loss) may lead to hypovolemic shock. Cardiac output drops. The patient's mental status can deteriorate to unconsciousness. Symptoms may progress to marked tachycardia and hypotension, with weak or absent peripheral pulses. The skin can become cool and mottled, or even cyanotic. Urine output drops below 10 ml/hour.

What tests show

No single diagnostic finding can confirm hypovolemia. Serum laboratory values may vary depending on the

---

I can't waste time

Recognizing hypovolemia

Avoid surprises. Watch for these often subtle signs of hypovolemia and impending hypovolemic shock:

- mental status deteriorates (from restlessness and anxiety to unconsciousness)
- thirst
- tachycardia
- delayed capillary refill time
- orthostatic hypotension progressing to marked hypotension
- urine output initially more than 30 ml/minute, then lower
- cool, pale skin on arms and legs
- weight loss.

underlying cause and other factors. Values usually suggest an increased concentration of blood. Typical laboratory findings include:

• normal or high (serum sodium level > 145 mEq/L) depending on the amount of fluid and sodium lost
• increased or normal hematocrit, depending on the amount of fluid lost
• decreased hemoglobin and hematocrit levels with hemorrhage
• elevated blood urea nitrogen (BUN) level
• increased urine specific gravity, as kidneys try to conserve fluid.

How hypovolemia is treated

Treatment of hypovolemia includes replacing lost fluids with fluids of the same concentration. Such replacement helps to regain normal blood pressure and to restore blood volume. Oral fluids are generally not enough to adequately treat hypovolemia. Isotonic fluids such as normal saline solution or lactated Ringer's solution are given I.V. to expand circulating volume.

Take the fluid challenge

Fluids may initially be administered as a fluid challenge, in which the patient receives large amounts of I.V. fluids in a short amount of time. For hypovolemic shock, an emergency condition, multiple fluid challenges are essential. Numerous I.V. infusions should be started using the shortest, largest-bore catheters possible, which offer less resistance to fluid flow than long, skinny catheters.

Infusions of normal saline solution or lactated Ringer's solution are given rapidly, often followed by an infusion of plasma proteins such as albumin. If a patient is hemorrhaging, he'll need blood transfusions. Drugs such as dopamine, a vasopressor agent, may be needed to support blood pressure.

In severe cases, the patient may require pneumatic antishock garments to support blood pressure. Oxygen therapy should be initiated to ensure sufficient tissue perfusion. Surgery may be required to control bleeding.

How you intervene

Nursing responsibilities for a hypovolemic patient include the following.

Intervene stat!

- Be sure the patient has a patent airway.
- Apply and adjust oxygen therapy as ordered.
- Lower the head of the bed to slow a declining blood pressure.
- If the patient is bleeding, apply direct continuous pressure to the area and elevate it, if possible. Assist with other interventions to stop bleeding.
- If the blood pressure doesn't respond to interventions as expected, look again for a site of bleeding that might have been missed. *Remember, a patient can lose a large amount of blood internally from a fractured hip or pelvis. In addition, fluids alone are often not enough to correct hypovolemic conditions. Vasopressors such as dopamine may be needed to raise blood pressure.*
- Maintain patent I.V. access. Use short, large-bore catheters to allow for faster infusion rates.
- Administer I.V. fluid, vasopressors, and blood as prescribed. An autotranfuser, which allows for reinfusion of the patient's own blood, may be required.
- Draw blood for typing and crossmatching, as ordered, to prepare for transfusion.
- Closely monitor the patient's mental status and vital signs, including orthostatic blood pressure measurements, when appropriate. Watch for arrhythmias.
- If available, monitor hemodynamics (cardiac output, CVP, PAP, and pulmonary artery wedge pressure), to judge how well the patient is responding to treatment. (See *Hemodynamic values in hypovolemic shock.*)
- Monitor the quality of peripheral pulses and skin temperature and appearance to assess for continued peripheral vascular constriction.
- Obtain and record results from diagnostic tests, such as a complete blood count, electrolyte levels, arterial blood gas (ABG) analyses, a 12-lead electrocardiogram, and chest X-rays.
- Offer emotional support to the patient and his family. (See *Teaching about hypovolemia.*)
- Encourage oral fluid intake as appropriate.

Hemodynamic values in hypovolemic shock

Hemodynamic monitoring helps you evaluate the patient's cardiovascular status in hypovolemic shock. Look for these values:

- central venous pressure below the normal range of 5 to 10 cm H_2O
- pulmonary artery pressure below the normal mean of 10 to 20 mm Hg
- pulmonary artery wedge pressure below the normal mean of 6 to 12 mm Hg
- cardiac output below the normal range of 4 to 8 L/minute.

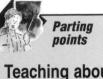

Parting points

Teaching about hypovolemia

Make sure you teach the patient the following points about hypovolemia and evaluate his learning:

- nature of the condition and its causes
- treatment and the importance of compliance
- avoiding orthostatic hypotension
- warning signs and symptoms and when they should be reported
- measuring own blood pressure and pulse rate
- prescribed medications.

• Insert a urinary catheter, as ordered, to measure urine output. Measure output hourly if indicated. (See *Documenting hypovolemia*.)

• Auscultate for breath sounds periodically to monitor for signs of fluid overload, a potential complication of I.V. therapy. Excess fluid in the lungs may cause a crackling sound on auscultation.

• Observe the patient for development of such complications as disseminated intravascular coagulation, myocardial infarction or adult respiratory distress syndrome.

• Weigh patient daily to monitor progress of treatment.

• Provide effective skin care to prevent skin breakdown.

Hypervolemia

Hypervolemia is an excess of isotonic fluid (water and sodium) in the extracellular compartment. Osmolality is usually not affected since fluid and solutes are gained in equal proportion. The body has compensatory mechanisms to deal with hypervolemia but, when they fail, the signs and symptoms of hypervolemia develop.

How it happens

Extracellular fluid volume may increase in either the interstitial or intravascular compartments. Usually, the body can compensate and restore fluid balance by fine-tuning circulating levels of aldosterone, antidiuretic hormone, and atrial natriuretic peptide to cause the kidneys to release additional water and sodium.

However, if hypervolemia is prolonged or severe, or if the patient has poor heart function, the body can't compensate for the extra volume and congestive heart failure (CHF) and pulmonary edema may result. Fluid will be forced out of the blood vessels and move into the interstitial space, causing edema of the tissues.

Elderly people (or any population with impaired renal or cardiovascular function) are especially prone to developing hypervolemia.

The rising tide

Hypervolemia results from retention or excessive intake of fluid or sodium or a shift in fluid from the interstitial

Chart smart

Documenting hypovolemia

With a patient who is hypovolemic, you'll be documenting:

- mental status
- vital signs
- strength of peripheral pulses
- appearance and temperature of skin
- I.V. therapy
- blood products infused
- doses of vasopressors used
- breath sounds and oxygen therapy in use
- hourly urine output
- lab results
- daily weight
- your interventions and the patient's response
- patient teaching.

space into the intravascular space. It may also result from acute or chronic renal failure with low urine output. Fluid or sodium may be retained because of:

- CHF
- cirrhosis of the liver
- nephrotic syndrome
- corticosteroid therapy
- hyperaldosteronism
- low intake of dietary protein.
   Excessive sodium or fluid intake may be caused by:
- I.V. replacement therapy using normal saline solution or lactated Ringer's solution
- blood or plasma replacement
- excessive dietary salt intake.
   Fluid shifts into the vasculature may be caused by:
- remobilization of fluids after burn treatment
- administration of hypertonic fluids, such as mannitol or hypertonic saline solution
- use of colloid oncotic fluids such as albumin.

What to look for

Since no single diagnostic test confirms hypervolemia, signs and symptoms are key to diagnosis. Cardiac output increases as the body tries to compensate for the excess volume. The pulse becomes rapid and bounding. Blood pressure, CVP, PAP, and pulmonary artery wedge pressure rise. As the heart fails, blood pressure and cardiac output drop. An S_3 gallop develops with heart failure. You'll see distended veins, especially in the hands and neck. If you have the patient raise his hand above the level of his heart, his hand veins will remain distended for more than 5 seconds. (See *Recognizing hypervolemia*.)

Edema's many faces

Edema results as the hydrostatic ("fluid-pushing") pressure builds in the vessels. Fluid is forced into the tissues. Edema may first be visible only in dependent areas such as the sacrum but then becomes generalized. Anasarca is the term used to describe severe, generalized edema. Edematous skin looks puffy, even around the eyes, and will feel cool or will "pit" when touched. The patient will

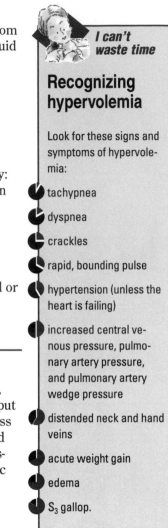

I can't waste time

Recognizing hypervolemia

Look for these signs and symptoms of hypervolemia:

- tachypnea
- dyspnea
- crackles
- rapid, bounding pulse
- hypertension (unless the heart is failing)
- increased central venous pressure, pulmonary artery pressure, and pulmonary artery wedge pressure
- distended neck and hand veins
- acute weight gain
- edema
- S_3 gallop.

gain weight as fluid is retained (each 17 oz of fluid gained translates to a 1-lb weight gain).

An increase in weight of 5% to 10% indicates a mild to moderate fluid gain, while an increase of more than 10% denotes a more severe fluid gain.

Overload!

Edema may also occur in the lungs. As the left side of the heart becomes overloaded and pump efficiency declines, fluid backs up into the lungs.

Hydrostatic pressure forces the fluid out of the pulmonary blood vessels (just like in other blood vessels) and into the interstitial and alveolar areas. Pulmonary edema results. In this condition, you'll hear crackles on auscultation. The patient will become short of breath and tachypneic with a frequent, sometimes frothy, cough. ABG results will reflect pulmonary edema. (See *How pulmonary edema develops,* page 70.)

What tests show

Diagnostic test results you may see include:
• low hematocrit level (from hemodilution)
• normal serum sodium level
• lower serum potassium and BUN levels (from hemodilution). If these levels are high, it may indicate renal failure or impaired renal perfusion
• ABG results will show a low oxygen level; with early tachypnea, the $Paco_2$ may be low, causing a drop in pH and respiratory alkalosis
• congestion in the lungs on chest X-rays.

How hypervolemia is treated

Treatment of hypervolemia includes restriction of sodium and fluid intake and administration of medications to prevent complications, such as CHF and pulmonary edema. The cause of the hypervolemia should also be treated. Diuretics are given to promote excess fluid loss from the body. (See *Evaluating pitting edema,* page 71.) If the patient has pulmonary edema, additional drugs, such as morphine and nitroglycerin, may be given to relieve air hunger and dilate blood vessels, which in turn reduces pulmonary congestion and the amount of blood returning

Now I get it!

How pulmonary edema develops

Excessive fluid volume that lasts a long time can cause pulmonary edema. The illustrations here show how that process occurs.

Normal
Normal pulmonary fluid movement depends on the equal force of two opposing pressures — hydrostatic pressure and plasma oncotic pressure from protein molecules in the blood.

Congestion
Abnormally high pulmonary hydrostatic pressure (indicated by increased pulmonary artery wedge pressure) forces fluid out of the capillaries and into the interstitial space, causing pulmonary congestion.

Edema
When the amount of interstitial fluid becomes excessive, fluid is forced into the alveoli. Pulmonary edema results. Fluid fills the alveoli and prevents the exchange of gases.

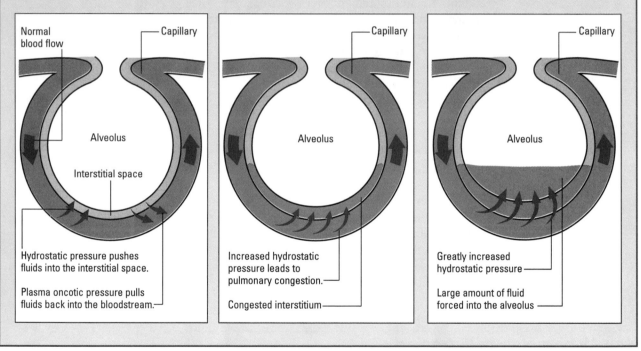

Normal blood flow — Capillary

Alveolus

Interstitial space

Hydrostatic pressure pushes fluids into the interstitial space.

Plasma oncotic pressure pulls fluids back into the bloodstream.

Capillary

Alveolus

Increased hydrostatic pressure leads to pulmonary congestion.

Congested interstitium

Capillary

Alveolus

Greatly increased hydrostatic pressure

Large amount of fluid forced into the alveolus

to the heart. CHF is treated with digoxin, which strengthens cardiac contractions and slows the heart rate. Oxygen and bedrest are also used to support the patient.

When the kidneys aren't working properly, diuretics may be inadequate to rid the body of extra fluid. The patient may require hemodialysis or continuous arteriovenous hemofiltration. (See *Understanding CAVH,* page 72.)

How you intervene

Caring for a patient with hypervolemia requires a number of nursing actions, including the following.

Assess

• Assess the patient's vital signs and hemodynamic status, noting his response to therapy. Watch for signs of hypovolemia due to overcorrection. *Remember that elderly, pediatric, and otherwise compromised patients are at higher risk for complications with therapy.*
• Monitor respiratory patterns for worsening distress, such as increased tachypnea or dyspnea.
• Watch for venous distention in the hands or neck.
• Record intake and output hourly.
• Listen to breath sounds regularly to assess for pulmonary edema. Note crackles or rhonchi.
• Follow ABG results and be alert for a drop in oxygen level or changes in acid-base balance.
• Monitor other laboratory test results for changes, including potassium (lost from the body with most diuretics) and hematocrit levels.
• Raise the head of the bed (if blood pressure allows) to facilitate breathing, and administer oxygen as ordered.
• Make sure the patient sticks to his fluid restriction if ordered. Alert the family and staff to ensure compliance. (See *Teaching about hypervolemia,* page 72.)
• Insert a urinary catheter as ordered before starting diuretic therapy.
• Maintain I.V. access as ordered for the administration of medications such as diuretics. If the patient is prone to hypervolemia, use a controller with any infusions to prevent inadvertent administration of too much fluid.
• Give prescribed diuretics and other medications and monitor for effectiveness and adverse reactions.
• Watch for edema.

Maintain

• Provide frequent mouth care.
• Obtain daily weight and evaluate trends.
• Provide skin care because edematous skin is prone to breakdown.
• Offer emotional support to the patient and his family.

Evaluating pitting edema

Edema can be evaluated using a scale of +1 to +4. Press your fingertip firmly into the skin over a bony surface for a few seconds. Then note the depth of the imprint your finger leaves on the skin.

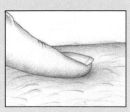

A slight imprint indicates +1 pitting edema.

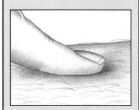

A deep imprint, with the skin slow to return to its original contour, indicates +4 pitting edema.

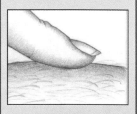

When the skin resists pressure but appears distended, the condition is called brawny edema. In brawny edema, the skin swells so much that fluid can't be displaced.

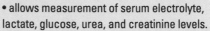

Now I get it!

Understanding CAVH

If your hypervolemic patient isn't responding to diuretics, his kidney function may be poor. Dialysis is typically the next step, but if your patient can't tolerate this procedure, continuous arteriovenous hemofiltration (CAVH) may be used.

What it does

By circulating blood through a special filter, CAVH removes plasma water and dissolved solutes while conserving cellular and protein components. Besides being efficient, CAVH offers these advantages:

• allows arterial blood sampling and arterial blood pressure control

• reduces frequency of hemodialysis treatments and need for a hemodialysis nurse

• maintains serum osmolality by avoiding rapid fluid removal

• circulates less blood out of the body than hemodialysis

• allows measurement of serum electrolyte, lactate, glucose, urea, and creatinine levels.

How it works

In CAVH, the patient's arterial blood pressure serves as a natural pump, driving blood through the arterial line. The illustration below shows the standard setup for CAVH. The patient's blood enters the hemofilter from an arterial line, flows through the hemofilter, and returns to the patient through a venous line. The filtered fluid, called ultrafiltrate, drains by gravity into a collection bag.

Filtration replacement fluid (less fluid than the amount removed) may be infused at the venous access port and returned to the patient along with the purified blood. This procedure allows the patient to gradually lose up to 15 L of fluid per day.

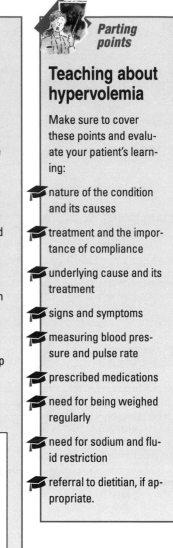

Parting points

Teaching about hypervolemia

Make sure to cover these points and evaluate your patient's learning:

• nature of the condition and its causes

• treatment and the importance of compliance

• underlying cause and its treatment

• signs and symptoms

• measuring blood pressure and pulse rate

• prescribed medications

• need for being weighed regularly

• need for sodium and fluid restriction

• referral to dietitian, if appropriate.

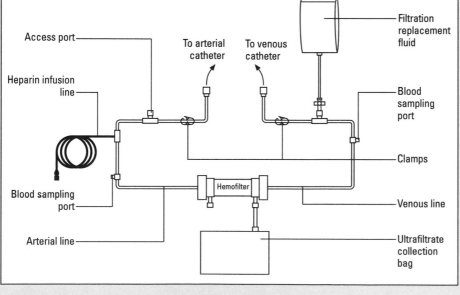

• Document your assessment and interventions. (See *Documenting hypervolemia.*)

Water intoxication

Water intoxication is a condition in which excess fluid moves from the extracellular space to the intracellular space. Here's the lowdown on this condition.

How it happens

Excessive low-sodium fluid in the extracellular space is considered hypotonic to the cells. The cells, in turn, are considered hypertonic. In that instance, fluid shifts — by osmosis — into the cells, which have comparatively less fluid and a greater concentration of solutes. That fluid shift causes swelling of the cells and occurs as a means of balancing the concentration of fluid between the two spaces, a condition called water intoxication.

Holding on to water

Water intoxication can be caused by syndrome of inappropriate antidiuretic hormone (SIADH). SIADH causes the body to hold on to electrolyte-free water despite low plasma osmolality (dilute plasma) and high fluid volume. It can result from central nervous system or pulmonary disorders, head trauma, certain medications, or tumors. (We'll talk more about SIADH when we discuss sodium imbalances in Chapter 5.)

The condition can occur with rapid infusions of hypotonic solutions, such as D_5W. Excessive use of tap water as a nasogastric tube irrigant or enema also increases water intake.

Psychogenic polydipsia is another cause. This occurs when, because of a psychological disturbance, a person continues to drink water or other fluids in large amounts, even when they're not needed. It's especially dangerous if the person's kidneys don't function well.

What to look for

The signs and symptoms of water intoxication reflect low sodium levels and increased intracranial pressure (ICP)

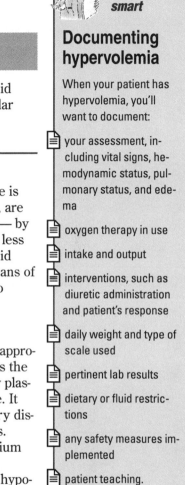

Chart smart

Documenting hypervolemia

When your patient has hypervolemia, you'll want to document:

- your assessment, including vital signs, hemodynamic status, pulmonary status, and edema
- oxygen therapy in use
- intake and output
- interventions, such as diuretic administration and patient's response
- daily weight and type of scale used
- pertinent lab results
- dietary or fluid restrictions
- any safety measures implemented
- patient teaching.

as brain cells swell. Symptoms begin with headache and personality changes. Be suspicious of any change in behavior or level of consciousness, such as confusion, irritability, or lethargy. There may also be nausea, vomiting, cramping, muscle weakness, or twitching.

Late signs of increased intracranial pressure include pupillary and vital sign changes, such as bradycardia and widened pulse pressure. A patient with water intoxication may develop seizures and coma. Any weight gain reflects additional cellular fluid.

What tests show

Diagnostic test results you may see include:
• serum sodium level < 125 mEq/L
• serum osmolality < 280 mOsm/kg.

How water intoxication is treated

Management of water intoxication includes restricting water intake (oral and parenteral) and avoiding the use of hypotonic I.V. solutions, such as D_5W, until serum sodium levels rise. Hypertonic solutions are used only in severe situations to draw fluid out of the cells. This requires close monitoring of the patient. The original cause of the intoxication should also be addressed.

How you intervene

The best treatment for water intoxication is prevention. However, if your patient develops water intoxication, you'll want to:
• Closely assess his neurologic status; be alert for deterioration.
• Monitor vital signs and intake and output to evaluate the patient's progress.
• Maintain oral and I.V. fluid restrictions, as prescribed.
• Alert the dietitian and the patient's family to the restrictions. Post a sign in the patient's room to alert staff to fluid restrictions. (See *Teaching about water intoxication*.)
• Insert and maintain I.V. access, as ordered; infuse hypertonic solutions with care, using a controller.
• Closely observe the patient's response to therapy.
• Weigh patient daily to detect excess water retention.

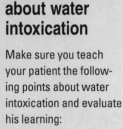

Parting points

Teaching about water intoxication

Make sure you teach your patient the following points about water intoxication and evaluate his learning:

🎓 nature of the condition and its causes

🎓 need for fluid restriction

🎓 warning signs and symptoms and when they should be reported

🎓 prescribed medications

🎓 need for being weighed regularly.

• Monitor laboratory test results, such as serum sodium.
• Provide a safe environment for the patient with an alteration in neurologic status and teach his family to do the same.
• Institute seizure precautions in severe cases.
• Document your assessment and interventions. (See *Documenting water intoxication.*)

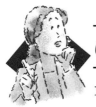

Quick quiz

1. Populations at risk for dehydration include:
    A. infants.
    B. adolescents.
    C. patients with SIADH.

Answer: A. Patients at risk for dehydration are those who have an impaired thirst mechanism or who can't respond to the thirst reflex. Infants fall into this category.

2. Checking for orthostatic hypotension allows the nurse to detect early signs of:
    A. hypovolemia.
    B. low serum osmolality.
    C. high serum osmolality.

Answer: A. Changes in blood pressure and pulse are two of the initial changes seen with hypovolemia.

3. Of the following, the first step you should take for a patient with hypovolemic shock is to:
    A. assess for dehydration.
    B. administer I.V. fluids.
    C. insert a urinary catheter.

Answer: B. Hypovolemic shock is an emergency that requires rapid infusions of I.V. fluids.

4. Signs of hypervolemia include:
    A. rapid, bounding pulse.
    B. clear, watery sputum.
    C. severe hypertension.

Answer: A. Excess fluid in the intravascular space causes a rapid, bounding pulse. When hypervolemia progresses, it can fill the lungs with fluid and cause pulmonary edema, as indicated by the presence of pink, frothy sputum.

Chart smart

Documenting water intoxication

When your patient has water intoxication, you'll want to document:

▤ all assessment findings

▤ intake and output, noting fluid restrictions

▤ safety measures

▤ types of seizure activity and treatment

▤ lab results

▤ daily weight

▤ nursing interventions and patient's response

▤ patient teaching.

5. Water intoxication can be caused by:
  A. administering too much hypertonic fluid.
  B. administering too much hypotonic fluid.
  C. encouraging fluid intake.

Answer: B. Administering too much hypotonic fluid can cause water to shift from the blood vessels into the cells, leading to water intoxication and cellular edema.

6. If your critically ill patient's fluid volume decreases, you would expect to see:
  A. high blood pressure and low oxygen saturation.
  B. increased cardiac output and distended neck veins.
  C. decreased CVP and pulmonary artery wedge pressure.

Answer: C. In general, with a decrease in circulating volume, the CVP and pulmonary artery wedge pressure will drop, as will blood pressure, cardiac output, and PAP.

Scoring

☆☆☆ If you answered all six items correctly, way to go! Your fluidity leaves us breathless!

☆☆ If you answered four or five correctly, great going! Your A-lines are Class A!

☆ If you answered three or fewer correctly, that's OK. We think your third-space fluid shifts are swell!

5

When sodium tips the balance

Just the facts

This chapter discusses the important role sodium plays in keeping the body functioning normally. In this chapter, you'll learn:

♦ how sodium contributes to fluid and electrolyte balance

♦ how the body regulates sodium balance

♦ what causes, signs, symptoms, and treatments are associated with sodium imbalances

♦ what you can do for your patient with a sodium imbalance.

A look at sodium

Sodium is one of the most important elements in the body and has many physiologic roles to play. It's the major cation (positively charged ion) and the most abundant solute in extracellular fluid. Almost all of the body's sodium content is found in this fluid. Sodium is often combined with chloride or bicarbonate.

The body needs sodium to maintain proper extracellular fluid osmolality (concentration). Sodium attracts fluid and helps preserve the extracellular fluid volume and fluid distribution in the body. It also helps transmit impulses in nerve and muscle fibers and combines with chloride and bicarbonate to regulate acid-base balance. Because the electrolyte compositions of serum and interstitial fluid are essentially equal, extracellular fluid sodium concentrations are measured in serum levels. The normal range of serum sodium is 135 to 145 mEq/L. As a comparison, the amount of sodium inside a cell is 10 mEq/L.

Balancing act

The sodium level in the body depends on what is eaten and how the intestines absorb it. Adults need a minimum of 2 g of sodium per day; however, the salty American diet provides at least 6 g per day. Even so, sodium levels stay fairly constant in the body because the more sodium is eaten, the more sodium is excreted by the kidneys. (See *Dietary sources of sodium*.)

Sodium is also excreted through the GI tract and in sweat. When you think "sodium," think "water" — the two are that closely related in the body. The normal range of serum sodium levels reflects the relationship between sodium and water. If sodium intake suddenly increases, extracellular fluid concentration also rises, and vice versa.

Not too much!

The body makes adjustments when the sodium level rises. Increased serum sodium causes increased thirst and the release of antidiuretic hormone (ADH) by the posterior pituitary gland. (For more information about ADH, see Chapter 1.) Antidiuretic hormone causes the kidneys to retain water, which "dilutes" the blood and normalizes serum osmolality.

When serum osmolality decreases and thirst and ADH secretion are suppressed, the kidneys excrete more water to restore normal osmolality. (See *Regulating sodium and water*.)

Aldosterone also regulates extracellular fluid sodium balance by way of a feedback loop. The adrenal cortex secretes aldosterone, which stimulates the renal tubules to conserve water and sodium when the body's sodium level is low, thus helping to normalize extracellular fluid sodium concentration.

The pump explained

Normally, sodium concentrations in extracellular fluid are very high compared to those in intracellular fluid. The body contains an active transport mechanism, called a

---

Dietary sources of sodium

Here are some major dietary sources of sodium:

- cheese
- salt
- seafood
- processed meats
- canned vegetables
- canned soups
- ketchup
- snack foods (pretzels and potato chips)

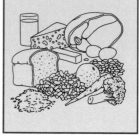

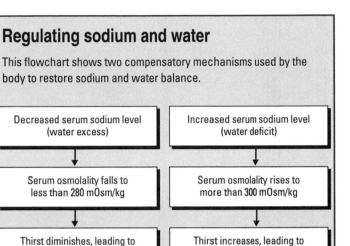

Regulating sodium and water

This flowchart shows two compensatory mechanisms used by the body to restore sodium and water balance.

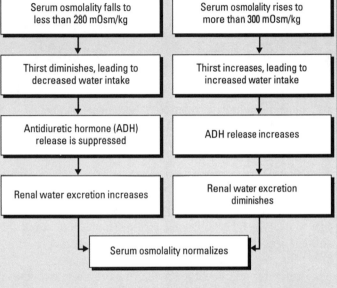

Decreased serum sodium level (water excess)	Increased serum sodium level (water deficit)
Serum osmolality falls to less than 280 mOsm/kg	Serum osmolality rises to more than 300 mOsm/kg
Thirst diminishes, leading to decreased water intake	Thirst increases, leading to increased water intake
Antidiuretic hormone (ADH) release is suppressed	ADH release increases
Renal water excretion increases	Renal water excretion diminishes

Serum osmolality normalizes

sodium pump or sodium-potassium pump, which helps maintain normal sodium levels. Here's how the pump works.

According to the laws of diffusion, a substance moves from an area of higher concentration to one of lower concentration. Sodium ions, normally most abundant outside the cells, want to diffuse inward, and potassium ions, normally most abundant inside the cells, want to diffuse outward. To combat this ionic diffusion and maintain normal sodium and potassium concentrations, a sodium pump is constantly at work in every body cell.

But moving sodium out of the cell and potassium back in can't happen without some help. Each ion links up with a "carrier" because it can't get through the cell wall alone. This movement requires energy, which comes from adenosine triphosphate (composed of phosphorus, another electrolyte), magnesium, and an enzyme. These substances help release sodium from the cell and draw potassium into the cell.

The sodium pump allows the body to carry out its essential functions and helps prevent cellular swelling due to too many ions inside the cell attracting excessive amounts of water. The pump also creates an electrical charge in the cell from the movement of ions, permitting transmission of neuromuscular impulses. (See *Sodium-potassium pump.*)

Hyponatremia

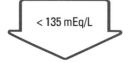

< 135 mEq/L

Hyponatremia, a common electrolyte imbalance, refers to a deficiency of sodium in relation to body water. In other words, body fluids are diluted. Severe hyponatremia can lead to seizures, coma, and permanent neurologic damage.

How it happens

Normally, the body gets rid of excess water by secreting less ADH, which causes diuresis. For that to happen, the nephrons need to be functioning normally, receiving and excreting excess water and reabsorbing sodium.

Hyponatremia develops when this regulatory function goes haywire. Serum sodium levels decrease, causing a decrease in serum concentration, and fluid shifts occur. When the blood vessels contain more water and less sodium, fluid moves by osmosis from the extracellular area into the more concentrated intracellular area. With more fluid in the cells and less in the blood vessels, cerebral edema and hypovolemia (fluid volume deficit) can occur. (See *Fluid movement in hyponatremia,* page 82.)

Deplete and dilute

Hyponatremia occurs from sodium loss, water gain (a condition called dilutional hyponatremia), or when a person doesn't take in enough sodium (depletional hyponatremia). It may be classified according to whether extracellular fluid volume is abnormally decreased (hypovolemic hyponatremia), abnormally increased (hypervolemic hypo-

Sodium-potassium pump

This illustration shows how the sodium-potassium pump carries ions when their concentrations change.

Normal placement
More sodium (Na) ions normally exist outside cells than inside. More potassium (K) ions exist inside cells than outside.

Increased permeability
Certain stimuli increase the membrane's permeability. Sodium ions diffuse inward; potassium ions diffuse outward.

Energy source
The cell links each ion with a carrier molecule that helps the ion return through the cell wall. Energy for the ion's return trip comes from adenosine triphosphate (ATP), magnesium (Mg), and an enzyme commonly found in cells.

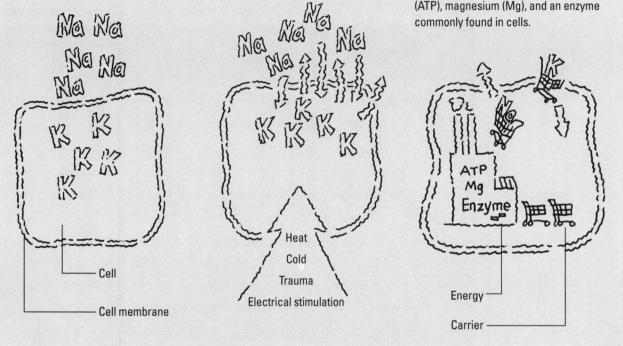

natremia), or equal to intracellular fluid volume (isovolumic hyponatremia).

Both sides lose

In hypovolemic hyponatremia, sodium loss is greater than water loss. Causes may be nonrenal or renal. Nonrenal causes include vomiting, diarrhea, fistulas, gastric suctioning, excessive sweating, cystic fibrosis, burns, and wound drainage. Renal causes include osmotic diuresis, salt-losing nephritis, adrenal insufficiency, and diuretic use.

Diuretics cause sodium loss and volume depletion from the blood vessels, resulting in thirst and retention of

Fluid movement in hyponatremia

This illustration shows fluid movement in hyponatremia. When serum osmolality decreases because of decreased sodium concentration, fluid moves by osmosis from the extracellular area to the intracellular area.

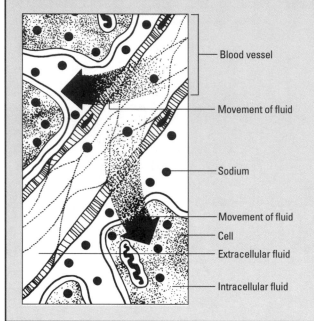

Blood vessel

Movement of fluid

Sodium

Movement of fluid

Cell

Extracellular fluid

Intracellular fluid

Drug culprits

Drugs may cause hyponatremia by potentiating the action of antidiuretic hormone (ADH) or by causing syndrome of inappropriate antidiuretic hormone secretion. Diuretics may also cause hyponatremia by inhibiting sodium reabsorption in the kidney.

Diuretics
• Furosemide
• Ethacrynic acid
• Bumetanide
• Thiazides

Antineoplastics
• Vincristine
• Cyclophosphamide

Antidiabetics
• Chlorpropamide
• Tolbutamide (rarely)

Sedatives
• Barbiturates
• Morphine

Antipsychotics
• Fluphenazine
• Thioridazine
• Thiothixene

Anticonvulsants
• Carbamazepine

water by the kidneys. (See *Drug culprits*.) Drinking large quantities of water can worsen hyponatremia. Sodium deficits will also be more pronounced if the patient is on a sodium-restricted diet. Diuretics can cause potassium loss, which is also linked to hyponatremia.

Both sides gain

In hypervolemic hyponatremia, both water and sodium increase in the extracellular area, but the water gain is more impressive. The serum sodium is diluted and edema also occurs. Causes include congestive heart failure (CHF), cirrhosis, nephrotic syndrome, and excessive administration of hypotonic I.V. fluids.

Only water gains

In isovolumic hyponatremia, total body sodium may be normal but may appear low because there's too much fluid

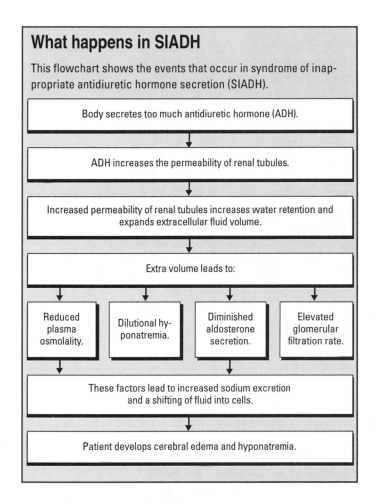

What happens in SIADH

This flowchart shows the events that occur in syndrome of inappropriate antidiuretic hormone secretion (SIADH).

Body secretes too much antidiuretic hormone (ADH).

↓

ADH increases the permeability of renal tubules.

↓

Increased permeability of renal tubules increases water retention and expands extracellular fluid volume.

↓

Extra volume leads to:

| Reduced plasma osmolality. | Dilutional hyponatremia. | Diminished aldosterone secretion. | Elevated glomerular filtration rate. |

↓

These factors lead to increased sodium excretion and a shifting of fluid into cells.

↓

Patient develops cerebral edema and hyponatremia.

in the body. Causes include glucocorticoid deficiency (causing inadequate fluid filtration by the kidneys), hypothyroidism (causing limited water excretion), and renal failure.

Disturbing the balance

Another cause of isovolumic hyponatremia is syndrome of inappropriate antidiuretic hormone secretion, which causes excessive release of ADH and disturbs fluid and electrolyte balance. This syndrome is a major cause of low sodium levels. ADH is released when the body doesn't need it, which results in water retention and sodium excretion. (See *What happens in SIADH*.)

Syndrome of inappropriate antidiuretic hormone secretion occurs with:

• cancers, especially oat cell carcinoma of the lung
• CNS disorders, such as trauma, tumors, or stroke
• pulmonary disorders, such as tumors, asthma, and chronic obstructive pulmonary disease
• medications, such as certain oral hypoglycemic agents, chemotherapy, and psychoactive drugs.

The patient is treated for the underlying cause of syndrome of inappropriate antidiuretic hormone as well as for hyponatremia. For instance, he'll receive cancer treatment if a tumor caused the syndrome or, if a medication is the cause, the drug will be stopped. The low sodium levels are treated with fluid restrictions (about a liter a day) and diuretics such as furosemide.

To increase water excretion, the patient may receive oral urea or a high salt diet to increase the solute excretion by the kidneys (water will follow). Medications such as demeclocycline or lithium may be used to block ADH in the renal tubule. If fluid restriction doesn't raise sodium levels, hypertonic saline solution may be given. (See *Key facts about hyponatremia*.)

What to look for

As you look for signs and symptoms of hyponatremia, remember that they may vary from patient to patient. They may also vary depending on how quickly the drop in sodium level occurred. If the drop was quick the patient will be more symptomatic than if the change was slow. Patients with sodium levels above 125 mEq/L may not show signs of hyponatremia — but, again, this depends on how fast sodium levels drop.

When signs do occur, they're primarily neurologic ones. The patient may complain of a headache or nausea and abdominal cramps. There may be muscle twitching, tremors, or weakness. Changes in mental status may start as a shortened attention span and progress to lethargy or confusion. If the sodium level drops to 110 mEq/L, the patient's neurologic status will deteriorate further, leading to stupor and even coma. He may also develop seizures.

Patients with hypovolemia may have poor skin turgor and dry, cracked mucous membranes. Assessment of vital signs shows a weak, rapid pulse and low blood pressure or orthostatic hypotension. Central venous pressure, pulmonary artery pressure, and pulmonary artery wedge pressure may be decreased.

Key facts about hyponatremia

☑ It's caused by inadequate sodium intake, excessive sodium loss, or water gain.

☑ Signs and symptoms vary greatly among patients.

☑ It's a very common electrolyte imbalance in hospitalized patients.

☑ Dilutional hyponatremia may be associated with hypervolemia; depletional hyponatremia, with hypovolemia.

☑ It always results in decreased serum osmolality. Fluid shifts into intracellular areas may cause neurologic symptoms related to cerebral edema.

☑ Altered level of consciousness usually accompanies serum sodium levels < 125 mEq/L and indicates that the patient's condition is deteriorating.

Patients with hypervolemia (fluid volume excess) may have edema, hypertension, weight gain, and rapid, bounding pulse. The central venous pressure and pulmonary artery pressure in these patients may be elevated. (See *Signs of hyponatremia*.)

What tests show

You'll probably note these diagnostic test results in your patient with hyponatremia:
• serum osmolality less than 280 mOsm/kg (dilute blood)
• serum sodium level less than 135 mEq/L (low sodium level in blood)
• urine specific gravity less than 1.010
• increased urine specific gravity and elevated urine sodium (> 20 mEq/L) in patients with syndrome of inappropriate antidiuretic hormone.

How hyponatremia is treated

In general, treatment varies with the cause and severity of hyponatremia. For example, hormone therapy may be necessary to treat underlying endocrine disorders.

For mild cases...

Therapy for mild hyponatremia associated with hypervolemia or isovolemia usually consists of restricted fluid intake and, possibly, oral sodium supplements. If hypovolemia is related to hyponatremia, isotonic I.V. fluids such as normal saline solution may be given to restore volume. High-sodium foods may also be offered to the patient.

For more severe cases...

When serum sodium levels fall below 110 mEq/L, treatment may include infusion of a hypertonic saline solution (such as 3% or 5% saline) in the intensive care unit. Monitor the patient carefully during the infusion for signs of circulatory overload or worsening neurologic status. A hypertonic saline solution causes water to shift out of cells, which may lead to intravascular volume overload and serious brain damage (osmotic demyelination), especially in the pons.

Fluid overload can be fatal if it's not treated. To prevent overload, the hypertonic sodium chloride solution is

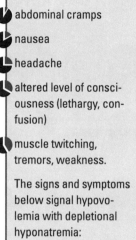

I can't waste time

Signs of hyponatremia

The signs and symptoms below signal hyponatremia:
• abdominal cramps
• nausea
• headache
• altered level of consciousness (lethargy, confusion)
• muscle twitching, tremors, weakness.

The signs and symptoms below signal hypovolemia with depletional hyponatremia:
• orthostatic hypotension
• poor skin turgor
• dry mucous membranes
• tachycardia.

The signs and symptoms below signal hypovolemia with dilutional hyponatremia:
• hypertension
• weight gain
• rapid, bounding pulse.

infused slowly and in small volumes. Furosemide is usually administered at the same time.

Hypervolemic patients shouldn't receive hypertonic sodium chloride solutions, except in rare instances of severe symptomatic hyponatremia. During treatment, monitor serum sodium and related diagnostic tests to follow the patient's progress.

How you intervene

Be sure to watch patients at risk for hyponatremia. They include those with CHF, cancer, or GI disorders with fluid losses. Review your patient's medications, noting those that are associated with hyponatremia. For patients who do develop hyponatremia, you'll want to take the following actions.

Monitor

• Monitor and record vital signs, especially blood pressure and pulse.
• Monitor neurologic status frequently. Report any deterioration in level of consciousness. Assess for lethargy, muscle twitching, seizures, and coma.
• Accurately measure and record intake and output.
• Weigh the patient daily to monitor the success of fluid restriction.
• Assess skin turgor at least every 8 hours.
• Watch for and report extreme changes in serum sodium and accompanying serum chloride levels. Also monitor other test results, such as urine specific gravity and serum osmolality.

Administer and maintain

• Restrict fluid intake as ordered, because this is the primary treatment for dilutional hyponatremia. Post a sign about fluid restriction in the patient's room, and be sure the staff, the patient, and his family are aware of the restrictions. (See *Teaching about hyponatremia*.)
• Administer oral sodium supplements, if prescribed, to treat mild hyponatremia. If the doctor has ordered increased dietary sodium, teach the patient about foods high in sodium.
• For severe hyponatremia, have a patent I.V. line in place for administration of isotonic or hypertonic sodium chloride solution. Administer prescribed I.V. isotonic or hyper-

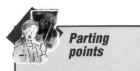

Parting points

Teaching about hyponatremia

Be sure to cover these topics with your patient, and then evaluate his learning:

🎓 explanation of hyponatremia, including causes and treatment

🎓 drug therapy and possible adverse effects

🎓 dietary changes and fluid restrictions, if any

🎓 signs and symptoms to report

🎓 need to monitor weight daily.

tonic saline solutions cautiously to avoid inducing hypernatremia, brain injury, or volume overload from excessive or too rapid an infusion. Watch closely for signs of hypervolemia (dyspnea, crackles, engorged neck or hand veins) and report them immediately. Use an infusion pump to ensure the patient receives only the prescribed volume of fluid.

• Keep the patient safe while he undergoes treatment. Provide a safe environment for a patient who has altered thought processes, and reorient him as needed. If seizures are likely, pad the bed's side rails and keep suction equipment and an airway handy. (See *Documenting hyponatremia*.)

Hypernatremia

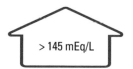

> 145 mEq/L

An excess of sodium relative to body water, hypernatremia occurs much less often than hyponatremia. Severe hypernatremia can lead to seizures, coma, and permanent neurologic damage.

How it happens

Thirst is the body's main defense against hypernatremia. The hypothalamus (with its osmoreceptors) is the brain's thirst center. High serum osmolality (increased solute concentrations in the blood) stimulates the hypothalamus and initiates the sensation of thirst.

The drive to respond to thirst is so strong that severe, persistent hypernatremia occurs only in people who can't drink voluntarily, such as infants, confused elderly patients, or unconscious patients. Hypothalamic disorders, such as a lesion on the hypothalamus, may cause a disturbance of the thirst mechanism, but this is rare.

Striving for balance

The body strives to maintain a normal sodium level by secreting antidiuretic hormone from the posterior pituitary gland. This hormone causes water to be retained, which helps to lower serum sodium levels.

The cells also play a role in maintaining sodium balance. When serum osmolality increases because of hypernatremia, fluid moves by osmosis from inside the cell to

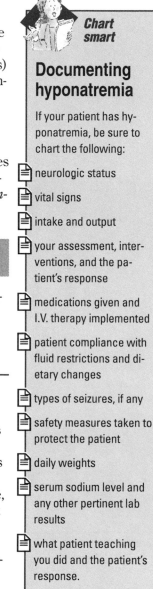

Chart smart

Documenting hyponatremia

If your patient has hyponatremia, be sure to chart the following:

📄 neurologic status

📄 vital signs

📄 intake and output

📄 your assessment, interventions, and the patient's response

📄 medications given and I.V. therapy implemented

📄 patient compliance with fluid restrictions and dietary changes

📄 types of seizures, if any

📄 safety measures taken to protect the patient

📄 daily weights

📄 serum sodium level and any other pertinent lab results

📄 what patient teaching you did and the patient's response.

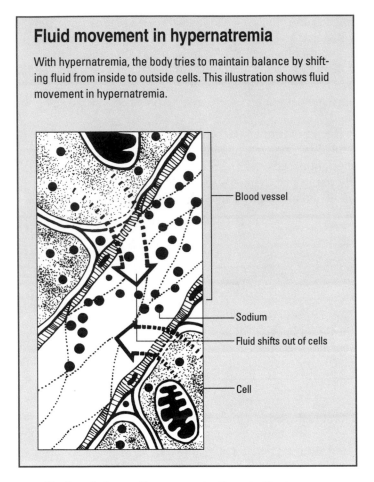

Fluid movement in hypernatremia

With hypernatremia, the body tries to maintain balance by shifting fluid from inside to outside cells. This illustration shows fluid movement in hypernatremia.

Blood vessel

Sodium

Fluid shifts out of cells

Cell

outside it to balance the concentrations in the two compartments. (For more information, see Chapter 1.)

As fluid leaves the cells, they may become dehydrated — especially the cells of the CNS. When this occurs, patients may show signs of neurologic impairment. They may also show signs of hypervolemia (fluid overload) from increased extracellular fluid volume in the blood vessels. (See *Fluid movement in hypernatremia*.)

Up with concentration

Hypernatremia may be caused by a water deficit — that is, more sodium relative to water in the body. It may also result from ingesting a larger-than-normal amount of sodium. (See *Key facts about hypernatremia*.) Regardless of the cause, body fluids become hypertonic (more concentrated).

Water deficit

A water deficit may occur alone or with a sodium loss (but more water will be lost than sodium). In either case, serum sodium levels are elevated. This elevation is more dangerous in debilitated patients and others with a deficient water intake.

Insensible water losses of several liters per day can result from fever and heat stroke, with older adults and athletes being equally susceptible. Large water losses also occur in patients with pulmonary infections, who lose water vapor from the lungs with hyperventilation, and in patients with extensive burns. Severe watery diarrhea is another cause of water loss and subsequent hypernatremia, and can be especially dangerous in children. Patients with hyperosmolar hyperglycemic nonketotic syndrome can also develop hypernatremia due to severe water losses from osmotic diuresis. Urea diuresis occurs with administration of high protein feedings without adequate water supplementation and can lead to hypernatremia.

Thirst to an extreme

Patients with diabetes insipidus have extreme thirst and enormous urinary losses, often more than 4 gal (15 L) per day. Usually, they can drink enough fluids to match the urinary losses; otherwise, severe dehydration and hypernatremia occur. Diabetes insipidus may result from a lack of ADH from the brain (central diabetes insipidus) or a lack of response from the kidneys to ADH (nephrogenic diabetes insipidus).

Central diabetes insipidus may result from a tumor or head trauma (injury or surgery) or be idiopathic (no known cause). It responds well to vasopressin (another name for ADH). Nephrogenic diabetes insipidus doesn't respond well to vasopressin and is more likely to occur with electrolyte imbalance, such as hypokalemia or with certain medications such as lithium.

Excessive sodium intake

Besides water losses from the body, relative sodium gains can also cause hypernatremia. High sodium intake may come from salt tablets, food, or medications containing a high sodium content such as sodium polystyrene sulfonate (Kayexalate).

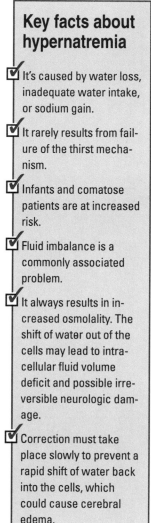

Key facts about hypernatremia

☑ It's caused by water loss, inadequate water intake, or sodium gain.

☑ It rarely results from failure of the thirst mechanism.

☑ Infants and comatose patients are at increased risk.

☑ Fluid imbalance is a commonly associated problem.

☑ It always results in increased osmolality. The shift of water out of the cells may lead to intracellular fluid volume deficit and possible irreversible neurologic damage.

☑ Correction must take place slowly to prevent a rapid shift of water back into the cells, which could cause cerebral edema.

Excessive parenteral administration of sodium solutions, such as hypertonic saline solutions or sodium bicarbonate preparations can also cause hypernatremia. Other causes of elevated sodium levels include inadvertent introduction of hypertonic saline solution into maternal circulation during therapeutic abortion, near drowning in salt water, and excessive amounts of adrenocortical hormones, as in Cushing's syndrome and hyperaldosteronism, which affects water and sodium balance.(See *Drugs associated with hypernatremia*.)

What to look for

The most important signs of hypernatremia will be neurologic because of the effects that fluid shifts have on brain cells. Remember that the body can tolerate a high sodium level that develops over time better than one that occurs rapidly. You may see restlessness or agitation, weakness, lethargy, confusion, stupor, seizures, and coma. (See *Signs of hypernatremia*.)

You may also observe signs of neuromuscular irritability such as twitching, and the patient may have a low grade fever and flushed skin. He'll complain of intense thirst from stimulation of the hypothalamus by increased osmolality.

Other symptoms vary depending on the cause of the high sodium levels. If a sodium gain has occurred, fluid may be drawn into the blood vessels and the patient will appear hypervolemic, with an elevated blood pressure, bounding pulse, and dyspnea.

Drugs associated with hypernatremia

The drugs below can cause high sodium levels. Ask your patient if he's taking any of them:

• antacids with sodium bicarbonate
• sodium bicarbonate injections (such as those given during cardiac arrest)
• I.V. sodium chloride preparations
• sodium polystyrene sulfonate (Kayexalate)
• salt tablets
• antibiotics such as ticarcillin disodium/ clavulanate potassium (Timentin).

Memory jogger

To help you remember some common signs and symptoms of hypernatremia, think of the word SALT.

S   skin flushed

A   agitation

L   low grade fever

T   thirst

If water loss occurs, fluid will leave the blood vessels and you'll notice signs of hypovolemia, such as dry mucous membranes, oliguria, and orthostatic hypotension (blood pressure drop and heart rate increase with position changes).

What tests show

Now that you know how hypernatremia progresses, you'll better understand the results of these common diagnostic findings in hypernatremia:
• serum sodium level greater than 145 mEq/L
• increased urine specific gravity (except in diabetes insipidus, where urine specific gravity is decreased)
• serum osmolality greater than 300 mOsm/kg.

How hypernatremia is treated

Treatment of hypernatremia varies with the cause. The underlying disorder needs to be corrected, and serum sodium levels and related diagnostic tests must be monitored. If hypernatremia is caused by too little water in the body, treatment may include oral fluid replacement. Be sure to replace fluids gradually, over 48 hours, to avoid shifting water into brain cells.

Remember, as sodium levels rise in the blood vessels, fluid shifts out of the cells — including the brain cells — to dilute the blood and equalize concentrations. If too much water is introduced into the body too quickly, water moves into brain cells and they get bigger, causing cerebral edema.

If the patient can't drink enough fluids, he'll need I.V. fluid replacement. He may receive salt-free solutions (such as dextrose 5% in water) to return serum sodium levels to normal, followed by infusion of half-normal saline solution to prevent hyponatremia and cerebral edema. Other treatments include restricting sodium intake and administering diuretics along with oral or I.V. fluid replacement to increase sodium loss.

Treatment for diabetes insipidus may include vasopressin, hypotonic I.V. fluids, and thiazide diuretics to decrease free water loss from the kidneys. The underlying cause should also be treated.

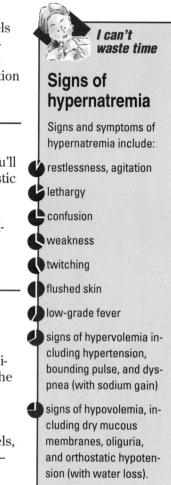

I can't waste time

Signs of hypernatremia

Signs and symptoms of hypernatremia include:
• restlessness, agitation
• lethargy
• confusion
• weakness
• twitching
• flushed skin
• low-grade fever
• signs of hypervolemia including hypertension, bounding pulse, and dyspnea (with sodium gain)
• signs of hypovolemia, including dry mucous membranes, oliguria, and orthostatic hypotension (with water loss).

How you intervene

Try to prevent hypernatremia in high-risk patients (such as those recovering from surgery near the pituitary gland) by observing them closely. Also check out medications they're taking that might cause hypernatremia. If your patient does develop hypernatremia, take these measures.

Assess, replenish, and restore

- Monitor and record vital signs, especially blood pressure and pulse.
- If the patient needs I.V. fluid replacement, monitor fluid delivery and his response to the therapy. Watch for signs of cerebral edema, and check his neurologic status frequently. Report any deterioration in level of consciousness.
- Carefully measure and record intake and output. Weigh the patient daily to check for body fluid loss.
- Assess skin and mucous membranes for signs of breakdown and infection.
- Monitor the patient's serum sodium level and report any increase. Monitor urine specific gravity and other laboratory test results.
- If the patient can't take oral fluids, recommend the I.V. route to the doctor. If the patient can drink and is alert and responsible, involve him in his treatment. Give him a target amount of fluid to drink each shift, mark cups with the volume they hold, leave fluids within easy reach, and provide paper and pen to record amounts. If the family will be helping the patient drink, be sure to give them specific instructions as well. (See *Teaching about hypernatremia*.)
- Insert and maintain a patent I.V., as ordered. Use a volumetric device to control delivery of I.V. fluids.
- Assist with oral hygiene. Lubricate the patient's lips frequently with a water-based lubricant, and provide mouthwash or gargle if he is alert. Good mouth care helps keep mucous membranes moist and decreases mouth odor.
- Provide a safe environment for confused or agitated patients. If seizures are likely, pad the bed's siderails and keep an artificial airway and suction equipment handy. Reorient the patient as needed, and reduce environmental stimuli. (See *Documenting hypernatremia*.)

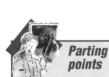

Parting points

Teaching about hypernatremia

Be sure to cover these points when teaching your patient with hypernatremia and to evaluate his learning:

- explanation of condition
- importance of maintaining sodium-restricted diet
- prescribed medications
- signs and symptoms and when to report them
- avoiding over-the-counter medications that contain sodium

Chart smart

Documenting hypernatremia

When documenting information about your patient with hypernatremia, you'll want to include:

- vital signs
- intake and output
- medications given and I.V. therapy implemented
- seizure precautions
- your assessments, including neurologic status
- notification of the doctor when the patient's condition changes
- nursing interventions and the patient's response
- teaching done, including fluid and dietary intake recommendations
- daily weights
- serum sodium level and other pertinent lab results.

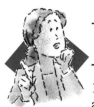

Quick quiz

1. Besides its responsibility for fluid balance, sodium is also responsible for:
    A. good eyesight and vitamin balance.
    B. bone structure.
    C. impulse transmission.

Answer: C. Sodium is the main extracellular cation responsible for regulating fluid balance in the body. It's also involved in impulse transmission in nerve and muscle fibers.

2. Symptoms of hyponatremia include:
    A. change in mental status, abdominal cramps, and muscle twitching.
    B. headache, rapid breathing, and high energy level.
    C. chest pain, fever, and pericardial rub.

Answer: A. The patient may also exhibit headache, nausea, coma, blood pressure changes, and tachycardia.

3. The minimum daily requirement of sodium for an average adult is:
    A. 2 g.
    B. 5 g.
    C. 8 g.

Answer: A. Although the minimum daily requirement is 2 g, the diets of many people in the United States include more than 6 g of sodium per day.

4. Increased serum sodium causes thirst and the release of:
    A. potassium into the cells.
    B. fluid into the interstitium.
    C. ADH into the bloodstream.

Answer: C. Higher levels of sodium in the blood prompts the release of ADH from the posterior pituitary.

5. The sodium-potassium pump transports sodium ions:
    A. into cells.
    B. out of cells.
    C. into and out of cells in equal amounts.

Answer: A. Normally most abundant outside of cells, sodium tends to diffuse inward. The sodium-potassium pump returns sodium to the extracellular area. Potassium ions tend to diffuse out of the cells and require transport back into the cell.

Scoring

☆☆☆ If you answered all five questions correctly, congratulations! You're a Sodium Somebody!

☆☆ If you answered three or four correctly, way cool. Have a cracker with peanut butter — on us!

☆ If you answered fewer than three correctly, don't fret. You're going to *love* the salt tablets we've got for you!

When potassium tips the balance

Just the facts

This chapter discusses the important role potassium plays in keeping the cells, nerves, and muscles functioning properly. In this chapter, you'll learn:

♦ how potassium contributes to fluid and electrolyte balance

♦ how the body regulates serum potassium levels

♦ how potassium imbalances are treated

♦ how to care for patients with potassium imbalances

♦ how to document care given to patients with potassium imbalances.

A look at potassium

The major cation (ion with a positive charge) in the intracellular fluid, potassium plays a critical role in many metabolic cell functions. Only 2% of the body's potassium is found in extracellular fluid; 98% is in intracellular fluid. That significant difference affects nerve impulse transmission.

Many diseases and injuries, and certain medications and therapies, can disturb potassium levels. Small, untreated alterations in serum potassium levels can seriously affect neuromuscular and cardiac functioning.

How it happens

Potassium has a direct impact on how well the body's cells, nerves, and muscles function by:
- maintaining cells' electrical neutrality and osmolality
- aiding neuromuscular transmission of nerve impulses
- assisting skeletal and cardiac muscle contraction and electrical conductivity
- affecting acid-base balance in relationship to the hydrogen ion (another cation). (See *Potassium's role in acid-base balance.*)

Normal serum (in the blood) potassium levels range from 3.5 to 5 mEq/L. In the cell, the potassium concentration (usually not measured) is much higher — 140 mEq/L. Potassium must be ingested daily because the body can't conserve it. The daily adult potassium dietary requirement is about 40 mEq; the average daily intake is 60 to 100 mEq. (See *Dietary sources of potassium.*) Extracellular fluid also gains potassium when cells are destroyed and release intracellular potassium, or when potassium shifts out of the intracellular fluid to the extracellular fluid.

Losing potassium

About 80% of the potassium taken in is excreted by the kidneys. Each liter of urine contains approximately 20 to 40 mEq of potassium. Any remaining potassium is excreted in feces and sweat.

Extracellular potassium loss also occurs when potassium moves from the extracellular fluid to the intracellular fluid or during cellular anabolism.

Three additional factors affect potassium levels — the sodium-potassium pump, renal regulation, and pH level.

The sodium-potassium pump is an active transport mechanism which requires energy to move ions across the cell membrane against a concentration gradient. The pump moves sodium from the cell into the extracellular fluid and maintains high intracellular potassium levels by pumping potassium into the cell.

Regulatin' those renals

The body also rids itself of excess potassium by way of the kidneys. As serum potassium levels rise, the renal tubules excrete more potassium, leading to increased potassium loss in the urine.

Sodium and potassium have a reciprocal relationship. The kidneys reabsorb sodium and excrete potassium

---

Dietary sources of potassium

Here are some major sources of potassium:

- Meats
- Vegetables, especially potatoes, mushrooms, tomatoes, and carrots
- Fruits, such as oranges, bananas, apricots, and cantaloupe
- Dried fruit, nuts, and seeds
- Chocolate

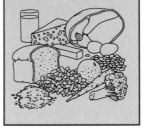

Potassium's role in acid-base balance

The illustration below shows the movement of potassium ions in response to changes in extracellular hydrogen ion concentration. Hydrogen ion concentration changes with acidosis and alkalosis.

Normal balance

Under normal conditions, the potassium ion (K) content in intracellular fluid (ICF) is much greater than in extracellular fluid (ECF). Hydrogen ion (H) concentration is low in both compartments.

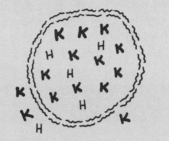

Acidosis

In acidosis, hydrogen ion content in ECF increases and the ions move into the ICF. To keep the ICF electrically neutral, an equal number of potassium ions (K) leave the cell, which creates a relative hyperkalemia.

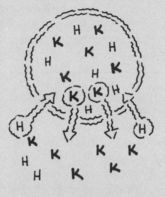

Alkalosis

In alkalosis, more hydrogen ions are present in the ICF than in the ECF. Therefore, hydrogen ions move from the ICF into the ECF. To keep the ICF electrically neutral, potassium ions move from the ECF into the ICF, creating a relative hypokalemia.

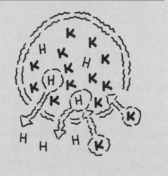

when the hormone aldosterone is secreted. The kidneys have no effective mechanism to combat loss of potassium and may excrete it even when the serum potassium level is low.

Moving freely

A change in pH may affect serum potassium levels because hydrogen ions and potassium ions freely exchange across plasma cell membranes. For example, in acidosis, excess hydrogen ions move into cells and push potassium into the extracellular fluid. Thus, acidosis can cause hyperkalemia as potassium moves out of the cell to maintain balance. Likewise, alkalosis can cause hypokalemia, as potassium moves into the cell to maintain balance.

Hypokalemia

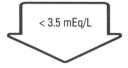

< 3.5 mEq/L

In hypokalemia, the serum potassium level drops below 3.5 mEq/L. Because the normal range for a serum potassium level is a narrow one (3.5 to 5 mEq/L), a slight decrease has profound consequences.

How it happens

Remember that the body can't conserve potassium. Inadequate intake and excessive output of potassium can cause a moderate drop in its level. Too little intake or too much output upsets the balance and causes a deficiency of total body potassium.

Conditions such as prolonged intestinal suction, recent ileostomy, and villous adenoma can cause excessive loss of total body potassium. In certain situations, potassium shifts from the extracellular space to the intracellular space. More potassium is *hiding* in the cells than usual, so less can be measured in the blood.

Not enough intake

A lack of potassium intake causes a drop in the level of potassium in the body. That could mean a person is not eating enough food containing potassium or is receiving potassium-deficient I.V. fluids.

Too much output

Intestinal fluids contain large amounts of potassium. Thus, severe GI fluid losses from suction, lavage, or prolonged vomiting can deplete the body's potassium supply. That can cause potassium levels to drop. Diarrhea, fistulas, or laxative abuse and severe diaphoresis also contribute to potassium loss.

In addition, potassium can be depleted through the kidneys. Diuresis that occurs with a newly functioning transplanted kidney can lead to hypokalemia. High glucose concentration in the urine causes osmotic diuresis and potassium is lost through the urine. Other potassium losses are seen in renal tubular acidosis, magnesium depletion, Cushing's syndrome, and periods of high stress.

Drugs can upset the balance

Drugs such as diuretics (especially thiazide and furosemide), corticosteroids, insulin, cisplatin and certain antibiotics (gentamicin, carbenicillin, and amphotericin B, for instance) also cause potassium to be lost from the body. (See *Drugs associated with hypokalemia*.)

Excessive secretion of insulin, whether endogenous or exogenous, may shift potassium into the cells. Insulin can be released from the body and cause hypokalemia in patients receiving large amounts of dextrose solutions. Potassium levels also drop when adrenergic agents, such as epinephrine or albuterol, are used to treat asthma.

Diseases wreak havoc, too

Conditions (such as vomiting) that lead to the loss of gastric acids can cause alkalosis and hypokalemia. Alkalosis moves potassium ions into the cell as hydrogen ions move out.

Other disorders associated with hypokalemia are hepatic disease, hyperaldosteronism, acute alcoholism, congestive heart failure (CHF), malabsorption syndrome, nephritis, and Barter's syndrome.

What to look for

The signs and symptoms of a low potassium level reflect how important the electrolyte is to normal body functions.

Neuromuscular alerts

Skeletal muscle weakness, especially in the legs, is a sign of a moderate loss of potassium. Weakness progresses and paresthesias develop. Leg cramps occur. Deep tendon reflexes may be decreased or absent. Paralysis could involve the respiratory muscles.

Drugs associated with hypokalemia

These drugs can deplete potassium and cause hypokalemia:

- diuretics, such as thiazide and furosemide
- certain antibiotics, such as gentamicin, carbenicillin, and amphotericin B
- laxative abuse
- corticosteroids
- insulin
- cisplatin
- adrenergic agents, such as albuterol and epinephrine.

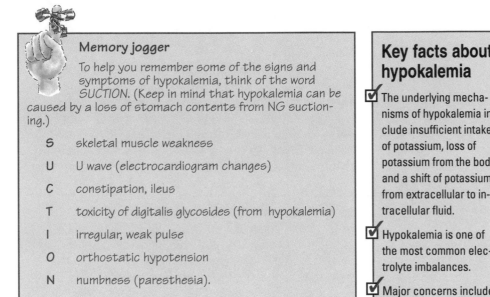

Memory jogger

To help you remember some of the signs and symptoms of hypokalemia, think of the word SUCTION. (Keep in mind that hypokalemia can be caused by a loss of stomach contents from NG suctioning.)

S   skeletal muscle weakness

U   U wave (electrocardiogram changes)

C   constipation, ileus

T   toxicity of digitalis glycosides (from hypokalemia)

I   irregular, weak pulse

O   orthostatic hypotension

N   numbness (paresthesia).

Because of potassium's effects on cell function, hypokalemia can lead to rhabdomyolysis, a breakdown of muscle fibers leading to myoglobin in the urine. As smooth muscle becomes affected by hypokalemia, the patient may develop anorexia, nausea, and vomiting.

Other problems

In addition, the patient may experience intestinal problems such as decreased bowel sounds, constipation, and paralytic ileus. He may also have difficulty concentrating urine (when hypokalemia is prolonged) and pass large volumes of urine. (See *Key facts about hypokalemia*.)

ECG alerts

Cardiac problems can result from a low potassium level. The pulse may be weak and irregular. The patient may have orthostatic hypotension. The electrocardiogram (ECG) may show a flattened T wave, a depressed ST segment, and a characteristic U wave. (See *Signs of hypokalemia*.)

Cardiac arrest can result from hypokalemia. A patient taking digitalis glycosides, especially if he is also taking a diuretic, should be watched closely for hypokalemia, which can potentiate the action of the digitalis glycoside preparation and cause toxicity. (See *Danger signs of hypokalemia,* page 102.)

Key facts about hypokalemia

☑ The underlying mechanisms of hypokalemia include insufficient intake of potassium, loss of potassium from the body, and a shift of potassium from extracellular to intracellular fluid.

☑ Hypokalemia is one of the most common electrolyte imbalances.

☑ Major concerns include arrhythmias (which may lead to cardiac arrest) and respiratory muscle weakness (which may lead to respiratory arrest).

☑ Serum potassium levels and electrocardiographic tracings are the best clinical indicators.

☑ Hypokalemia may precipitate digitalis toxicity; patients receiving potassium-wasting diuretics and digitalis glycosides require close monitoring.

☑ Hypokalemia commonly accompanies alkalosis.

What tests show

The following test results may help confirm the diagnosis of hypokalemia:
• serum potassium level less than 3.5 mEq/L
• elevated pH and bicarbonate levels
• slightly elevated serum glucose level
• characteristic ECG changes.

How hypokalemia is treated

Treatment of hypokalemia focuses on restoring a normal potassium balance, preventing serious complications, and removing or treating the underlying causes. Treatment varies depending on the severity of the imbalance.
• The patient should be placed on a high potassium diet.
• Increased dietary potassium may not be sufficient to treat less acute hypokalemia; the patient may need oral potassium supplements using potassium salts. Potassium chloride is preferred.
• Patients who have severe hypokalemia or who can't take oral supplements may need I.V. potassium replacement therapy. Whether through a peripheral or central catheter, I.V. potassium must be administered with care to prevent serious complications.

OK, now it's balanced

Once the serum potassium level is back to normal, the patient may receive a sustained-release oral potassium supplement as well as increased dietary potassium. Patients taking diuretics may be switched to a potassium-sparing diuretic to prevent excessive urinary loss of potassium.

How you intervene

Careful monitoring and skilled interventions can help prevent hypokalemia and spare your patient from its associated complications. For patients at risk for developing hypokalemia or who have hypokalemia already, you'll want to perform these actions.

Assess and monitor

• Monitor vital signs, especially pulse and blood pressure. Hypokalemia can cause orthostatic hypotension.

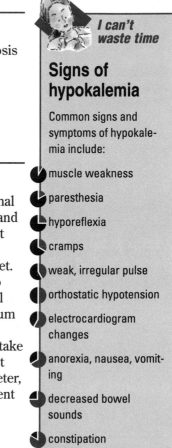

I can't waste time

Signs of hypokalemia

Common signs and symptoms of hypokalemia include:

muscle weakness

paresthesia

hyporeflexia

cramps

weak, irregular pulse

orthostatic hypotension

electrocardiogram changes

anorexia, nausea, vomiting

decreased bowel sounds

constipation

polyuria.

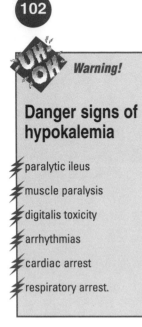

Warning!

Danger signs of hypokalemia

- paralytic ileus
- muscle paralysis
- digitalis toxicity
- arrhythmias
- cardiac arrest
- respiratory arrest.

• Assess the heart rate and rhythm and ECG tracings in the severely hypokalemic patient whose serum potassium level less than 3 mEq/L.

• Assess the patient's respiratory rate, depth, and pattern. Hypokalemia may weaken or paralyze respiratory muscles. Notify the doctor at once if respirations become shallow and rapid. Keep a manual resuscitation bag at the bedside of a severely hypokalemic patient. (See *When treatment doesn't work.*)

• Monitor serum potassium levels. Changes in serum potassium levels can lead to serious cardiac complications.

• Assess for clinical evidence of hypokalemia, especially in patients receiving diuretics or digitalis glycosides. A patient who has hypokalemia and who takes digitalis glycosides is at increased risk for digitalis toxicity.

• Monitor and document fluid intake and output. About 40 mEq of potassium is lost in each liter of urine. Diuresis can put the patient at a risk for potassium loss.

•Check for signs of hypokalemia-linked metabolic alkalosis, including irritability and paresthesia.

I.V. guidelines

• Insert and maintain patent I.V. access as ordered. When choosing a vein, remember that I.V. potassium prepara-

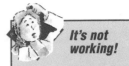

It's not working!

When treatment doesn't work

If you're having trouble trying to raise a patient's potassium level, step back and take a look at the entire fluid and electrolyte picture.

• Is the patient still diuresing or suffering losses from the GI tract or the skin? If so, he's losing fluid and potassium.

• Is the patient's magnesium level normal, or does he need supplementation? Keep in mind, low magnesium levels make it hard for the kidneys to conserve potassium.

Guidelines for I.V. potassium administration

Here are some guidelines for administering I.V. potassium and for monitoring patients receiving I.V. potassium. Remember that I.V. replacement of potassium is necessary only if hypokalemia is severe or if the patient can't take oral potassium supplements.

Administration

• When adding the potassium preparation to an I.V. solution, mix well. Don't add to a container in the hanging position; the potassium will pool and the patient will receive a highly concentrated bolus.

• To avoid or lessen toxic effects, I.V. infusion concentrations shouldn't exceed 40 to 60 mEq/L. Rates are usually 10 mEq/hour, sometimes 20 mEq/hour. More rapid infusions may be used in severe cases, although rapid infusion requires closer monitoring of the car-

diac status. The maximum adult dose generally should not exceed 200 mEq/24 hours, unless prescribed.

• Use infusion devices when administering potassium solutions to control flow rate.

• NEVER administer potassium by I.V. push or bolus; doing so may cause cardiac arrhythmias, and possibly, cardiac arrest.

Patient monitoring

• Monitor the patient's cardiac rhythm during rapid I.V. potassium administra-

tion to avoid toxic effects from inadvertent hyperkalemia. Report any irregularities immediately.

• Evaluate the results of treatment by checking serum potassium levels and assessing the patient for signs of toxicity, such as muscle weakness or paralysis.

• Watch the I.V. site for signs and symptoms of infiltration, phlebitis, or tissue necrosis.

• Monitor the patient's urine output and notify the doctor of inadequate volume. Urine output should be >30 ml/hour to avoid hyperkalemia.

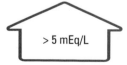

Parting points

Teaching about hypokalemia

Be sure to cover the following teaching topics and evaluate your patient's learning:

- explanation of hypokalemia, including its signs, symptoms, and complications
- causes and risk factors
- prevention of future episodes
- medication, including dosages and possible adverse effects
- need for a potassium-rich diet
- warning signs and symptoms to report to the doctor.

tions can be irritating to peripheral veins and may cause discomfort.
- Administer I.V. potassium replacement solutions as prescribed. (See *Guidelines for I.V. potassium administration*.)
- Monitor heart rate and rhythm and ECG tracings of patients receiving potassium infusions of more than 5 mEq/hour or a concentration of more than 40 mEq/L of fluid.
- Administer I.V. potassium infusions cautiously. Make sure that infusions are diluted and mixed thoroughly in adequate amounts of fluid.
- Watch the I.V. infusion site for infiltration or pain; highly concentrated solutions may cause discomfort and irritation.
- Never give potassium by I.V. push or as a bolus. It could be fatal.
- To prevent gastric irritation from oral potassium supplements, administer the supplements in at least 4 oz of fluid or with food.
- Slow release tablets should not be crushed to avoid a quick load of potassium entering the body.
- Dosing with oral supplements should be done as carefully as with I.V. administration.
- Provide a safe environment for the patient who is weak from hypokalemia. Explain any activity restrictions imposed. (See *Teaching about hypokalemia*.)
- Check for signs of constipation, such as abdominal distention and decreased bowel sounds. Although medication may be prescribed to combat constipation, don't use laxatives that promote potassium loss. (See *Documenting hypokalemia*.)
- Emphasize the importance of taking potassium supplements as prescribed, especially when also taking digitalis glycosides or diuretics. If appropriate, teach the patient to recognize and report signs of digitalis toxicity, such as pulse irregularities, anorexia, nausea, and vomiting.
- Make sure the patient can identify the signs and symptoms of hypokalemia.

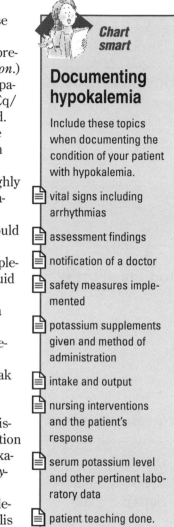

Chart smart

Documenting hypokalemia

Include these topics when documenting the condition of your patient with hypokalemia.

- vital signs including arrhythmias
- assessment findings
- notification of a doctor
- safety measures implemented
- potassium supplements given and method of administration
- intake and output
- nursing interventions and the patient's response
- serum potassium level and other pertinent laboratory data
- patient teaching done.

Hyperkalemia

> 5 mEq/L

Hyperkalemia occurs when the serum potassium level rises above 5 mEq/L. Because the normal serum potassium range is so narrow (3.5 to 5 mEq/L), a slight increase can have profound consequences. Although less common than hypokalemia, hyperkalemia is more serious. Hyperkalemia is often induced by other treatments.

How it happens

Remember, potassium is gained through intake and lost by excretion. If either is altered, hyperkalemia can result. (See *Key facts about hyperkalemia*.)

    The kidneys, which excrete potassium, are vital in preventing a toxic buildup of this electrolyte. Acid-base imbalances can alter potassium balance as well. Acidosis moves potassium outside the cell as hydrogen ions shift into the cell. Cell injury results in release, or spilling, of potassium into the serum, which is reflected in the patient's laboratory test results.

Too much intake

Increased dietary intake of potassium (especially with decreased urine output) can cause the potassium level to rise. Excessive use of salt substitutes (most of which use potassium as a substitute for sodium) further compounds the situation. Potassium supplements, whether in oral or I.V. form, raise the potassium level. Excessive doses can lead to hyperkalemia.

Watch transfusions and drugs

Because the serum concentration increases as donated blood is stored longer, a patient's potassium level may rise if given a large volume of blood nearing its expiration date.

    Certain medications are associated with high potassium levels, such as beta blockers (which inhibit potassium shifts into cells), potassium-sparing diuretics such as spironolactone, and some antibiotics such as penicillin G potassium. Use of chemotherapy, which causes cell death (and sometimes renal injury), can lead to hyperkalemia.

    Angiotensin converting enzyme inhibitors and nonsteroidal anti-inflammatory drugs are thought to cause hyperkalemia by effecting aldosterone secretion, which promotes potassium excretion in the kidneys. When administering any medication that can cause renal injury (such as aminoglycosides), be on the lookout for hyperkalemia. (See *Drugs associated with hyperkalemia*.)

Key facts about hyperkalemia

☑ Underlying mechanisms responsible for hyperkalemia include increased intake of potassium, decreased urinary excretion of potassium, and shift of potassium out of the cells to extracellular fluid.

☑ Hyperkalemia may be the most dangerous of the electrolyte disorders.

☑ Serum potassium levels > 7 mEq/L may cause serious cardiac arrhythmias leading to cardiac arrest.

☑ Signs and symptoms are often nonspecific; serum potassium levels and electrocardiogram tracings are often the best clinical indicators.

☑ Hyperkalemia frequently accompanies metabolic acidosis.

Drugs associated with hyperkalemia

• excessive potassium
• spironolactone
• beta blockers
• some antibiotics
• chemotherapy
• nonsteroidal anti-inflammatory drugs
• angiotensin converting enzyme inhibitors.

Too little output

Potassium excretion is diminished with acute or chronic renal failure. Any disease that can cause kidney damage (diabetes, sickle cell disease, or systemic lupus erythematosus, for instance) can lead to hyperkalemia. Addison's disease and hypoaldosteronism can decrease potassium excretion from the body.

Injury moves it out

Potassium can leave the cell when the cell has been injured by burns, severe infection, trauma, crush injuries, or intravascular hemolysis.

Chemotherapy causes cell lysis and release of potassium. Metabolic acidosis and insulin deficiency decrease the movement of potassium into cells. (See *Make sure the results are real.*)

What to look for

Signs and symptoms of hyperkalemia reflect its effects on neuromuscular and cardiac functioning in the body. Paresthesia, an early sign, and irritability signal hyperkalemia. (See *Signs of hyperkalemia,* page 106.)

Neuromuscular alerts

Hyperkalemia may cause skeletal muscle weakness that, in turn, may lead to flaccid paralysis. Muscle weakness tends to spread from the legs to the trunk and involves respiratory muscles. Hyperkalemia also causes smooth muscle hyperactivity, particularly in the GI tract, which can result in nausea, abdominal cramping, and diarrhea, an early sign.

Cardiac alerts

Other possible complications include a decreased heart rate, irregular pulse, decreased cardiac output, hypotension and, possibly, cardiac arrest.

The tall, tented T wave is a prominent ECG characteristic of the patient with hyperkalemia. Other ECG changes include a flattened P wave, prolonged PR interval, widened QRS complex, and depressed ST segment. The condition can also lead to heart block, ventricular arrhythmias, and asystole. The more serious arrhythmias become especially dangerous when the serum potassium level reaches 7 mEq/L or more.

Make sure the results are real

When you see a high serum potassium result and it just doesn't seem to make sense, be sure that it's a true result. If the sample was drawn using poor technique, the results may be falsely high. Some of the causes of high potassium levels that don't truly reflect the patient's serum potassium level include:

• drawing the sample above an I.V. infusion containing potassium
• using a recently exercised extremity for the venipuncture site
• causing hemolysis (cell damage) as the specimen is obtained.

What tests show

The following test results help confirm the diagnosis and determine the severity of hyperkalemia:
- serum potassium level greater than 5 mEq/L
- decreased arterial pH, indicating acidosis
- ECG abnormalities. (See *Key facts about hyperkalemia.*)

How hyperkalemia is treated

Treatment for hyperkalemia is aimed at lowering the potassium level as well as treating its cause. The severity of hyperkalemia dictates how it will be treated.

For mild cases...

Mild hyperkalemia may be treated with loop diuretics to increase potassium loss from the body or to resolve any acidosis present. Dietary potassium is restricted. Medications associated with high potassium level should be readjusted or stopped. Underlying disorders leading to the high potassium level are treated.

For moderate to severe cases...

With moderate to severe hyperkalemia, other measures may be undertaken. Sometimes diuretics are not effective in a patient with renal failure. In acute symptomatic hyperkalemia, hemodialysis may be required.

Sodium polystyrene sulfonate (Kayexalate), a cation-exchange resin, is a common treatment for hyperkalemia. Sorbitol, or another osmotic substance, should be included with this medication to promote its excretion. Kayexalate can be given orally or through an NG tube, or as a retention enema (may require repeated treatments). The onset of action may take several hours; the duration of action is about 4 to 6 hours. As the medication sits in the intestines, sodium moves across the bowel wall into the blood, and potassium moves out of the blood into the intestines. Loose stools remove potassium from the body.

Emergency measures

More severe hyperkalemia is treated as an emergency. Closely monitor the patient's cardiac status. ECGs are obtained to follow progress.

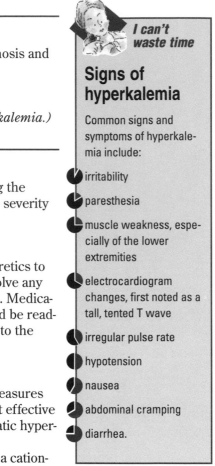

I can't waste time

Signs of hyperkalemia

Common signs and symptoms of hyperkalemia include:
- irritability
- paresthesia
- muscle weakness, especially of the lower extremities
- electrocardiogram changes, first noted as a tall, tented T wave
- irregular pulse rate
- hypotension
- nausea
- abdominal cramping
- diarrhea.

To counteract the myocardial effects of hyperkalemia, administer 10% calcium gluconate (usually 10 ml) I.V. over 3 minutes. The patient must be connected to a cardiac monitor. Calcium gluconate is not a treatment for hyperkalemia itself. The high potassium must still be treated because the effects of calcium last only a short time.

A patient with acidosis may receive sodium bicarbonate (usually 50 mEq) I.V., which helps decrease serum potassium level by temporarily shifting potassium into the cells. The drug becomes effective within 15 to 30 minutes and lasts 1 to 3 hours.

Another way to move potassium into the cells and lower the serum level is to administer regular insulin (10 units) I.V. The drug becomes active within 15 to 60 minutes and lasts 4 to 6 hours. It is given concurrently with I.V. hypertonic dextrose (10% to 50%).

How you intervene

Patients at risk of hyperkalemia require frequent monitoring of serum potassium and other electrolyte levels. Those at risk include patients with acidosis, renal failure, and those receiving potassium-sparing diuretics, oral potassium supplements, or I.V. potassium preparations. If a patient develops hyperkalemia, take these nursing actions.

Assess

• Assess vital signs. Anticipate cardiac monitoring if the patient's serum potassium level is more than 6 mEq/L. A patient with ECG changes may need aggressive treatment to prevent cardiac arrest.
• Monitor the patient's intake and output. Report an output of less than 30 ml/hour. An inability to excrete potassium adequately may lead to dangerously high potassium levels. (See *The next step*.)
• Prepare to administer a slow calcium gluconate I.V. infusion in acute cases to counteract the myocardial depressant effects of hyperkalemia.
• Assess for clinical signs of hypoglycemia, including muscle weakness, syncope, hunger, and diaphoresis in patients receiving repeated insulin and glucose treatment.
• Keep in mind when giving Kayexalate that serum sodium levels may rise. Watch for signs of CHF.

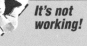

It's not working!

The next step

If you're unable to bring down your patient's potassium level as expected, consider the following questions:

• Is the patient receiving antacids? Antacids containing magnesium or calcium can interfere with ion exchange resins.
• Is the patient's renal status worsening?
• Is the patient on medications that raise the potassium level?
• Is the patient receiving old banked blood during transfusions?

• Monitor bowel sounds and the number and character of bowel movements.
• Monitor serum potassium level and related laboratory results.

Administer and follow up

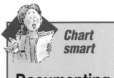

Documenting hyperkalemia

When your patient has hyperkalemia, you'll want to document the following information:

☐ vital signs including arrhythmias

☐ assessment findings

☐ doctor notification

☐ medications administered

☐ interventions and the patient's response

☐ safety measures implemented

☐ serum potassium level and other pertinent lab results

☐ intake and output

☐ patient teaching done.

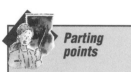

Parting points

Teaching about hyperkalemia

Be sure to cover the following topics and to evaluate your patient's learning

🎓 explanation of hyperkalemia, including its signs and symptoms, and potential complications

🎓 prevention of future episodes of hyperkalemia

🎓 medication, including dosage and potential for hypokalemia

🎓 need for a potassium-restricted diet and importance of avoiding salt substitutes

🎓 warning signs and symptoms to report to the doctor.

• Administer prescribed medications and monitor for their effectiveness and adverse effects.
• Encourage the patient to retain sodium polystyrene sulfonate enemas for 30 to 60 minutes. Monitor for hypokalemia when administering this agent on 2 or more consecutive days.
• Try an indwelling urinary catheter, with the balloon inflated after insertion into the rectum, to assist with enema retention in a patient with diarrhea who can't retain the liquid.
• Prepare a patient who has acute hyperkalemia that doesn't respond to other therapies for possible dialysis.
• Implement safety measures for the patient with muscle weakness. Tell the patient to request assistance before attempting to get out of bed and walk. Continue to evaluate muscle strength.
• Administer prescribed antidiarrheal medications and monitor the patient's response.
• Help the patient select foods that won't stimulate peristalsis. (See *Teaching about hyperkalemia*.)
• Check the donation date of blood. Obtain fresh blood for the hyperkalemic patient who needs a transfusion.
• Be alert for signs of hypokalemia after treatment.
• Document all care given and the patient's response. (See *Documenting hyperkalemia*.)
• Explain the signs of hyperkalemia, including muscle weakness, diarrhea, and pulse irregularities. Urge the patient to report such signs to the doctor.
• Describe the signs of hypokalemia to patients taking medications to lower serum potassium levels.

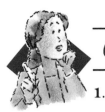

Quick quiz

1. Potassium is responsible for:
    A. building muscle mass.
    B. building bone structure and strength.
    C. maintaining the heartbeat.

Answer: C. Potassium is vital for proper cardiac function because it facilitates cardiac muscle contraction and electrical conductivity. Alterations in the serum potassium level should be recognized and treated as early as possible.

2. When the hormone aldosterone is secreted, the kidneys reabsorb:
    A. sodium.
    B. potassium.
    C. magnesium.

Answer: A. The kidneys reabsorb sodium and excrete potassium when aldosterone is secreted.

3. Neuromuscular signs and symptoms of hypokalemia include:
    A. confusion and irritability.
    B. diminished deep tendon reflexes.
    C. Parkinsonian-type tremors.

Answer: B. Deep tendon reflexes may be decreased or absent in hypokalemia. Leg cramps may also occur. Paralysis could involve the respiratory muscles.

4. Medications to be given when treating severe hyperkalemia include:
    A. sodium succinate and mannitol.
    B. mannitol and regular insulin.
    C. 10% calcium gluconate and regular insulin.

Answer: C. Calcium gluconate helps to stabilize cardiac cell membranes, though it doesn't lower a high potassium level itself. Regular insulin, in conjunction with hypertonic dextrose, causes potassium to move into the cells, thus lowering the serum potassium level.

5. A hallmark ECG characteristic of the patient with hyperkalemia is the presence of:
    A. irregular PR intervals.
    B. narrowed QRS complexes.
    C. tall, tented T waves.

Answer: C. A tall, tented T wave is a hallmark of hyperkalemia, a condition that can also lead to heart block, ventricular arrhythmias, and asystole.

Scoring

☆☆☆   If you answered all five questions correctly, wow! You're Top Banana!

☆☆   If you answered three or four correctly, super! You're Captain of the Banana Boat.

☆   If you answered fewer than three correctly, hang in there. This banana bunch is for you!

When magnesium tips the balance

Just the facts

In this chapter, you'll learn:

♦ why magnesium is so important

♦ why your patient's serum magnesium level might be a challenge to interpret

♦ how a below-normal serum magnesium level can arise and how to detect and manage this imbalance

♦ what causes an above-normal serum magnesium level and what to do if this imbalance occurs.

A look at magnesium

After potassium, magnesium is the most abundant cation (positively charged ion) in the intracellular fluid. The bones contain about 60% of the body's magnesium; extracellular fluid contains less than 1%. Intracellular fluid holds the rest.

What magnesium does

Magnesium performs many important functions in the body. For example, it:
• promotes enzyme reactions within the cell during carbohydrate metabolism
• helps the body produce and use adenosine triphosphate for energy
• takes part in protein synthesis
• influences vasodilation, helping the cardiovascular system function normally

• helps sodium and potassium ions cross the cell membrane (this explains why magnesium affects sodium and potassium ion levels both inside and outside the cell).

Regulating muscle movements

Magnesium also regulates muscle contractions, making it especially vital to the neuromuscular system. By acting on the myoneural junctions — the sites where nerve and muscle fibers meet — magnesium affects the irritability and contractility of cardiac and skeletal muscle.

What's calcium got to do with it?

There's one more function of magnesium worth remembering: It influences the body's calcium level through its effect on parathyroid hormone. Parathyroid hormone, you might recall, is the hormone that maintains a constant calcium concentration in extracellular fluid.

Interpreting magnesium levels

You'll need to keep the magnesium-calcium connection in mind when assessing a patient's lab values. But that's not the only thing you'll need to consider.

Your patient's serum magnesium value *itself* may be misleading. Normally, the body's total serum magnesium level is 1.5 to 2.5 mEq/L.

But the level may not accurately reflect your patient's *actual* magnesium stores. That's because most magnesium is found within cells, where it measures about 40 mEq/L. In serum, magnesium levels are relatively low.

Ties that bind

Here's another reason why interpreting a patient's serum magnesium level can pose a challenge. More than half of circulating magnesium moves in a free, ionized form. Another 30% binds with a protein — mostly albumin — and the remainder binds with other substances.

Ionized magnesium is physiologically active and must be regulated to maintain homeostasis. However, this form alone can't be measured, so a patient's measured concentrations reflect the total amount of circulating magnesium.

To complicate matters, magnesium levels are linked to albumin levels. A patient with a low serum albumin level will have a low total serum magnesium level — even if the level of ionized magnesium remains unchanged.

That's why serum albumin needs to be measured along with serum magnesium.

Serum calcium and certain other lab values also come into play when assessing and treating magnesium imbalances. And because magnesium is mainly an intracellular electrolyte, changes in the levels of other intracellular electrolytes, such as potassium and phosphorus, can affect serum magnesium levels, too.

How the body regulates magnesium

The gastrointestinal (GI) and urinary systems regulate magnesium through the processes of absorption, excretion, and retention — specifically by dietary intake and excretion in the urine and feces. A well-balanced diet should provide roughly 25 mEq (or about 300 to 350 mg) of magnesium daily. (See *Dietary sources of magnesium.*) Of this amount, about 40% is absorbed in the small intestine.

The body's balancing act

The body tries to adjust to any changes in the magnesium level. For instance, if the serum magnesium level drops, the GI tract may absorb more magnesium and to excrete more in the feces.

The kidneys, for their part, balance magnesium by altering its reabsorption at the proximal tubule and loop of Henle. So if a person's serum magnesium level climbs, the kidneys excrete the excess in the urine. Diuretics heighten this effect. The reverse occurs, too: If magnesium levels fall, the kidneys conserve magnesium. That conservation is so efficient that the daily loss of circulating ionized magnesium can be restricted to just 1 mEq.

> **Dietary sources of magnesium**
>
> Most healthy people can get all the magnesium they need by eating a well-balanced diet that includes foods rich in magnesium. Here are the "lucky 7" foods high in magnesium:
> - chocolate
> - dry beans and peas
> - green, leafy vegetables
> - meats
> - nuts
> - seafood
> - whole grains.
>
>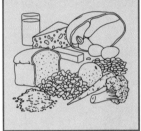

Hypomagnesemia

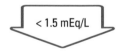

A serum magnesium level below 1.5 mEq/L indicates hypomagnesemia. Although sometimes overlooked, this imbalance is relatively common. In fact, it affects about 10% of all hospitalized patients. As you might expect, critically ill patients have the highest incidence.

Most symptoms of hypomagnesemia occur when the magnesium level drops below 1 mEq/L. At its worst, hypomagnesemia can lead to:
- respiratory muscle paralysis
- complete heart block
- coma.

Key facts about hypomagnesemia

☑ The condition is often overlooked in critically ill patients, who are at increased risk.

☑ Common risk factors include chronic alcoholism.

☑ Symptoms mainly reflect increased neuromuscular excitation.

☑ The condition is commonly linked to hypocalcemia and hypokalemia.

☑ ECG changes may reflect hypomagnesemia, hypocalcemia, or hypokalemia.

How it happens

Any condition that impairs either of the body's magnesium regulators — the GI and urinary systems — can lead to a magnesium shortage. These conditions fall into four main categories:
- poor dietary intake of magnesium
- poor magnesium absorption by the GI tract
- excessive magnesium loss from the GI tract
- excessive magnesium loss from the urinary tract. (See *Key facts about hypomagnesemia.*)

Wages of alcohol

Chronic alcoholics are at risk for hypomagnesemia because they tend to eat a poor diet. What's worse, alcohol overuse causes the urinary system to excrete more magnesium than normal. Alcoholics can also lose magnesium through poor intestinal absorption or from frequent or prolonged vomiting.

At risk!

Patients who can't take magnesium orally are at high risk for developing a magnesium deficiency unless they get adequate supplementation. Patients on prolonged I.V. fluid therapy or total parenteral nutrition that contains insufficient magnesium are also at risk.

Absorption problems

If a patient's dietary intake seems adequate but the serum magnesium level remains low, poor GI absorption may be the culprit. For instance, malabsorption syndromes, steatorrhea, ulcerative colitis, and Crohn's disease can diminish magnesium absorption. Surgery to treat these disorders can also reduce absorption. Bowel resection, for example, reduces potential absorption sites by decreasing the surface area within the GI tract.

Other conditions that can cause hypomagnesemia from poor GI absorption include cancer, pancreatic insufficiency, and excessive calcium or phosphorus in the GI tract.

GI problems

Fluids in the GI tract (especially the lower part) contain magnesium. That's why a person who loses a great deal of these fluids — say, from prolonged diarrhea or drainage caused by a fistula — can be deficient in magnesium. A person who abuses laxatives or who has a nasogastric tube connected to suction is also at risk. In the latter case, the lost magnesium comes from the upper, not lower, GI tract.

In acute pancreatitis, magnesium forms soaps with fatty acids. This process takes some of the magnesium out of circulation, causing serum levels to drop.

Urinary problems

Greater excretion of magnesium in the urine can also lead to a low serum level. Conditions that boost urinary excretion of magnesium include:
• primary aldosteronism (overproduction of aldosterone, an adrenal hormone)
• hyperparathyroidism (hyperfunction of the parathyroid glands)
• diabetic ketoacidosis
• use of amphotericin B, cisplatin, cyclosporine, pentamidine, or aminoglycoside antibiotics, such as tobramycin or gentamicin
• prolonged administration of loop or thiazide diuretics.
(See *Drugs associated with hypomagnesemia.*)

Other causes

Magnesium levels may also drop dramatically in patients with:
• sepsis
• serious burns
• wounds requiring debridement.

What to look for

Signs and symptoms of hypomagnesemia can range from mild to life-threatening and involve the:
- central nervous system (CNS)
- neuromuscular system
- cardiovascular system
- GI system.

Generally speaking, your patient's signs and symptoms may resemble those you'd see with a potassium or calcium imbalance. However, you can't always count on detecting hypomagnesemia from clinical findings alone. Occasionally, a patient remains symptom-free even though his serum magnesium level measures less than 1.5 mEq/L. (See *Identifying hypomagnesemia*.)

Irritating the CNS

A low serum magnesium level irritates the CNS. Such irritation can lead to:
- seizures
- altered level of consciousness
- confusion
- depression
- delusions
- hallucinations
- emotional lability.

When magnesium moves out

To compensate for a low serum magnesium level, magnesium moves out of the cells. This exodus can take an especially high toll on the neuromuscular system. As cells become magnesium-starved, skeletal muscles grow weak and nerves and muscles become hyperirritable.

The three Ts and hyper-DTRs

Watch your patient for neuromuscular signs of hypomagnesemia, such as:
- tremors
- twitching
- tetany
- hyperactive deep tendon reflexes (DTRs). (See *Grading deep tendon reflexes*.)

Respiratory muscles may be affected, too, resulting in breathing difficulties. Some patients also experience laryngeal stridor, foot or leg cramps, and paresthesia.

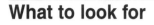
I can't waste time

Identifying hypomagnesemia

Consult the list of signs and symptoms below whenever you need to assess your patient for hypomagnesemia.

CNS: altered level of consciousness, confusion, hallucinations

Neuromuscular: muscle weakness, leg and foot cramps, hyperactive deep tendon reflexes, tetany, Chvostek's and Trousseau's signs

Cardiovascular: tachycardia, hypertension, characteristic ECG changes

GI: dysphagia, anorexia, nausea, vomiting.

Grading deep tendon reflexes

If you suspect your patient has hypomagnesemia, you'll want to test his deep tendon reflexes to determine whether his neuromuscular system is irritable — a clue that his magnesium level is too low. When grading your patient's deep tendon reflexes, use the following scale:

0	Absent
+	Present but diminished
++	Normal
+++	Increased but not necessarily abnormal
++++	Hyperactive, clonic

To record the patient's reflex activity, draw a stick figure and mark the strength of the response at the proper locations. This figure indicates normal deep tendon reflex activity.

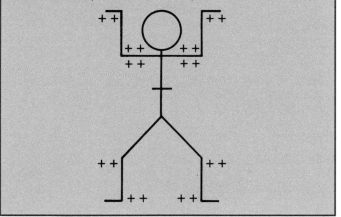

Check these signs

If you suspect hypomagnesemia, you'll also want to test your patient for:
• Chvostek's sign — facial twitching when the facial nerve is tapped
• Trousseau's sign — carpal spasm when the upper arm is compressed. (For more information about these signs, see Chapter 8.)

Hard on the heart

You'll recall that magnesium promotes cardiovascular function. So if you're thinking that hypomagnesemia must affect the heart and blood vessels, you're right. A drop in the magnesium level can irritate the myocardium — with potentially disastrous consequences.

Wrongful rhythms

Myocardial irritability can lead to cardiac arrhythmias, which can cause the cardiac output to drop. Arrhythmias are especially likely to develop in patients with coexisting potassium and calcium imbalances. (See *Hypomagnesemia,* page 130.) Arrhythmias triggered by a low serum magnesium level include:

- premature ventricular contractions
- supraventricular tachycardia
- ventricular tachycardia
- ventricular fibrillation.

Because of the arrhythmia risk, patients with severe hypomagnesemia (serum levels below 1 mEq/L) should undergo continuous cardiac monitoring.

General ECG changes that can occur with a low serum magnesium level include:

- prolonged PR interval
- prolonged QRS complex
- broad, flattened T wave
- depressed ST segment
- prolonged QT interval
- prominent U wave.

The plot may turn toxic

If your patient with hypomagnesemia is receiving a cardiac glycoside such as digoxin, assess closely for signs and symptoms of digitalis toxicity — another condition

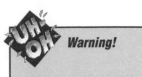

Warning!

Danger signs of low magnesium

Suspect that your patient with hypomagnesemia is *really* in trouble if he has any of these late-developing danger signs:

- digitalis toxicity
- laryngeal stridor
- seizures
- respiratory muscle weakness
- cardiac arrhythmias
- cardiac arrest.

Memory jogger

You'll recall that starvation is a possible cause of a below-normal serum magnesium level. The word STARVED can help you remember some signs and symptoms of hypomagnesemia. Each of its letters stands for a typical clinical finding.

S	seizures
T	tetany
A	anorexia and arrhythmias
R	rapid heart rate
V	vomiting
E	emotional lability
D	deep tendon reflexes increased

that can trigger arrhythmias. A low magnesium level may increase the body's retention of a cardiac glycoside. Suspect digitalis toxicity if your patient has:
- anorexia
- nausea
- vomiting
- arrhythmias
- yellow-tinged vision.

Tough times for the GI tract

Without sufficient serum magnesium, a patient may suffer such GI problems as:
- dysphagia (difficulty swallowing)
- anorexia
- nausea and vomiting.

These conditions can lead to poor dietary magnesium intake or loss of magnesium through the GI tract, in turn worsening the patient's condition.

What tests show

Diagnostic test results that point to hypomagnesemia include:
- a serum magnesium level below 1.5 mEq/L (possibly with a below-normal serum albumin level)
- other electrolyte abnormalities, such as a below-normal serum potassium or calcium level
- characteristic ECG changes
- elevated serum levels of cardiac glycosides in a patient receiving one of those drugs.

How hypomagnesemia is treated

Treatment of hypomagnesemia depends on the underlying cause and the patient's clinical findings. For patients with mild magnesium shortages, dietary replacement and teaching alone may correct the imbalance. Some doctors also prescribe oral supplements such as magnesium oxide tablets. Because it may take a few days to replenish magnesium stores inside the cell, magnesium replacement may continue for several days after the serum magnesium level returns to normal.

Patients with more severe hypomagnesemia may need I.V. or deep I.M. injections of magnesium sulfate. (See *Check the label.*)

Check the label

When you prepare a magnesium sulfate injection, keep in mind that the drug comes in various concentrations, such as 10%, 12.5%, and 50%. Check the label (such as the one shown here) to be sure you're using the correct concentration. The label shows other dosage information as well.

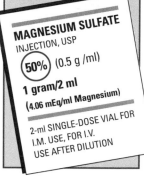

MAGNESIUM SULFATE
INJECTION, USP
(50%) (0.5 g /ml)
1 gram/2 ml
(4.06 mEq/ml Magnesium)
2-ml SINGLE-DOSE VIAL FOR I.M. USE, FOR I.V. USE AFTER DILUTION

How you intervene

The best treatment for hypomagnesemia is prevention, so keep a watchful eye on patients at risk for this imbalance, such as those who can't tolerate oral intake. For patients who have already been diagnosed with hypomagnesemia, take the following actions.

Assess

• Assess the patient's mental status and report changes.
• Evaluate the patient's neuromuscular status regularly by checking for hyperactive DTRs, tremors, tetany, and Chvostek's or Trousseau's signs.
• Assess dysphagia before the patient is given food, oral fluids, or oral medications. Hypomagnesemia may impair the ability to swallow.

Monitor

• Monitor and record your patient's vital signs. Report findings that indicate hemodynamic instability.
• Monitor the patient's respiratory status. A magnesium deficiency can cause laryngeal stridor and compromise the airway.
• Connect your patient to a cardiac monitor if his magnesium level is under 1 mEq/L. Watch the rhythm strip closely for arrhythmias.

Prepare

• Institute seizure precautions.
• If a seizure occurs, report the type of seizure, its length, and the patient's behavior during the seizure. Reorient him as needed.
• Keep emergency equipment nearby for airway protection.

Maintain and administer

• Ensure your patient's safety at all times.
• Reorient the patient as needed.
• To ease your patient's anxiety, tell him what to expect before each procedure. (See *Teaching about low magnesium*.)
• Establish I.V. access and maintain a patent I.V. line in case your patient needs I.V. magnesium replacement or I.V. fluids.

Parting points

Teaching about low magnesium

When teaching a patient about his hypomagnesemia, include the following points and evaluate his learning:

🎓 explanations about hypomagnesemia, its risk factors, and its treatment

🎓 prescribed medications

🎓 avoidance of drugs that deplete magnesium in the body, such as diuretics and laxatives

🎓 consumption of high-magnesium diet

🎓 danger signs and when to report them

🎓 referral to appropriate support groups such as Alcoholics Anonymous.

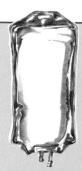

Infusing magnesium sulfate

If the doctor prescribes magnesium sulfate to boost your patient's serum magnesium level, you'll need to take some special precautions. Read on for details.

• Using an infusion pump, administer magnesium sulfate *slowly* — no faster than 150 mg/minute. Injecting a bolus dose too rapidly can trigger cardiac arrest.

• Monitor your patient's vital signs during magnesium sulfate therapy. Every 15 minutes, check for signs and symptoms of excess magnesium, such as hypotension and respiratory distress.

• Check the patient's serum magnesium level after each bolus dose or at least every 6 hours if he has a continuous I.V. drip.

• Stay especially alert for an above-normal serum magnesium level if your patient's renal function is impaired.

• Place the patient on continuous cardiac monitoring. Observe him closely, especially if he's also receiving a cardiac glycoside.

• Monitor urine output before, during, and after magnesium sulfate infusion. Notify the doctor if output measures less than 100 ml over 4 hours.

• Keep calcium gluconate on hand to counteract adverse reactions. Also have resuscitation equipment nearby. Be prepared to use it if the patient goes into cardiac or respiratory arrest.

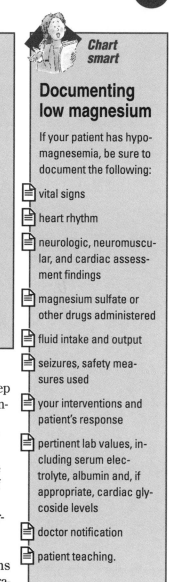

Chart smart

Documenting low magnesium

If your patient has hypomagnesemia, be sure to document the following:

📄 vital signs

📄 heart rhythm

📄 neurologic, neuromuscular, and cardiac assessment findings

📄 magnesium sulfate or other drugs administered

📄 fluid intake and output

📄 seizures, safety measures used

📄 your interventions and patient's response

📄 pertinent lab values, including serum electrolyte, albumin and, if appropriate, cardiac glycoside levels

📄 doctor notification

📄 patient teaching.

• When preparing an infusion of magnesium sulfate, keep in mind that I.V. magnesium sulfate comes in various concentrations (such as 10%, 12.5%, and 50%). Clarify a doctor's order that specifies only the number of ampules or vials to give. A proper order states how many grams or milliliters of a particular concentration to administer, the volume of desired solution for dilution, and the length of time for infusion. (See *Infusing magnesium sulfate.*)

• Administer magnesium supplements as needed and ordered.

• During magnesium replacement, check the cardiac monitor frequently and assess the patient closely for signs of too much magnesium, such as hypotension and respiratory distress. Keep calcium gluconate at the bedside in case such signs occur.

• Maintain an accurate record of your patient's fluid intake and output. Report any decrease in urine output. (See *Documenting low magnesium.*)

Hypermagnesemia

> 2.5 mEq/L

How it happens

Having too much magnesium in the serum can be just as bad as having too little. Hypermagnesemia is defined as a serum magnesium level that exceeds 2.5 mEq/L.

Hypermagnesemia results from the conditions opposite those that bring on a magnesium shortage. Its main causes are impaired magnesium excretion, as from renal dysfunction, and excessive magnesium intake.

Retaining too much

Renal dysfunction is the most common cause of hypermagnesemia. Just as some renal conditions boost magnesium excretion to cause *hypo*magnesemia, others can make the body retain too much magnesium, causing *hyper*magnesemia. Causes of poor renal excretion of magnesium include:
• advancing age, which tends to reduce renal function
• renal failure
• Addison's disease
• adrenocortical insufficiency
• untreated diabetic ketoacidosis. (See *Key facts about high magnesium.*)

Too much intake

Magnesium build-up is common in patients with renal failure who use magnesium-containing antacids or laxatives. (See *Drugs associated with hypermagnesemia.*)
  Other causes of excessive magnesium intake include:
• hemodialysis with a magnesium-rich dialysate
• total parenteral nutrition solutions that contain too much magnesium
• continuous infusion of magnesium sulfate to treat disorders, such as seizures, pregnancy-induced hypertension, or preterm labor. (The fetus of a woman receiving magnesium sulfate may develop a higher serum magnesium level, too.)

What to look for

Just as an abnormally low serum magnesium level overstimulates the neuromuscular system, an abnormally high

Key facts about high magnesium

☑ The condition is relatively uncommon.

☑ The most common risk factor for hypermagnesemia is renal insufficiency, especially in patients who take drugs that contain magnesium.

☑ Serious signs and symptoms include respiratory muscle paralysis and complete heart block, possibly leading to cardiac arrest.

one depresses it. So expect neuromuscular signs and symptoms opposite those of hypomagnesemia, such as:
• decreased muscle and nerve activity
• hypoactive deep tendon reflexes
• generalized weakness (for instance, a patient who has a weak hand grasp or difficulty repositioning himself in bed); in severe cases, weakness progressing to flaccid paralysis
• sometimes nausea and vomiting. (See *Signs of hypermagnesemia.*)

Drowsy patient? Suspect high magnesium

Because excess magnesium depresses the CNS, the patient may appear drowsy and lethargic. His level of consciousness may even diminish to the point of coma.

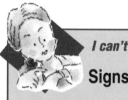

I can't waste time

Signs of hypermagnesemia

Use this chart to compare total serum magnesium levels with the typical signs and symptoms that may appear.

Total serum magnesium level	Signs and symptoms
3 mEq/L	• Feelings of warmth • Flushed appearance • Mild hypotension • Nausea and vomiting
4 mEq/L	• Diminished deep tendon reflexes • Muscle weakness
5 mEq/L	• Somnolence • ECG changes • Bradycardia • Worsening hypotension
7 mEq/L	• Loss of deep tendon reflexes
8 mEq/L	• Respiratory compromise
12 mEq/L	• Heart block • Coma
15 mEq/L	• Respiratory arrrest
20 mEq/L	• Cardiac arrest

Drugs associated with hypermagnesemia

Be sure to monitor your patient's serum magnesium level closely if he's receiving any of these medications:

• antacids, such as Di-Gel, Gaviscon, Gelusil, Maalox, Mylanta, Riopan, or Tempo
• certain laxatives, such as milk of magnesia, Haley's M-O, magnesium citrate, or magnesium sulfate (Epsom salts)
• magnesium supplements, such as magnesium oxide or magnesium sulfate.

Hypermagnesemia can pose a danger to the respiratory system — and to life itself — if it weakens the respiratory muscles. Typically, such muscle weakness manifests as slow, shallow, depressed respirations. Eventually, the patient may suffer respiratory arrest and require mechanical ventilation.

A high serum magnesium level may also trigger serious heart problems — among them a weak pulse, bradycardia, heart block, and cardiac arrest. Arrhythmias may lead to diminished cardiac output.

ECG changes, along with a serum magnesium value above 2.5 mEq/L, can help confirm the diagnosis of hypermagnesemia. (See *How electrolyte imbalances affect ECGs*, pages 127 to 130.)

A high serum magnesium level also causes vasodilation, which lowers the blood pressure and may make your patient feel flushed and warm all over.

What tests show

To help confirm the diagnosis of hypermagnesemia, look for a serum magnesium level above 2.5 mEq/L and these telltale ECG changes: prolonged PR interval, widened QRS complex, and tall T wave.

How hypermagnesemia is treated

Once hypermagnesemia is confirmed, the doctor orders measures to correct both the magnesium imbalance and its underlying cause.

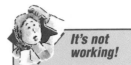

It's not working!

If treatment doesn't work

If, despite treatment, your patient's lab reports continue to show that his serum magnesium level is above normal, what should you do?

Your first step is to notify the doctor. Expect to prepare the patient for peritoneal dialysis or hemodialysis using magnesium-free dialysate. The patient needs to get rid of the excess magnesium fast — especially if his renal function is failing.

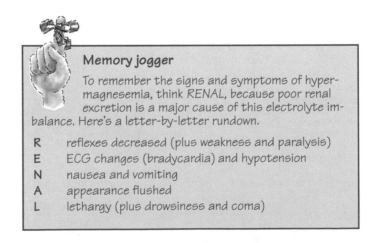

Memory jogger

To remember the signs and symptoms of hypermagnesemia, think RENAL, because poor renal excretion is a major cause of this electrolyte imbalance. Here's a letter-by-letter rundown.

R   reflexes decreased (plus weakness and paralysis)
E   ECG changes (bradycardia) and hypotension
N   nausea and vomiting
A   appearance flushed
L   lethargy (plus drowsiness and coma)

Fluid up, mag level down

If the patient has normal renal function, expect the doctor to order oral or I.V. fluids. Increased fluid intake raises the patient's urine output, ridding his body of excess magnesium. If the patient doesn't respond to increased fluid intake, the doctor may order a loop diuretic to promote magnesium excretion.

What if it gets worse?

In an emergency, expect to give calcium gluconate, a magnesium antagonist. (You'll probably give 10 to 20 ml of a 10% solution.) Some patients with magnesium toxicity also need mechanical ventilation to relieve respiratory depression.

Patients who have severe renal dysfunction may need hemodialysis with magnesium-free dialysate to lower the serum magnesium level. (See *If treatment doesn't work.*)

How you intervene

Whenever possible, take steps to prevent hypermagnesemia by identifying high-risk patients. Those at risk include:
- the elderly
- those with renal insufficiency or failure
- pregnant women in preterm labor or with pregnancy-induced hypertension
- neonates whose mothers received magnesium sulfate during labor
- patients receiving magnesium sulfate to control seizures
- patients with a high intake of magnesium or magnesium-containing products, such as antacids or laxatives.

If your patient already has hypermagnesemia, you may need to take the following actions.
- Monitor your patient's vital signs frequently. Stay especially alert for hypotension and respiratory depression — clues to hypermagnesemia. (See *Teaching about hypermagnesemia.*)
- Observe for signs of diminishing respiratory function. Notify the doctor immediately if the patient's respiratory status deteriorates.
- Check for flushed skin and diaphoresis.
- Assess the patient's neuromuscular system, including deep tendon reflexes and muscle strength. (See *Testing the patellar reflex,* page 126.)

Parting points

Teaching about hypermagnesemia

Be sure to cover the following topics and to evaluate your patient's learning:

- explanation of hypermagnesemia
- risk factors
- hydration requirements
- dietary modification, if indicated
- prescribed medications
- warning signs and symptoms
- need to avoid medications containing magnesium
- dialysis, if needed.

Testing the patellar reflex

One way to gauge your patient's magnesium status is to test her patellar reflex, one of the deep tendon reflexes affected by the serum magnesium level. To test the reflex, strike the patellar tendon just below the patella with the patient sitting or lying supine, as shown. Look for leg extension or contraction of the quadriceps muscle in the front of the thigh.

If the patellar reflex is absent, notify the doctor immediately. This finding may mean your patient's serum magnesium level is 7 mEq/L or higher.

Sitting
Have the patient sit on the side of the bed with her legs dangling freely, as shown here. Then test the reflex.

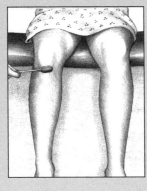

Supine
Flex the patient's knee at a 45-degree angle, and place your nondominant hand behind it for support. Then test the reflex.

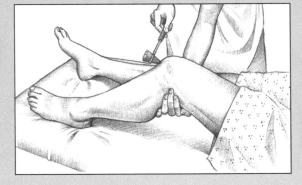

• Check lab results and report abnormal ones. Keep a close eye on serum electrolytes as well as other lab values that reflect renal function, such as blood urea nitrogen and creatinine levels.
• Evaluate for changes in mental status. If the patient's level of consciousness decreases, institute safety measures. Reorient the patient if he's confused.

Prepare

• Prepare the patient for continuous cardiac monitoring. Assess ECG tracings for the changes typically seen with hypermagnesemia.
• Be prepared to administer resuscitation drugs, maintain a patent airway, and provide calcium gluconate, as ordered, in case of a hypermagnesemia emergency.
• Prepare the patient for dialysis, as ordered, if his magnesium level becomes dangerously high.

Maintain

• Establish I.V. access and maintain a patent I.V. line.
• Provide adequate fluids, both I.V. and oral if prescribed, to help your patient's kidneys excrete excess magnesium.

(Text continues on page 131.)

How electrolyte imbalances affect ECGs

Electrical impulses move through the heart's conduction system to create rhythmic contractions. Normal electrical activity in the heart depends on normal serum electrolyte concentrations.

The electrolytes sodium, potassium, and calcium, with the help of magnesium, shift back and forth across myocardial cell membranes. That shifting of electrolytes causes alternating periods of activity (depolarization) and rest (repolarization), which allow for normal myocardial function. Imbalances of electrolytes cause trademark changes in electrocardiogram (ECG) readings and in altered myocardial function. This special section details changes in two critical electrolytes.

Hypermagnesemia

Magnesium

Hypermagnesemia may be caused by excessive magnesium administration and renal failure. The condition can cause a prolonged PR interval and the ECG changes shown below. If left untreated, hypermagnesemia may lead to sinoatrial or atrioventricular (AV) heart block and, finally, to cardiac arrest.

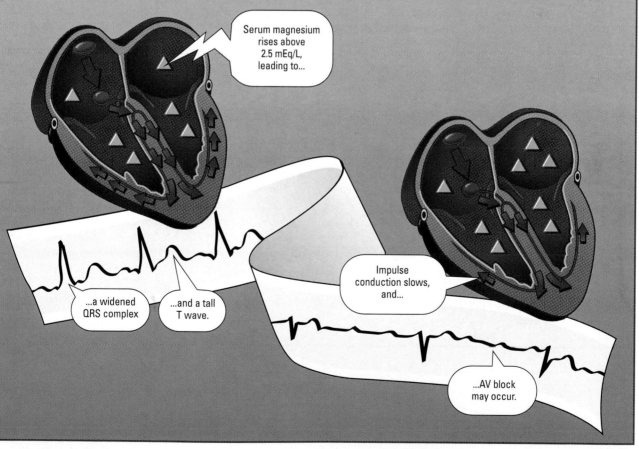

(continued)

Hyperkalemia

Potassium

Hyperkalemia may be caused by renal failure or by excessive potassium administration. Excess potassium alters the heart's electrical activity and leads to a depression of conduction. Among the earliest signs of hyperkalemia (> 5.5 mEq/L) is a tall, tented T wave, as shown here. Atrioventricular or ventricular block may develop. Other possible ECG abnormalities include a flattened P wave, a prolonged PR interval, a widened QRS complex as ventricular conduction slows, and a depressed ST segment.

Left untreated, severe hyperkalemia (> 9 mEq/L) causes the disappearance of the P wave, widening of the QRS complex, and the formation of sine waves. Hyperkalemia may end in lethal arrhythmias.

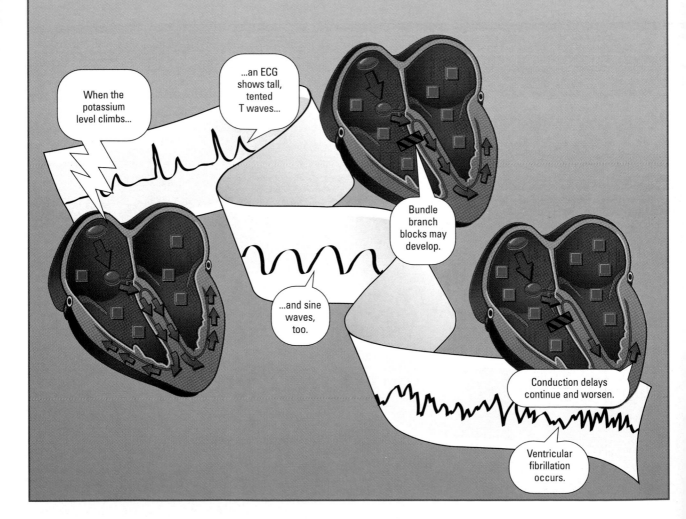

Hypokalemia

Potassium

Hypokalemia (serum potassium < 3.5 mEq/L) can be caused by diuresis or by the loss of other body fluids. An abnormally low potassium level affects the heart's electrical activity. Ventricular repolarization is prolonged. ECG changes include a prominent U wave—a hallmark of hypokalemia.

As the potassium level decreases, ectopic impulses form and conduction disturbances increase. Atrial and ventricular arrhythmias may develop. As ectopy becomes more frequent, the patient is at risk for potentially fatal arrhythmias. Examples of hypokalemic ECG changes are shown here.

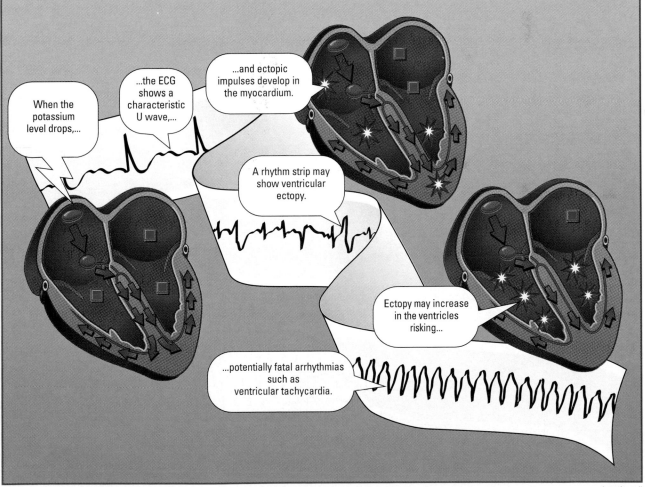

(continued)

Hypomagnesemia

Magnesium

Hypomagnesemia (serum magnesium < 1.5 mEq/L) may be caused by malnutrition or excessive loss of body fluids. Its effects on the electrical activity of the heart include ECG changes (shown below), such as a slightly prolonged QRS complex, a prolonged QT interval (which increases myocardial vulnerability to a stimulus), and ST segment depression.

Dangerously low magnesium levels make myocardial cells more excitable, which may trigger such life-threatening arrhythmias as ventricular tachycardia, torsades de pointes, and ventricular fibrillation.

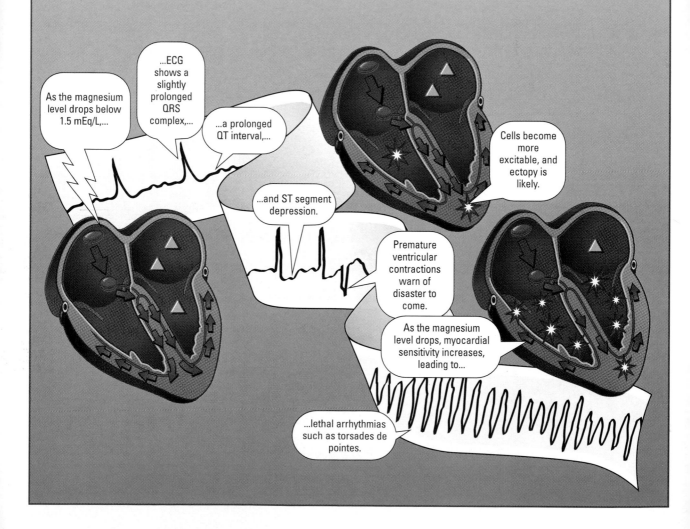

Remember, though, when giving large volumes of fluids, you need to keep accurate intake and output records and watch closely for signs of fluid overload and kidney failure. Both conditions can arise quickly. (See *Documenting high magnesium.*)

• Avoid giving your patient medications that contain magnesium. To make sure no other staff members give them, flag the patient's chart and medication administration record with a note that says, "No magnesium products."

• Restrict the patient's dietary magnesium intake as needed.

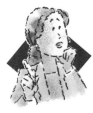

Quick quiz

1. Magnesium is an important electrolyte because it:
A. helps control urine volume.
B. promotes the production of growth hormone.
C. facilitates neuromuscular transmission.

Answer: C. Magnesium acts at the myoneural junction and is vital to nerve and muscle activity.

2. Your patient with Crohn's disease develops tremors while receiving total parenteral nutrition. Suspecting she might have hypomagnesemia, you assess her neuromuscular system. You would expect to see:
A. Homans' sign.
B. Chvostek's sign.
C. hypoactive deep tendon reflexes.

Answer: B. In a patient with probable hypomagnesemia, expect to see Chvostek's sign — facial twitching when the facial nerve is tapped — because hypomagnesemia increases neuromuscular excitability.

3. When teaching your patient with hypomagnesemia about a proper diet, you should recommend that he consume plenty of:
A. seafood.
B. fruits.
C. corn products.

Answer: A. Magnesium is found in seafood as well as in chocolate, dry beans and peas, green leafy vegetables, meats, nuts, and whole grains.

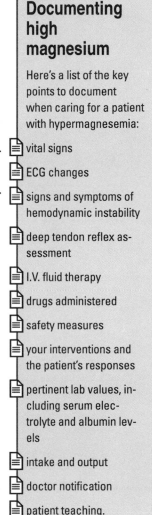

Chart smart

Documenting high magnesium

Here's a list of the key points to document when caring for a patient with hypermagnesemia:

▤ vital signs

▤ ECG changes

▤ signs and symptoms of hemodynamic instability

▤ deep tendon reflex assessment

▤ I.V. fluid therapy

▤ drugs administered

▤ safety measures

▤ your interventions and the patient's responses

▤ pertinent lab values, including serum electrolyte and albumin levels

▤ intake and output

▤ doctor notification

▤ patient teaching.

4. The doctor prescribes I.V. magnesium sulfate for your patient with hypomagnesemia. Before giving the magnesium preparation, you review the doctor's order to make sure it specifies:

    A.   the number of grams or milliliters to give.
    B.   the number of ampules to give.
    C.   the number of vials to give.

Answer: A. Magnesium sulfate comes in several different concentrations. The doctor's order should specify the number of grams or milliliters of a particular concentration, plus either the amount of solution to use for dilution or the length of the infusion.

5. Your patient is diagnosed with hypermagnesemia. To treat this imbalance, the doctor is likely to order:

    A.   magnesium citrate.
    B.   magnesium sulfate diluted in fluids.
    C.   oral and I.V. fluids.

Answer: C. Both oral and I.V. fluids may be used to treat hypermagnesemia. By causing diuresis, the fluids promote excretion of excess magnesium by the kidneys.

6. Your hemodialysis patient needs a laxative. When you see that the doctor has ordered magnesium citrate, you decide to question the order because:

    A.   this magnesium salt would be too strong for the patient.
    B.   magnesium administration could worsen the patient's condition.
    C.   magnesium citrate must be given orally.

Answer: B. Magnesium citrate is a poor laxative choice for a patient with a renal impairment whose kidneys can't excrete magnesium properly. The patient could develop hypermagnesemia.

Scoring

✰✰✰   If you answered all six questions correctly, you should be twitching with pride. You're a magnesium magician!

✰✰   If you answered four or five correctly, excellent! You're ready to become a magnesium magician's assistant!

✰   If you answered fewer than three correctly, not to worry. You're now enrolled as a first-year learner in Magical Magnesium College of Fine Electrolytes.

When calcium tips the balance

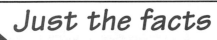

Just the facts

This chapter describes how to care for patients who have a deficiency or an excess of calcium. In this chapter, you'll learn:

◆ how calcium works in the body

◆ what the relationship is between calcium and albumin

◆ how parathyroid hormone helps to regulate calcium levels

◆ how to assess for signs of calcium imbalance

◆ how to care for patients with hypocalcemia and hypercalcemia.

A look at calcium

Calcium is a positively charged ion, or cation, found in both the extracellular fluid and the intracellular fluid. Ninety-nine percent of the body's calcium is found in the bones and the teeth. Only 1% of the mineral is found in serum and in soft tissue. That 1% is what matters when measuring calcium levels in the blood.

What it does

Calcium is involved in numerous body functions. Together with phosphorus, calcium is responsible for the formation and structure of bones and teeth. It helps to maintain cell structure and function and plays a role in cell membrane permeability and impulse transmission.

This cation affects the contraction of cardiac muscle, smooth muscle, and skeletal muscle. Calcium also participates in the blood-clotting process.

Measuring calcium

Calcium can be measured in two ways. The most commonly ordered test is a total serum calcium level, which measures the total amount of calcium in the blood. The normal value for total serum calcium is 8.9 to 10.1 mg/dl.

The second test measures the various forms of calcium in extracellular fluid. About 41% of all extracellular calcium is bound to protein; 9% is bound to citrate or other organic ions. About half is ionized (or free) calcium, the only active form of calcium. Ionized calcium carries out most of the ion's physiologic functions. The normal ionized calcium level is 4.5 to 5.1 mg/dl.

Because nearly half of all calcium is bound to the protein albumin, serum protein abnormalities can influence total serum calcium levels. For example, in hypoalbuminemia, the total serum calcium level decreases. However, ionized calcium levels — the more important of the two levels — remain unchanged. So when considering total serum calcium levels, you should also take into consideration serum albumin levels. (See *Calculating calcium and albumin levels.*)

How the body regulates calcium

Calcium levels are affected by the body's stores of the ion and by dietary intake. The recommended minimum daily requirement for calcium is 800 to 1,000 mg/day for adults. Requirements vary in childhood and pregnancy and when a person is being treated for osteoporosis.

Calcium is found in large quantities in dairy products but can also be found in green, leafy vegetables. (See *Dietary sources of calcium.*) Calcium is absorbed in the small intestine and is excreted in the urine and feces.

Bones help out

Several factors influence calcium levels in the body. The first is parathyroid hormone. When serum calcium levels are low, the parathyroid glands release parathyroid hormone, which draws calcium from the bones and promotes

---

Dietary sources of calcium

Here's a list of the most common dietary sources of calcium:
- bone meal
- dairy products, such as milk, cheese, and yogurt
- leafy green vegetables
- legumes
- molasses
- nuts
- whole grains.

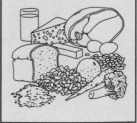

Calculating calcium and albumin levels

For every 1 g/dl drop in serum albumin in a noncritically ill patient, total calcium decreases by 0.8 mg/dl. To see what your patient's calcium level would be if his serum albumin level was normal — and to help determine if treatment is justified — just do a little math.

Correcting a level
The normal albumin level is 4 g/dl. The formula for correcting a patient's calcium level is:

Total serum calcium + 0.8 (4 − albumin level)

=

corrected calcium

Sample problem
For example, if a patient's serum calcium level is 8.2 mg/dl and his albumin level is 3 g/dl, what would his corrected calcium be?

$$8.2 + 0.8 (4 - 3) = 9 \text{ mg/dl}$$

The corrected calcium is in a normal range and would most likely not be treated.

the transfer of calcium (along with phosphorus) into the plasma. That transfer increases serum calcium levels.

Parathyroid hormone also promotes kidney reabsorption of calcium and stimulates the intestines to absorb the mineral. Phosphorus is excreted at the same time. In hypercalcemia, where too much calcium exists in the blood, the body suppresses the release of parathyroid hormone.

Enter calcitonin

Calcitonin also helps to regulate calcium levels. Calcitonin, a hormone, is produced in the thyroid gland and acts as an antagonist to parathyroid hormone.

When calcium levels are too high, the thyroid releases calcitonin. High levels of the hormone inhibit bone resorption, which causes a decrease in the amount of calcium available from bone. That causes a decrease in the serum calcium level.

Memory jogger

To help you remember the roles of calcitonin and parathyroid hormone, think of this memory jogger: *Parathyroid pulls, calcitonin keeps.*

Parathyroid hormone pulls calcium out of the bone. Calcitonin keeps it there.

Calcitonin also decreases absorption of calcium and enhances its excretion by the kidneys.

And now, vitamin D

Another factor that influences calcium levels is vitamin D. Vitamin D can be ingested with foods, particularly dairy products, or synthesized by the skin when exposed to ultraviolet light.

Vitamin D (the active form, not the inactive one) promotes calcium absorption through the intestines, calcium resorption from bone, and kidney reabsorption of calcium, all of which raise the serum calcium level. (See *Calcium in balance*.)

Calcium in balance

Extracellular calcium levels are normally kept constant by several interrelated processes that move calcium ions into and out of extracellular fluid. Calcium enters the extracellular space through resorption of calcium ions from bone, through the absorption of dietary calcium in the GI tract, and through reabsorption of calcium from the kidneys. Calcium leaves extracellular fluid mainly through excretion in the feces and urine and through its deposition in bone tissues. The illustration shows how calcium moves throughout the body.

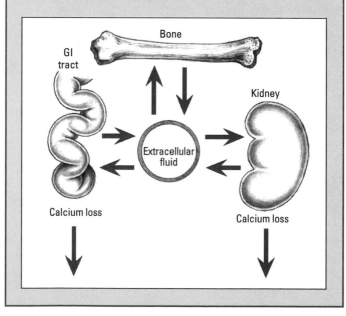

Phosphorus follows

Phosphorus also affects serum calcium levels. Phosphorus inhibits calcium absorption in the intestines, the opposite effect of vitamin D. When calcium levels are low and the kidneys retain calcium, phosphorus is excreted.

An inverse relationship between calcium and phosphorus exists in the body. When calcium levels rise, phosphorus levels drop. The opposite is also true: When calcium levels drop, phosphorus levels rise.

Serum pH helps...inversely

The serum pH also has an inverse relationship with the ionized calcium level. If the serum pH level rises (the blood becomes alkaline), more calcium binds with protein and the ionized calcium level drops. Thus, a patient with alkalosis may appear hypocalcemic.

The opposite is true for acidosis. When the pH level drops, less calcium binds to protein and the ionized calcium level rises. When all those regulatory efforts fail to control the level of calcium in the body, two conditions may result: hypocalcemia or hypercalcemia.

Hypocalcemia

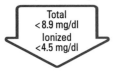
Total
< 8.9 mg/dl
Ionized
< 4.5 mg/dl

Hypocalcemia occurs when the serum calcium falls below the normal values. The condition is reflected in a serum calcium level below 8.9 mg/dl or an ionized calcium level below 4.5 mg/dl.

How it happens

Hypocalcemia can occur when a person doesn't take in enough calcium, when the body doesn't absorb the mineral properly, or when excessive amounts of calcium are lost from the body. A decreased level of ionized calcium can also cause hypocalcemia.

When you need calcium

Inadequate intake of calcium can put a patient at risk for hypocalcemia. Alcoholics, with their typically poor nutritional intake, poor calcium absorption, and low magnesium level (magnesium affects parathyroid hormone secretion), are especially prone.

A breast-fed infant can have low calcium and vitamin D levels if his mother's intake of those nutrients is inadequate. The elderly may also lack calcium in their diet, may suffer from poor absorption (especially in postmenopausal women lacking estrogen), and may be significantly less active than when they were younger. Inactivity causes loss of calcium from the bone and osteoporosis, in which serum levels may be normal but bone stores of the mineral are depleted. In addition, anyone who doesn't receive sufficient exposure to sunlight may suffer from vitamin D deficiency and subsequently lower calcium levels.

When malabsorption hits

Hypocalcemia can result when calcium isn't absorbed properly from the GI tract, a condition often caused by malabsorption. Malabsorption can result from increased intestinal motility from severe diarrhea, laxative abuse, or chronic malabsorption syndrome.

Absorption is also affected by a lack of vitamin D in the diet. Renal failure may harm the kidneys' ability to activate vitamin D. Anticonvulsants, such as phenobarbital and phenytoin (Dilantin), can interfere with vitamin D metabolism and calcium absorption.

A high phosphorus level in the intestines can interfere with absorption, as can a reduction in gastric acidity, which decreases the solubility of calcium salts.

Excess calcium loss

Pancreatic insufficiency can cause malabsorption of calcium and a subsequent loss of calcium in the feces. Acute pancreatitis can cause hypocalcemia as well, although the mechanism is not well understood. Parathyroid hormone is thought to be involved, or possibly the combining of free fatty acids and calcium in pancreatic tissue.

Hypocalcemia can also occur when secretion of parathyroid hormone is reduced or eliminated. Thyroid surgery, surgical removal of the parathyroid gland, removal of a parathyroid tumor, or injury or disease of the parathyroid gland (such as hypoparathyroidism) can all lead to that reduction or elimination of parathyroid hormone secretion.

Hypocalcemia can also result from medications such as calcitonin and mithramycin because these drugs decrease calcium resorption from bone.

Drugs associated with hypocalcemia

Drugs that can cause hypocalcemia include:

- anticonvulsants, especially phenytoin and phenobarbital
- calcitonin
- drugs that lower serum magnesium (like cisplatin, gentamicin)
- Disodium EDTA (disodium edetate)
- loop diuretics
- mithramycin
- phosphates (oral, I.V., rectal).

Kidneys take out calcium

The kidneys may excrete excess calcium and cause hypocalcemia. Diuretics, especially loop diuretics such as furosemide (Lasix) and ethacrynic acid (Edecrin), increase renal excretion of calcium as well as water and other electrolytes.

Edetate disodium (E.D.T.A.), used in the treatment of lead poisoning, can combine with calcium and carry the calcium out of the body when excreted. Other causes of hypocalcemia include severe burns and infections. Burned or diseased tissues trap calcium ions from extracellular fluid, thereby reducing serum calcium levels.

Still *more causes*

Hypomagnesemia (low magnesium level) can affect the function of the parathyroid gland and cause a decrease in calcium reabsorption in the GI tract and the kidneys. Drugs that lower serum magnesium levels, such as cisplatin and gentamicin, may decrease calcium absorption from bone. (See *Drugs associated with hypocalcemia*.)

Remember also that a low serum albumin level (hypoalbuminemia) can cause low calcium levels. Hyperphosphatemia (a high level of phosphorus in the blood) can cause calcium levels to fall as phosphorus levels rise. Excess phosphorus combines with calcium to form salts, which are then deposited in tissues.

When phosphates are administered orally, I.V., or rectally, the phosphorus binds with calcium and serum calcium levels drop. Infants receiving cow's milk feedings are predisposed to hypocalcemic tetany because of the high concentration of phosphorus in cow's milk.

Alkalosis can cause calcium to bind to albumin, thereby decreasing ionized calcium levels. Citrate, added to stored blood to prevent clotting, binds with calcium and renders it unavailable for use. Therefore, patients receiving massive blood transfusions are at risk for hypocalcemia. That risk holds true for pediatric patients as well. (See *Key facts about hypocalcemia*.)

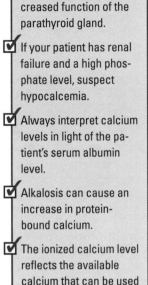

Key facts about hypocalcemia

☑ The most common cause of hypocalcemia is decreased function of the parathyroid gland.

☑ If your patient has renal failure and a high phosphate level, suspect hypocalcemia.

☑ Always interpret calcium levels in light of the patient's serum albumin level.

☑ Alkalosis can cause an increase in protein-bound calcium.

☑ The ionized calcium level reflects the available calcium that can be used in key calcium functions.

What to look for

Signs and symptoms of hypocalcemia reflect calcium's effects on nerve transmission and muscle and heart function. The neurologic effects of a low calcium level include

Checking for Trousseau's and Chvostek's signs

Testing for Trousseau's and Chvostek's signs can aid in the diagnosis of tetany and hypocalcemia. Here's how to check for these important signs.

Trousseau's sign
To check for Trousseau's sign, apply a blood pressure cuff to the patient's upper arm and inflate it to a pressure 20 mm Hg above the systolic pressure. Trousseau's sign may appear after 1 to 4 minutes. The patient will experience carpopedal spasm — an adducted thumb, flexed wrist and metacarpopha-langeal joints, and extended interphalangeal joints (with fingers together) — indicating tetany, a major sign of hypocalcemia.

Chvostek's sign
You can induce Chvostek's sign by tapping the patient's facial nerve adjacent to the ear. A brief contraction of the upper lip, nose, or side of the face indicates Chvostek's sign.

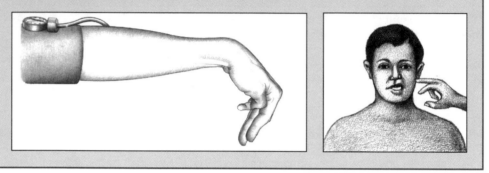

anxiety, confusion, and irritability. Those symptoms can progress to seizures.

Neuromuscular symptoms may develop. The patient may experience paresthesia of the toes, fingers, or face, especially around the mouth. He may also experience twitching, muscle cramps, or tremors. Laryngeal and abdominal muscles are particularly prone to spasm. An increase in nerve excitability can lead to tetany. At such times, you may be able to elicit positive Trousseau's or Chvostek's signs. (See *Checking for Trousseau's and Chvostek's signs.*)

More signs

Fractures may occur more easily in a patient who is hypocalcemic for an extended period. The patient may also have brittle nails or dry skin and hair.

Other signs of hypocalcemia include:
- diarrhea
- hyperactive deep tendon reflexes
- diminished response to digitalis glycosides

- decreased cardiac output and subsequent arrhythmias
- prolonged ST segment on ECG
- QT interval on ECG, which invites a form of ventricular tachycardia called "torsades de pointes."

What tests show

The following test results can help doctors diagnose hypocalcemia as well as determine the severity of the deficiency:
- total serum calcium level less than 8.9 mg/dl
- an ionized calcium level below 4.5 mg/dl
- characteristic ECG changes.

How hypocalcemia is treated

Treatment for hypocalcemia focuses on correcting the imbalance as quickly and as safely as possible. The underlying cause should be addressed to prevent recurrence.

Acute hypocalcemia requires immediate correction by administering either calcium gluconate or calcium chloride, both given I.V. While calcium chloride contains three times as much available calcium as calcium gluconate, the latter is given more frequently. Magnesium replacement may also be needed, since hypocalcemia often doesn't respond to calcium therapy alone. (See *Administering I.V. calcium safely,* page 142.)

Chronic hypocalcemia requires vitamin D supplements to facilitate GI absorption of calcium. Oral calcium supplements also help increase calcium levels.

The patient's diet should also be adjusted to allow for an adequate intake of calcium, vitamin D, and protein. In cases where the patient also has a high phosphorus level, aluminum hydroxide antacids may be given to bind with excess phosphorus. (See *When treatment doesn't work.*)

How you intervene

Carefully assess a patient at an increased risk for hypocalcemia, especially if the patient has had parathyroid surgery or received massive blood transfusions. Assess the breast-feeding mother for adequate vitamin D intake and exposure to sunlight.

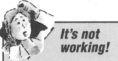

It's not working!

When treatment doesn't work

If treatment for hypocalcemia doesn't seem to be working, consider the following.

- Check the magnesium level. Low magnesium must be corrected before I.V. calcium will increase serum calcium levels.
- Check the phosphate level. If the phosphate level is too high, calcium will not be absorbed. Reduce the phosphate level first.
- Mix I.V. calcium in dextrose solutions only. Normal saline may cause calcium to be excreted.

Administering I.V. calcium safely

Be prepared to administer parenteral calcium to a patient who has symptomatic hypocalcemia. Always clarify whether the doctor orders calcium *gluconate* or calcium *chloride.* Doses vary according to the specific drug. Note the type and dosage of each calcium preparation carefully. Follow these steps when administering calcium.

Preparing
Dilute the prescribed I.V. calcium preparation in dextrose 5% in water. Never dilute calcium in solutions containing bicarbonate; precipitation will occur. Avoid giving the patient calcium diluted in normal saline solution because the sodium chloride will increase renal calcium loss.

Administering
Always administer I.V. calcium slowly, according to the doctor's order or established protocol. Never give it rapidly because it may result in syncope, hypotension, and cardiac arrhythmias. Initially, calcium may be given as a slow I.V. bolus. If hypocalcemia persists, the initial bolus may be followed by a slow I.V. drip using an infusion pump.

Monitoring
Overcorrection may lead to hypercalcemia. Watch for signs of hypercalcemia, including anorexia, nausea, vomiting, lethargy, and confusion. Institute cardiac monitoring and observe for cardiac arrhythmias, especially in patients receiving digitalis glycosides. Observe the I.V. site for signs of infiltration; calcium can cause tissue sloughing and necrosis. Closely monitor serum calcium levels.

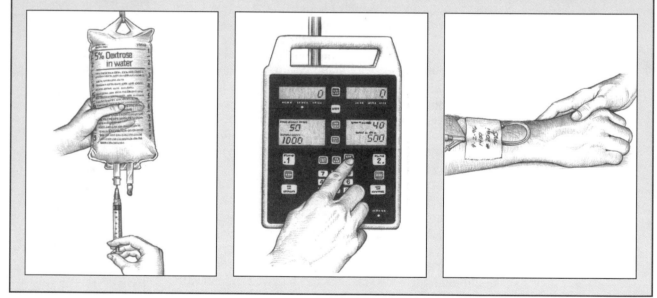

When assessing a patient you suspect has hypocalcemia, obtain a full health history. Be sure to assess the effects of symptoms on the patient's ability to perform activities of daily living.

Obtain a complete medical history. Note if the patient has ever had neck surgery. Hypoparathyroidism may develop immediately or several years after neck surgery. Ask a patient who has chronic hypocalcemia if he has a history of fractures. Also obtain a list of medications the patient is taking, because the list may help you determine the underlying cause of hypocalcemia.

Calcium by the bed

If your patient is recovering from parathyroid or thyroid surgery, keep calcium gluconate at the bedside. A handy supply of the drug ensures a quick response to signs of a sudden drop in calcium levels. If the patient develops hypocalcemia, here's what you can do.

Monitor

• Monitor vital signs, and assess the patient frequently. Monitor respiratory status, including rate, depth, and rhythm. Be alert for stridor, dyspnea, or crowing.
• If the patient shows overt signs of hypocalcemia, keep a tracheotomy tray and a handheld resuscitation bag at the bedside in case laryngospasm occurs.
• Place your patient on a cardiac monitor, and evaluate him for changes in heart rate and rhythm. Notify the doctor if arrhythmias, such as ventricular tachycardia or heart block, develop.
• Evaluate for the presence of Chvostek's sign or Trousseau's sign. (See *Teaching about hypocalcemia*.)

Maintain and administer

• Monitor a patient receiving I.V. calcium for arrhythmias, especially if he is also taking digitalis glycoside preparations. Calcium and digitalis glycosides exert similar effects on the heart.
• Insert and maintain a patent I.V. for calcium therapy.
• Administer I.V. calcium replacements carefully. Ensure the patency of the I.V., because infiltration can cause tissue necrosis and sloughing.
• Administer oral replacements as ordered. Give calcium supplements 1 to 1½ hours after meals. If GI upset occurs, give the medication with milk.

Follow-up

• Monitor pertinent laboratory test results, including not only calcium levels but also albumin levels and those of other electrolytes such as magnesium. Remember to check the ionized calcium level after every 4 units of blood transfused.

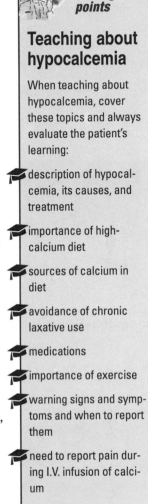

Parting points

Teaching about hypocalcemia

When teaching about hypocalcemia, cover these topics and always evaluate the patient's learning:

• description of hypocalcemia, its causes, and treatment
• importance of high-calcium diet
• sources of calcium in diet
• avoidance of chronic laxative use
• medications
• importance of exercise
• warning signs and symptoms and when to report them
• need to report pain during I.V. infusion of calcium
• possible use of female hormones in patients with osteoporosis.

• Encourage the older patient to take calcium supplements as ordered and also to exercise as much as he can tolerate, to prevent calcium loss from bones.
• Take precautions for seizures, such as padding the side rails.
• Reorient a confused patient. Provide a calm, quiet environment.
• Document all care given to the patient and all observations made. (See *Documenting hypocalcemia*.)

Hypercalcemia

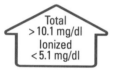

Total
> 10.1 mg/dl
Ionized
< 5.1 mg/dl

Hypercalcemia is a condition in which the serum calcium level rises above 10.1 mg/dl and the ionized serum calcium level rises above 5.1 mg/dl. The condition occurs when the rate of calcium entry into extracellular fluid exceeds the rate of calcium excretion by the kidneys.

How it happens

Any situation that causes an increase in the total serum or ionized calcium level can lead to hypercalcemia. The condition is usually caused by an increase in the resorption of calcium from bone.

There are two major causes of hypercalcemia — hyperparathyroidism and cancer. In hyperparathyroidism, the body excretes more parathyroid hormone than normal, which greatly strengthens the effects of the hormone. Calcium resorption from bone and reabsorption from the kidneys are also increased, as is calcium absorption from the intestines.

Malignant invasion

Cancer, the second most common cause of hypercalcemia, causes bone destruction as malignant cells invade the bones and may cause the release of a substance similar to parathyroid hormone. That hormone causes an increase in serum calcium levels.

When that happens, the kidneys can become overwhelmed and unable to excrete all that excess calcium,

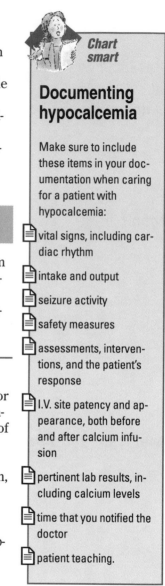

Chart smart

Documenting hypocalcemia

Make sure to include these items in your documentation when caring for a patient with hypocalcemia:

◻ vital signs, including cardiac rhythm

◻ intake and output

◻ seizure activity

◻ safety measures

◻ assessments, interventions, and the patient's response

◻ I.V. site patency and appearance, both before and after calcium infusion

◻ pertinent lab results, including calcium levels

◻ time that you notified the doctor

◻ patient teaching.

Drugs associated with hypercalcemia

Here's a list of medications that can cause hypercalcemia:

- excess calcium preparations (oral or I.V.)
- calcium-containing antacids
- lithium
- thiazide diuretics
- vitamin D
- vitamin A.

which in turn keeps calcium levels elevated. A patient who has squamous cell carcinoma of the lung is especially prone to hypercalcemia, as is a patient with myeloma or breast cancer.

Hypercalcemia can also be caused by an increase in the absorption of calcium in the GI tract or by a decrease in the excretion of calcium by the kidneys. Those mechanisms may occur alone or in combination.

Hyperthyroidism can cause an increase in calcium release as more calcium is resorbed from bone. Multiple fractures or prolonged immobilization can also cause an increase in calcium release from bone.

Hypophosphatemia and acidosis (which increases calcium ionization) are linked with hypercalcemia. Certain medications are also associated with the condition. For instance, abuse of calcium-containing antacids, receiving an overdose of calcium (from calcium medications given during cardiopulmonary resuscitation, for example), or excessive vitamin D ingestion can each prompt an increase in serum calcium levels. (See *Drugs associated with hypercalcemia.*)

Vitamin A overdose can lead to increased bone resorption of calcium. Use of lithium or thiazide diuretics can decrease calcium excretion by the kidneys. Milk-alkali syndrome, a condition in which calcium and alkali are combined, also raises calcium levels. (See *Key facts about hypercalcemia.*)

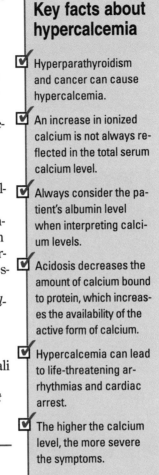

Key facts about hypercalcemia

☑ Hyperparathyroidism and cancer can cause hypercalcemia.

☑ An increase in ionized calcium is not always reflected in the total serum calcium level.

☑ Always consider the patient's albumin level when interpreting calcium levels.

☑ Acidosis decreases the amount of calcium bound to protein, which increases the availability of the active form of calcium.

☑ Hypercalcemia can lead to life-threatening arrhythmias and cardiac arrest.

☑ The higher the calcium level, the more severe the symptoms.

What to look for

Signs and symptoms of hypercalcemia are intensified if the condition develops acutely. Symptoms are also more severe at calcium levels greater than 15 mg/dl.

Many symptoms stem from the effects of excess calcium in cells, which causes a decrease in cell membrane excitability, especially in the tissues of the skeletal muscle, the heart muscle, and the nervous system.

The patient with hypercalcemia may complain of fatigue or exhibit confusion or personality changes. Lethargy can progress to coma in severe cases.

Affecting the muscles

As calcium levels rise, the patient develops muscle weakness, hyporeflexia, and decreased muscle tone. Hypercalcemia may lead to hypertension.

Because heart muscle and the cardiac conduction system are affected by hypercalcemia, arrhythmias such as bradycardia can lead to cardiac arrest. ECG tests may reveal a shortened QT interval and a shortened ST segment. Also look for digitalis toxicity in patients receiving digitalis glycoside preparations.

Affecting other systems

Hypercalcemia can also lead to GI symptoms, often the first signs noticed by the patient. (See *Signs of hypercalcemia.*) The patient may experience anorexia, nausea, or vomiting. Bowel sounds are decreased. Constipation can occur because of calcium's effect on smooth muscle and subsequent decrease in GI motility. Abdominal pain and paralytic ileus may result.

As the kidneys work overtime to remove excess calcium, renal problems may develop. The patient may experience polyuria and subsequent dehydration. Hypercalcemia can also cause kidney stones and other calcifications. Renal failure may be the end result. In addition, the patient may develop pathologic fractures and bone pain. (See *Danger signs of hypercalcemia.*)

What tests show

If you suspect hypercalcemia in a patient, look for the following results of diagnostic tests:
- serum calcium level greater than 10.1 mg/dl
- ionized calcium level above 5.1 mg/dl
- digitalis toxicity
- X-rays revealing pathologic fractures
- characteristic ECG changes.

How hypercalcemia is treated

If hypercalcemia produces no symptoms, treatment may consist only of managing the underlying cause. Dietary intake of calcium may be reduced and medications or infusions containing calcium stopped. Treatment for asympto-

I can't waste time

Signs of hypercalcemia

The signs and symptoms of hypercalcemia include:

- anorexia, nausea, vomiting
- behavioral changes, including confusion
- bone pain
- constipation, abdominal pain
- characteristic ECG changes
- hypertension
- lethargy
- muscle weakness, decreased deep-tendon reflexes
- polyuria, extreme thirst.

matic hypercalcemia also includes measures to increase the excretion of calcium and to decrease bone resorption of it.

Hydrate!

Increasing the excretion of calcium can be achieved by hydrating the patient, which encourages diuresis and increases excretion of the mineral. Normal saline solution is normally used for hydration in these cases. Sodium in the solution inhibits renal tubular reabsorption of calcium.

Loop diuretics, such as furosemide (Lasix) and ethacrynic acid (Edecrin), also promote calcium excretion. Thiazide diuretics are not used for hypercalcemia because they inhibit calcium excretion.

In life-threatening hypercalcemia, measures to increase calcium excretion may include hemodialysis or peritoneal dialysis with a solution that contains little or no calcium.

Back to the bones

Measures to inhibit bone resorption of calcium may also be used to help reduce calcium levels in extracellular fluids. Corticosteroids administered I.V. and then orally can block bone resorption and decrease calcium absorption from the GI tract.

Etidronate disodium, commonly used in the treatment of hypercalcemia, inhibits the action of osteoclasts in bone, thereby reducing bone resorption. This medication takes full effect in 2 to 3 days. Pamidronate disodium, a drug similar to etidronate disodium, can also be used to inhibit bone resorption. Mithramycin, a chemotherapy drug, can decrease bone resorption of calcium and is used mostly when the patient's hypercalcemia is due to cancer. Calcitonin inhibits bone resorption as well, but its effects are short-lived. (See *When treatment doesn't work.*)

How you intervene

Be sure to monitor patients at risk for hypercalcemia, such as those who have cancer or parathyroid disorders, are immobile, or are receiving calcium supplements. For a patient who develops hypercalcemia, you'll want to take these actions.

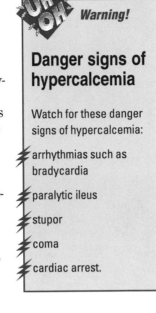

Warning!

Danger signs of hypercalcemia

Watch for these danger signs of hypercalcemia:

- arrhythmias such as bradycardia
- paralytic ileus
- stupor
- coma
- cardiac arrest.

It's not working!

When treatment doesn't work

If your patient doesn't seem to be responding to treatment for hypercalcemia, make sure he's not still taking vitamin D supplements.

Keep in mind that calcitonin may be given to decrease calcium levels rapidly, but the effects are only temporary.

Monitor

• Monitor vital signs and assess the patient frequently.
• Observe for arrhythmias that may develop. Assess neurologic and neuromuscular function and report any changes.
• Monitor the patient's fluid intake and output.
• Monitor serum electrolyte levels, especially calcium, to determine the effectiveness of treatment and to detect new imbalances that might result from therapy.

Maintain and administer

• Insert and maintain I.V. access. Normal saline solution is usually administered at a rate of 200 to 500 ml/hour. Monitor for signs of pulmonary edema, such as crackles and dyspnea.
• If administering diuretics, make sure the patient is properly hydrated first so as not to cause volume depletion.
• Encourage the patient to drink 3 to 4 liters of fluid daily, unless contraindicated, to stimulate calcium excretion from the kidneys and to decrease the risk of calculi formation. (See *Teaching about hypercalcemia.*)
• Strain the urine for calculi. Assess for flank pain, which can indicate the presence of renal calculi.
• If the patient is receiving digitalis glycosides, watch for signs of toxicity, such as anorexia, nausea, vomiting, or an irregular heart rate.
• Ambulate the patient as soon as possible to prevent calcium from being released by the bones.
• Handle a patient who has chronic hypercalcemia gently, to prevent pathologic fractures. Reposition bedridden patients frequently. Perform active or passive range of motion exercises to prevent complications of immobility.
• Provide a safe environment. Keep side rails raised as needed, keep the bed in its lowest position, keep the wheels locked, and make sure the patient's belongings and call button are within reach. Reorient a confused patient.
• Offer emotional support to the patient and his family throughout treatment. Overt signs of hypercalcemia can be emotionally distressing for all involved.
• Chart all care given and the patient's response. (See *Documenting hypercalcemia.*)

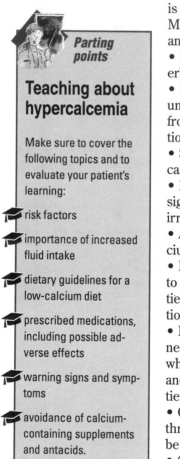

Parting points

Teaching about hypercalcemia

Make sure to cover the following topics and to evaluate your patient's learning:

- risk factors
- importance of increased fluid intake
- dietary guidelines for a low-calcium diet
- prescribed medications, including possible adverse effects
- warning signs and symptoms
- avoidance of calcium-containing supplements and antacids.

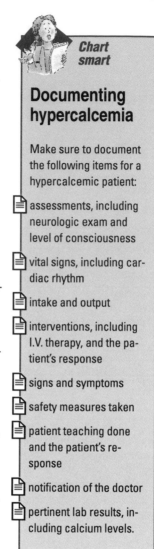

Chart smart

Documenting hypercalcemia

Make sure to document the following items for a hypercalcemic patient:

- assessments, including neurologic exam and level of consciousness
- vital signs, including cardiac rhythm
- intake and output
- interventions, including I.V. therapy, and the patient's response
- signs and symptoms
- safety measures taken
- patient teaching done and the patient's response
- notification of the doctor
- pertinent lab results, including calcium levels.

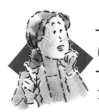

Quick quiz

1. Albumin affects calcium levels by:
   A. blocking phosphorus absorption, which prevents calcium excretion.
   B. binding with calcium, which makes the calcium ineffective.
   C. inhibiting magnesium uptake, which prevents calcium absorption.

Answer: B. Albumin binds with calcium and renders it ineffective.

2. The most common cause of hypocalcemia involves a dysfunction of:
   A. antidiuretic hormone.
   B. growth hormone.
   C. parathyroid hormone.

Answer: C. Parathyroid hormone promotes reabsorption of calcium from the bone to the serum. When the secretion of parathyroid hormone is decreased, hypocalcemia results.

3. Your patient is hypercalcemic. As part of his treatment, you would expect to:
   A. administer I.V. sodium bicarbonate.
   B. administer vitamin D.
   C. hydrate the patient.

Answer: C. Hydrating a patient with oral or I.V. fluids will increase the urinary excretion of calcium and help to lower serum calcium levels.

4. Hypercalcemia would be most likely to develop in:
   A. a 60-year-old man who has squamous cell carcinoma of the lung.
   B. an 80-year-old woman who has heart failure and is taking furosemide (Lasix).
   D. a 25-year-old trauma patient who has received massive blood transfusions.

Answer: A. Squamous cell carcinoma of the lung can lead to hypercalcemia. Loop diuretics, such as Lasix, can cause a loss of calcium from the kidneys. A preservative (citrate) contained in stored blood binds with ionized calcium and causes hypocalcemia.

5. You are told during shift report that your patient has a positive Chvostek's sign. You would expect lab tests to reveal:

    A.   total serum calcium of less than 8.9 mEq/L.
    B.   total serum calcium of greater than 10.1 mEq/L.
    C.   ionized calcium of greater than 5.1 mg/dl.

Answer: A. Chvostek's sign, along with Trousseau's sign, is associated with hypocalcemia. Only A indicates that condition.

Scoring

☆☆☆ If you answered all five questions correctly, we're impressed! We wonder, have you been hanging out in Professor Chvostek's lab?

☆☆ If you answered three or four questions correctly, oh my! Have you been reading Professor Trousseau's diary, by chance?

☆ If you answered fewer than three questions correctly, that's fine. We've got a great seat for you at the Chvostek-Trousseau lecture series!

When phosphorus tips the balance

Just the facts

This chapter describes how to recognize and correct phosphorus imbalances. In this chapter, you'll learn:

♦ what role phosphorus plays in the body

♦ how the body regulates phosphorus

♦ what hypophosphatemia and hyperphosphatemia are and how to manage them.

A look at phosphorus

Phosphorus is the primary anion, or negatively charged ion, found in the intracellular fluid. It is contained in the body as phosphate. (Often, the two words — phosphorus and phosphate — are used interchangeably.) About 85% of phosphorus exists in bone and teeth, combined in a 1:2 ratio with calcium. About 14% is in soft tissue, and less than 1% is in extracellular fluid.

The role phosphorus plays

An essential element of all body tissues, phosphorus is vital to a variety of body functions. It plays a crucial role in cell membrane integrity (phospholipids make up the cell membranes), muscle function, neurologic function, and the metabolism of carbohydrate, fat, and protein. Phosphorus is a primary ingredient in 2,3-diphosphoglycerate (2,3-DPG), a compound in red blood cells (RBCs) that facilitates oxygen delivery from RBCs to the tissues. Phosphorus is also involved in the buffering of acids and bases.

In addition, phosphorus promotes energy transfer to cells through the formation of energy-storing substances such as adenosine triphosphate (ATP). It's also important for white blood cell (WBC) phagocytosis and for platelet function. Finally, along with calcium, phosphorus is an essential component of bones and teeth.

Serum levels don't tell the whole story

Normal serum phosphorus levels in adults range from 2.5 to 4.5 mg/dl (or 1.8 to 2.6 mEq/L). In comparison, normal phosphorus concentration in the cells is 100 mEq/L. Because phosphorus is located primarily within the cells, serum levels may not always reflect the total amount of phosphorus in the body.

Keeping levels regulated

The total amount of phosphorus in the body is related to dietary intake, hormonal regulation, kidney excretion, and transcellular shifts. The daily adult dietary requirement for phosphorus is 800 to 1,200 mg. Phosphorus is readily absorbed through the GI tract, and the amount absorbed is proportional to the amount ingested. (See *Dietary sources of phosphorus.*)

Most ingested phosphorus is absorbed through the jejunum. The kidneys excrete about 90% of phosphorus as they regulate serum levels. (The GI tract excretes the rest.) If dietary intake of phosphorus increases, the kidneys increase excretion to maintain normal levels of phosphorus. A low-phosphorus diet causes the kidneys to reabsorb more phosphorus in the proximal tubules in order to conserve it.

Calcium and PTH

The parathyroid gland controls hormonal regulation of phosphorus levels by affecting the activity of parathyroid hormone. (See *Parathyroid hormone and phosphorus.*) Changes in calcium concentration, rather than changes in phosphorus levels, affect release of parathyroid hormone. You may recall that phosphorus balance is closely related to that of calcium.

Normally, calcium and phosphorus have an inverse relationship: If one is elevated, the other is decreased. When the serum calcium level is low, the phosphorus level is elevated. Parathyroid hormone is released, causing an increase in calcium and phosphorus resorption from bone and raising both the calcium and phosphorus levels. Phosphorus absorption from the intestines is also increased. (Activated vitamin D — calcitriol — also enhances its absorption in the intestines.)

Parathyroid hormone then acts on the kidneys to increase excretion of phosphorus. The renal effect of

---

Dietary sources of phosphorus

Major dietary sources of phosphorus include the following:

- cheese
- dried beans
- eggs
- fish
- milk, milk products
- nuts and seeds
- organ meats (brain, liver)
- poultry
- whole grains.

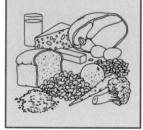

Parathyroid hormone and phosphorus

This illustration shows how parathyroid hormone (PTH) affects serum phosphorus (P) levels — by increasing phosphorus release from bone, increasing phosphorus absorption from the intestines, and decreasing phosphorus reabsorption in the renal tubules.

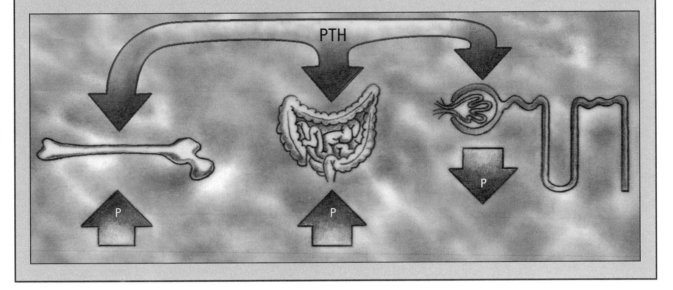

parathyroid hormone outweighs its other effects on the serum phosphorus level, particularly that of returning the phosphorus level to normal. Reduced parathyroid hormone levels allow for phosphorus reabsorption by the kidneys. As a result, serum levels rise.

Shifts affect serum levels

Certain conditions cause phosphorus to move, or shift, in and out of cells. Insulin moves not only glucose but also phosphorus into the cell. Alkalosis results in the same kind of phosphorus shift. Those shifts affect serum phosphorus levels.

Hypophosphatemia

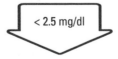

< 2.5 mg/dl

Hypophosphatemia occurs when the serum phosphorus level falls below 2.5 mg/dl (or 1.8 mEq/L). Although this condition often indicates a deficiency of phosphorus, it can occur in a variety of circumstances when total body phosphorus stores are normal. In severe hypophosphatemia (serum phosphorus levels less than 1 mg/dl), the body cannot support its energy needs. The condition may lead to organ failure.

How it happens

Three underlying mechanisms can lead to hypophosphatemia: a shift of phosphorus from extracellular fluid to intracellular fluid, a decrease in intestinal absorption of phosphorus, and an increased loss of phosphorus through the kidneys. Some causes of hypophosphatemia may involve more than one mechanism.

Several factors may cause phosphorus to shift from extracellular fluid into the cell. Here are the most common causes.

Hyperventilation

Respiratory alkalosis can stem from a number of conditions that produce hyperventilation, including sepsis, alcohol withdrawal, heat stroke, and acute salicylate poisoning. Although the mechanism that prompts respiratory alkalosis to induce hypophosphatemia is unknown, the response is a shift of phosphorus into the cells and a resulting decrease in serum phosphorus levels.

Insulin drives it into the cell

Hyperglycemia, an elevated serum glucose level, causes the release of insulin, which transports glucose and phosphorus into the cells. The same effect may occur when administering insulin to a diabetic patients or in significantly malnourished patients, such as those who are elderly, debilitated, or alcoholic or those who have anorexia nervosa. (See *Key facts about hypophosphatemia.*)

After initiation of enteral or parenteral feeding, and when phosphorus supplementation is not sufficient, phosphorus shifts into the cells. Called "refeeding syndrome," that shift usually occurs 3 or more days after feedings begin. Patients recovering from hypothermia can also develop hypophosphatemia as phosphorus moves into the cells.

Absorption problems

Malabsorption syndromes, starvation, and prolonged or excessive use of phosphorus-binding antacids are among the many causes of impaired intestinal absorption of phosphorus. Since vitamin D contributes to intestinal absorption of

---

Key facts about hypophosphatemia

☑ Because phosphorus is used to make high-energy adenosine triphosphate, hypophosphatemia may lead to low energy stores, which in turn may lead to muscle weakness and other clinical effects.

☑ Neurologic effects usually follow severe hypophosphatemia.

☑ An increased risk of infection is possible because of decreased metabolic functioning of leukocytes.

☑ Alcoholism is a significant risk factor.

phosphorus, inadequate vitamin D intake or synthesis can inhibit phosphorus absorption. Diarrhea or laxative abuse can also result in increased GI loss of phosphorus.

Don't forget the kidneys

Diuretic use is the most common cause of phosphorus loss through the kidneys. Thiazides, loop diuretics, and acetazolamide are the diuretics that most often cause hypophosphatemia. (See *Drugs associated with hypophosphatemia*.) The second most common cause is diabetic ketoacidosis in patients who have poorly controlled blood glucose levels. In diabetic ketoacidosis, an osmotic diuresis is induced from high glucose levels. This results in a significant loss of phosphorus from the kidneys. Ethanol affects phosphorus reabsorption in the kidney so that more phosphorus is excreted in the urine.

A buildup of parathyroid hormone, which occurs with hyperparathyroidism and hypocalcemia, also leads to hypophosphatemia. Finally, hypophosphatemia occurs in patients who have extensive burns. Although the mechanism is unclear, the condition is suspected to occur in response to the extensive diuresis of salt and water that typically occurs during the first 2 to 4 days after a burn injury. Respiratory alkalosis and carbohydrate administration may also play a role here.

> **Drugs associated with hypophosphatemia**
>
> The following drugs are commonly associated with hypophosphatemia:
>
> • acetazolamide, thiazide diuretics (chlorothiazide and hydrochlorothiazide), loop diuretics (furosemide and bumetanide), and other diuretics
> • antacids, such as aluminum hydroxide, aluminum carbonate, calcium carbonate, and magnesium oxide
> • insulin
> • laxatives.

What to look for

The characteristics of hypophosphatemia are apparent in many organ systems. Signs and symptoms may develop acutely due to rapid decreases in phosphorus or gradually as the result of slow, chronic decreases in phosphorus.

Hypophosphatemia affects the musculoskeletal, central nervous, cardiac, and hematologic systems. Because phosphorus is required to make high-energy ATP, many of the signs and symptoms of hypophosphatemia are related to low energy stores.

Getting weak

With hypophosphatemia, muscle weakness, malaise, and anorexia occur. The patient may experience a weakened hand grasp, slurred speech, or dysphagia. He also may develop myalgia (tenderness or pain in the muscles).

Respiratory failure may result from weakened respiratory muscles and poor contractility of the diaphragm. Respirations will appear shallow and ineffective. In later stages, the patient may be cyanotic. *Keep in mind that a mechanically ventilated patient with hypophosphatemia may be difficult to wean from the ventilator.*

Rhabdomyolysis (skeletal muscle destruction) can occur with altered muscle cell activity in severe hypophosphatemia. Muscle enzymes such as creatine kinase are released from the cells into the extracellular fluid. Loss of bone density, osteomalacia (softening of the bones), and bone pain may also occur with prolonged hypophosphatemia. Fractures can result.

Neuroeffects

Without enough phosphorus, the body can't make enough ATP, a cornerstone of energy metabolism. As a result, central nervous system cells can malfunction, causing paresthesia, irritability, apprehension, and confusion. The neurologic effects of hypophosphatemia may progress to seizures and coma. (See *Signs of hypophosphatemia.*)

Weak heartbeats

The heart's contractility is decreased due to low energy stores of ATP. As a result, the patient may develop hypotension and a low cardiac output. Severe hypophosphatemia may lead to cardiomyopathy, which can be reversed with treatment.

Oxygen delivery drop-off

A drop in production of 2,3-DPG causes a decrease in oxygen delivery to tissues. Because hemoglobin has a stronger affinity for oxygen than for other gases, oxygen is less likely to be given up to the tissues as it circulates through the body. As a result, less oxygen is delivered to the myocardium, which can cause chest pain.

Hypophosphatemia may also cause hemolytic anemia because of changes in the structure and function of red blood cells.

Patients with hypophosphatemia have an increased susceptibility to infection because of the effect of low levels of ATP in white blood cells. Lack of ATP results in a decreased functioning of leukocytes. Chronic hypophosphatemia also affects platelet function, resulting in bruising and bleeding, particularly mild GI bleeding.

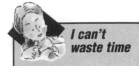

I can't waste time

Signs of hypophosphatemia

The following assessment findings commonly occur in patients with hypophosphatemia:

- anorexia
- bleeding or bruising
- confusion, irritability, apprehension
- fever, inflammation, or other signs of infection
- generalized muscle weakness (difficulty speaking, dysphagia, weak hand grasp)
- hypotension
- malaise
- muscle or bone pain
- paresthesia
- rapid, shallow respirations.

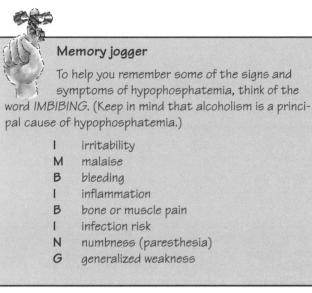

Memory jogger

To help you remember some of the signs and symptoms of hypophosphatemia, think of the word *IMBIBING*. (Keep in mind that alcoholism is a principal cause of hypophosphatemia.)

I   irritability
M   malaise
B   bleeding
I   inflammation
B   bone or muscle pain
I   infection risk
N   numbness (paresthesia)
G   generalized weakness

What tests show

The following diagnostic test results may indicate hypophosphatemia or a related condition:
• serum phosphorus level of less than 2.5mg/dl (or 1.8 mEq/L)
• elevated creatine kinase level if rhabdomyolysis is present
• X-ray studies that reveal the skeletal changes typical of osteomalacia or bone fractures.

How hypophosphatemia is treated

Treatment varies with the severity and cause of hypophosphatemia and includes treating the underlying cause and correcting the imbalance with phosphorus replacement and a high phosphorus diet. The route of replacement therapy depends on the severity of the imbalance.

For mild to moderate...

Treatment for mild-to-moderate hypophosphatemia includes a diet high in phosphorus-rich foods, such as eggs, nuts, whole grains, meat, fish, poultry, and milk or milk products. However, if calcium is contraindicated or milk is not tolerated, oral phosphorus supplements are indicated. Oral supplements include Neutra-Phos and Neutra-Phos-K and can be used for moderate hypophosphatemia. Dosage limitations are related to the adverse effects, most notably nausea and diarrhea. (See *When dietary changes aren't working*.)

It's not working!

When dietary changes aren't working

If your patient's phosphorus-rich diet hasn't raised serum phosphorus levels as you had hoped, it's time to ask the following questions.

• Is a GI problem making phosphorus digestion difficult?
• Is your patient using phosphate-binding antacids?
• Is your patient abusing alcohol?
• Is your patient continuing the use of thiazide diuretics?
• Is your patient complying with the treatment regimen for diabetes?

For more severe...

In severe hypophosphatemia or in cases of a nonfunctioning GI tract, I.V. phosphorus replacement is the recommended route. Two I.V. preparations, potassium phosphate and sodium phosphate, are used. Dosage is guided by the patient's response to treatment and serum phosphorus levels.

Potassium phosphate should be administered slowly (no more than 10 mEq/hour). Adverse effects of I.V. replacement for hypophosphatemia include hyperphosphatemia and hypocalcemia.

How you intervene

If your patient is beginning total parenteral nutrition or is otherwise at risk for developing hypophosphatemia, monitor for signs and symptoms of this imbalance. If the patient has already developed hypophosphatemia, your nursing care should focus on careful monitoring, safety measures, and interventions to restore normal serum phosphorus levels. (See *Teaching about low phosphorus.*) Report changes in the patient's condition to the doctor and take these other actions.

Assess and monitor

• Monitor vital signs. Remember that hypophosphatemia can lead to respiratory failure, low cardiac output, confusion, seizures, or coma.
• Assess the patient's level of consciousness and neurologic status each time you check his vital signs. Document your observations and the patient's neurologic status on a flow sheet so changes can be noted immediately, even on other shifts. (See *Documenting low phosphorus.*)
• Monitor the rate and depth of respirations, especially in a patient who has severe hypophosphatemia. Report signs of hypoxia, such as confusion, restlessness, increased respiratory rate and, in later stages, cyanosis. Where possible, take steps to prevent hyperventilation in the patient, since this worsens respiratory alkalosis and can further lower phosphorus levels. Follow arterial blood gas results to monitor the effectiveness of ventilation. Wean ventilator patients slowly.
• Monitor the patient for evidence of heart failure related to reduced myocardial functioning. Such evidence includes crackles, shortness of breath, decreased blood pressure, and elevated heart rate.

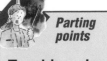

Parting points

Teaching about low phosphorus

Make sure you cover the following points with your patient and that you evaluate his learning:

➤ description of hypophosphatemia and its risk factors, prevention, and treatment

➤ medications ordered

➤ need to consult with a dietitian

➤ need for high-phosphorus diet

➤ avoidance of phosphorus-containing over-the-counter antacids

➤ warning signs and symptoms and when to report them

➤ need to maintain follow-up appointments.

• Monitor the patient's temperature at least every 4 hours. Check WBC counts. Follow strict aseptic technique in changing dressings. Report any signs of infection.

• Assess the patient frequently for evidence of decreasing muscle strength, such as weak hand grasps or slurred speech, and document your findings regularly.

Assess, administer, and maintain

• Administer prescribed phosphorus supplements. Keep in mind that oral supplements may cause diarrhea. To improve the taste of those medications, mix them with ice water or juice.

• Insert an I.V. line, as ordered, and maintain its patency. Infuse phosphorus solutions slowly, using an infusion device to control the rate. During infusions, watch for signs of hypocalcemia, hyperphosphatemia, and I.V. infiltration. Potassium phosphate can cause tissue sloughing and necrosis.

• Administer analgesics as ordered.

• Maintain bedrest if ordered for the patient's safety. Keep the bed in its lowest position, with the wheels locked and the side rails raised. If the patient is at risk for seizures, pad the side rails and keep an artificial airway at the patient's bedside.

Follow-up

• Orient the patient as needed. Keep clocks, calendars, and familiar personal objects within his sight.

• Inform the patient and his family that confusion caused by the low phosphorus level is only temporary and will most likely decrease with therapy.

• Record the patient's fluid intake and output.

• Carefully monitor serum electrolytes, especially calcium and phosphorus levels, as well as other pertinent laboratory results. Report abnormalities.

• Assist with ambulation and activities of daily living if necessary, and keep essential objects near the patient to prevent accidents.

Chart smart

Documenting low phosphorus

When caring for a patient with hypophosphatemia, be sure to document the following:

🗎 I.V. therapy, including condition of I.V. site, medication, dose, patient's response

🗎 muscle strength

🗎 neurologic status, including level of consciousness, restlessness, apprehension

🗎 notification of the doctor

🗎 patient teaching

🗎 respiratory assessment

🗎 safety measures to protect patient

🗎 seizures, if any

🗎 serum electrolytes and other pertinent laboratory data

🗎 vital signs

🗎 your interventions and the patient's response.

Hyperphosphatemia

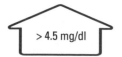

> 4.5 mg/dl

Hyperphosphatemia occurs when the serum phosphorus level exceeds 4.5 mg/dl (or 2.6 mEq/L) and usually reflects the kidneys' inability to excrete excessive phosphorus. The condition often occurs in combination with an increased release of phosphorus from damaged cells. Hyperphosphatemia is considered severe when the serum phosphorus level reaches 6.0 mg/dl or higher.

How it happens

Hyperphosphatemia results from a number of underlying mechanisms, including impaired renal excretion of phosphorus, a shift of phosphorus from the intracellular fluid to the extracellular fluid, or an increased dietary intake of phosphorus.

Kidney filter fails

Hyperphosphatemia most commonly results from renal failure due to the kidneys' inability to excrete excess phosphorus.

When the glomerular filtration rate begins to drop below 30 ml/minute, the kidneys can't filter excess phosphorus adequately. Since the kidneys are responsible for the bulk of phosphorus excretion, their inability to filter phosphorus leads to an elevated serum phosphorus level.

Hypoparathyroidism

A risk after thyroid or parathyroid surgery, hypoparathyroidism impairs synthesis of parathyroid hormone. When less parathyroid hormone is synthesized, less phosphorus is excreted from the kidneys. The result? Elevated serum phosphorus levels.

Puttin' on the transcellular shift

Several conditions can cause phosphorus to shift from the intracellular fluid to the extracellular fluid. Acid-base imbalances, such as respiratory acidosis and diabetic ketoacidosis, are common examples. Anything that causes cellular destruction can also result in a transcellular shift of phosphorus.

Destruction of cells can trigger the release of intracellular phosphorus into the extracellular fluid, causing serum phosphorus levels to rise. Chemotherapeutic treatment, for example, causes significant cell destruction, as do muscle necrosis and rhabdomyolysis, conditions that can stem from infection, heat stroke, and trauma.

Increased intake of phosphorus

Infants fed cow's milk are predisposed to hyperphosphatemia because the milk contains higher concentrations of phosphorus than breast milk. Excessive intake of phosphorus can result from overadministration of phosphorus supplements or of phosphorus-containing laxatives or enemas (such as Fleet enemas).

Excessive intake of vitamin D can result in increased absorption of phosphorus and lead to an elevated serum phosphorus level. (See *Drugs associated with hyperphosphatemia*.) Poor renal function heightens the risk of hyperphosphatemia due to increased intake of phosphorus.

What to look for

Hyperphosphatemia causes few clinical problems by itself. However, phosphorus and calcium levels have an inverse relationship: If one is high, the other is low. Because of this see-saw relationship, hyperphosphatemia may lead to hypocalcemia, which can be life-threatening.

Muscles and nerves

The patient may develop numbness or tingling (paresthesia) in the fingertips and around the mouth, which may increase in severity and spread proximally along the limbs and to the face. Muscle spasm, cramps, pain, and weakness may also occur and may be severe enough to prevent the patient from performing normal activities. In addition, the patient may exhibit hyperreflexia and positive Chvostek's and Trousseau's signs.

> ### Memory jogger
>
> To help you remember some of the signs and symptoms of hyperphosphatemia, think of the word *CHEMO*. (Keep in mind that chemotherapy can lead to hyperphosphatemia.)
>
> C cardiac irregularities
> H hyperreflexia
> E eating poorly
> M muscle weakness
> O oliguria

Drugs associated with hyperphosphatemia

The following drugs may cause hyperphosphatemia:

- enemas such as Fleet enemas
- laxatives containing phosphorus or phosphate
- vitamin D supplements
- oral phosphorus supplements such as Neutro-Phos
- parenteral phosphorus supplements, such as sodium phosphate or potassium phosphate.

A look at calcification

When the serum phosphorus level is high, phosphorus binds with calcium to form an insoluble compound called calcium phosphate. The compound is deposited in the heart, lungs, kidneys, eyes, skin, and other soft tissues. Called calcification, the deposit of calcium phosphate interferes with normal organ and tissue function. The illustration shows some of the effects of calcification.

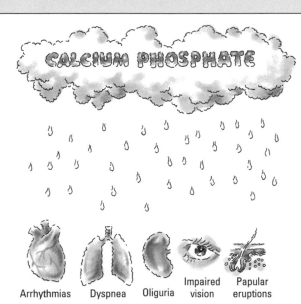

Arrhythmias Dyspnea Oliguria Impaired vision Papular eruptions

I can't waste time

Signs of hyperphosphatemia

The following assessment findings commonly occur in patients with hyperphosphatemia caused by hypocalcemia and soft tissue calcification:

- anorexia
- decreased mental status
- hyperreflexia
- hypocalcemic ECG changes
- muscle weakness, cramps, spasm
- nausea and vomiting
- papular eruptions
- paresthesia
- presence of Chvostek's or Trousseau's sign
- tetany
- visual impairment, conjunctivitis.

Neurologic symptoms include decreased mental status and seizures. Electrocardiogram (ECG) changes include a prolonged QT interval and ST segment. The patient may experience anorexia, nausea, and vomiting. Bone development may also be affected.

Calcification cues

When the phosphorus level rises, phosphorus binds with calcium, forming an insoluble compound called calcium phosphate. Organ dysfunction can result when calcium phosphate precipitates, or is deposited, in the heart, lungs, kidneys, corneas, or other soft tissues. Called calcification, this process usually occurs as a result of chronically elevated phosphorus levels. (See *A look at calcification*.)

With calcification, the patient may experience arrhythmias, an irregular heart rate, and decreased urine output. Corneal haziness, conjunctivitis, and impaired vision may occur, and papular eruptions may develop on the skin. (See *Signs of hyperphosphatemia*.)

What tests show

The following diagnostic test results may indicate hyperphosphatemia or a related condition, such as hypocalcemia:
• serum phosphorus level above 4.5 mg/dl (or 2.6 mEq/L)
• serum calcium level below 8.9 mg/dl
• X-ray studies that may reveal skeletal changes due to osteodystrophy (defective bone development) in chronic hyperphosphatemia
• increased blood urea nitrogen and creatinine levels, which reflect worsening renal function
• ECG changes characteristic of hypocalcemia.

How hyperphosphatemia is treated

An elevated serum phosphorus level may be treated with drugs and other therapeutic measures. In addition, treatment is aimed at correcting the underlying disorder, if one exists.

Try a low-phosphorus diet

If a patient's elevated serum phosphorus level is due to excessive phosphorus intake, the condition may be easily remedied by reducing phosphorus intake. Therapeutic measures include reducing dietary intake of phosphorus and eliminating the use of phosphorus-based laxatives and enema. (See *When dietary changes aren't enough.*)

Decreasing absorption

Drug therapy may assist in decreasing absorption of phosphorus in the GI system. Drug therapy may include aluminum, magnesium, or calcium gel or phosphate-binding antacids. In patients with underlying renal insufficiency or renal failure, use of magnesium antacids may result in hypermagnesemia and should be avoided.

Keep in mind that a mildly elevated phosphorus level may benefit a patient with renal failure. High phosphorus levels allow more oxygen to move from the RBCs to tissues, which can help avoid hypoxemia and limit the effects of chronic anemia on oxygen delivery.

Treat what's underneath

Treatment of the underlying cause of respiratory acidosis or diabetic ketoacidosis can lower serum phosphorus levels. In a diabetic patient, the administration of insulin caus-

It's not working!

When dietary changes aren't enough

If your patient's low-phosphorus diet hasn't changed his serum phosphorus level, it's time to ask the following questions.

• Is the patient taking the medication (phosphorus-binding antacids) as directed?
• Is the patient continuing to use phosphate-containing laxatives or enemas?
• Are the patient's kidneys functioning?
• Has the underlying cause of hyperphosphatemia been corrected?

es phosphorus to shift back into the cell, which can result in a decrease in serum phosphorus levels.

When the situation worsens

In severe hyperphosphatemia, I.V. saline solution may be given to promote renal excretion of phosphorus. However, this treatment requires that the patient have functional kidneys and be able to tolerate the increased load of sodium and fluid.

As a final therapeutic intervention, hemodialysis or peritoneal dialysis may be initiated if the patient has chronic renal failure or an extreme case of acute hyperphosphatemia with symptomatic hypocalcemia.

How you intervene

Identify patients at risk for hyperphosphatemia and monitor them carefully. Use care when administering phosphorus in I.V. infusions, enemas, and laxatives because the extra phosphorus may cause hyperphosphatemia. If your patient has already developed hyperphosphatemia, your nursing care should focus on careful monitoring, safety measures, and interventions to restore normal serum phosphorus levels. Follow these steps to provide care for the patient.

• Monitor vital signs, keeping in mind the signs and symptoms of hypocalcemia. If you note any signs of worsening hypocalcemia, such as numbness or tingling of the fingers or mouth area, hyperactive reflexes, or muscle cramps, notify the doctor promptly. (See *Teaching about high phosphorus.*) Also notify the doctor if you detect signs or symptoms of calcification, including oliguria, visual impairment, conjunctivitis, irregular heart rate or palpitations, and papular eruptions.

• Monitor fluid intake and output. If urine output falls below 30 ml/hour, notify the doctor immediately. Decreased output can seriously affect renal clearance of excessive serum phosphorus.

• Carefully monitor serum electrolyte levels, especially calcium and phosphorus. Report changes immediately. Also monitor BUN and serum creatinine levels, as hyperphosphatemia can impair renal tubules when calcification occurs.

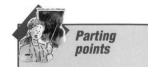

Parting points

Teaching about high phosphorus

Before your patient heads home, cover these topics with him and evaluate his learning:

◢ causes and treatment

◢ prescribed medications

◢ avoidance of preparations that contain phosphorus

◢ avoidance of high-phosphorus foods

◢ warning signs and symptoms

◢ referrals to dietitian and social services, if indicated.

• Keep a flowsheet of daily laboratory test results for a patient at risk. Include BUN and serum phosphorus, calcium, and creatinine levels, as well as fluid intake and output. Keep the flowsheet on a clipboard so changes can be detected immediately. (See *Documenting hyperphosphatemia*.)

Administer and follow-up

• Administer prescribed medications, monitor their effectiveness, and assess for possible adverse reactions. Give antacids with meals to increase their effectiveness in binding phosphorus.
• Prepare the patient for possible dialysis if hyperphosphatemia is severe.
• If a patient's condition results from chronic renal failure or if his treatment includes a low-phosphorus diet, consult a dietitian to assist the patient in complying with dietary restrictions.

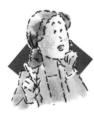

Quick quiz

1. If your patient has hyperphosphatemia, he may also have the secondary electrolyte disturbance:
    A. hypermagnesemia.
    B. hypocalcemia.
    C. hypernatremia.

Answer: B. Phosphorus and calcium have an inverse relationship: If the serum phosphorus levels are elevated, then the serum calcium levels are decreased.

2. In a patient with hyperphosphatemia and renal failure, avoid giving the phosphate-binding antacid:
    A. aluminum hydroxide.
    B. calcium carbonate.
    C. magnesium oxide.

Answer: C. Administering a magnesium antacid in a patient with renal failure can result in hypermagnesemia.

3. Many of the signs and symptoms of hypophosphatemia are related to:
    A. low energy stores.
    B. hypercalcemia.
    C. extensive diuresis.

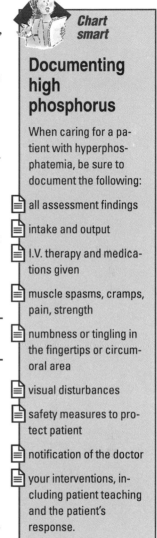

Chart smart

Documenting high phosphorus

When caring for a patient with hyperphosphatemia, be sure to document the following:

▤ all assessment findings

▤ intake and output

▤ I.V. therapy and medications given

▤ muscle spasms, cramps, pain, strength

▤ numbness or tingling in the fingertips or circumoral area

▤ visual disturbances

▤ safety measures to protect patient

▤ notification of the doctor

▤ your interventions, including patient teaching and the patient's response.

Answer: A. The body needs phosphorus to make high energy ATP, which provides all the cells — especially muscles — with energy.

4. The binding of phosphorus and calcium in a patient with hyperphosphatemia can lead to:
   A. increased calcium release by the kidneys.
   B. widespread calcification of tissues.
   C. decreased calcium uptake by the pituitary gland.

Answer: B. Hyperphosphatemia results in hypocalcemia. The calcium and phosphorus bind together and are deposited in the tissues, resulting in calcification.

5. You are advised that your alcoholic patient will be receiving his first infusion of total parenteral nutrition (TPN) tonight. Before hanging the first solution, you'll want to make sure:
   A. the patient's serum phosphorus level is normal.
   B. the patient isn't allergic to phosphorus.
   C. the patient's urine output is greater than 30 ml/ hour.

Answer: A. A low serum phosphorus level can drop further below normal if a patient receives TPN. The high glucose load causes phosphorus to shift into the cells.

6. Your patient's ability to be weaned from mechanical ventilation would be most likely affected by a serum phosphorus level:
   A. greater than 8 mg/dl.
   B. between 2 and 4 mg/dl.
   C. lower than 1 mg/dl.

Answer: C. Severe hypophosphatemia can lead to respiratory muscle weakness and impaired contractility of the diaphragm, which compromises the patient's ability to breathe spontaneously.

Scoring

☆☆☆ If you answered all six items correctly, wow! You're phospho-fabulous!

☆☆ If you answered four or five correctly, way to go! How about a lovely plate of baked halibut?

☆ If you answered three or fewer correctly, that's OK. Here's a delicious egg-and-cheese sandwich. Enjoy!

When chloride tips the balance

Just the facts

This chapter discusses chloride and how to care for patients who have either a deficit or an excess of this abundant anion. In this chapter, you'll learn:

♦ why chloride is important in the body

♦ how chloride and sodium are related

♦ how the body regulates the chloride level

♦ how to recognize and treat high and low chloride levels.

A look at chloride

Chloride is the most abundant anion (negatively charged ion) in extracellular fluid. It moves in and out of the cells with sodium and potassium and combines with major cations (positively charged ions) to form sodium chloride, hydrochloric acid, potassium chloride, calcium chloride, and other important compounds. High levels of chloride are found in cerebrospinal fluid, but the anion can also be found in bile and in gastric and pancreatic juices.

All about chloride

Because of its negative charge, chloride travels with positively charged sodium and helps maintain serum osmolality and water balance. Chloride and sodium also work together to form cerebrospinal fluid. The choroid plexus, a tangled mass of tiny blood vessels inside the ventricles of the brain, depends on these two electrolytes to attract water and to form the fluid component of cerebrospinal fluid.

In the stomach, chloride is secreted by the gastric mucosa as hydrochloric acid, providing the acid medium conducive to digestion and enzyme activation. Chloride helps maintain acid-base balance and assists in carbon dioxide transport in the red blood cells.

On the level

Serum chloride levels normally range between 96 and 106 mEq/L. By comparison, the chloride level inside a cell is 4 mEq/L. Chloride levels remain relatively stable with age. Because chloride balance is closely associated with sodium balance, the levels of both electrolytes usually change in direct proportion to one another.

Chloride control

Chloride regulation depends on intake and excretion of chloride and reabsorption of chloride ions in the kidneys. The daily chloride requirement for adults is 750 mg. Most diets provide sufficient chloride in the form of salt (usually as sodium chloride) but also in the same foods that contain sodium. (See *Dietary sources of chloride.*)

Most chloride is absorbed in the intestines with only a small portion lost in the feces. Chloride is produced mainly in the stomach as hydrochloric acid, so chloride levels can be influenced by GI disorders.

Linked electrolytes

Because chloride and sodium are closely linked, a change in one electrolyte level causes a comparable change in the other. Chloride levels can also be indirectly affected by aldosterone secretion, which causes sodium reabsorption by the renal tubules. As positively charged sodium ions are reabsorbed, negatively charged chloride ions are passively reabsorbed, due to their electrical attraction to sodium.

Acids and bases

Regulation of chloride levels also involves acid-base balance. Chloride is reabsorbed and excreted in direct opposition to bicarbonate. When chloride levels change, the body attempts to keep its positive-negative balance by making corresponding changes in the levels of bicarbonate (another negatively charged ion) in the kidneys. (Remember, bicarbonate is alkaline.)

Dietary sources of chloride

Dietary sources of chloride include:

- fruits
- vegetables
- salt, salty foods
- processed meats
- canned vegetables.

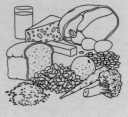

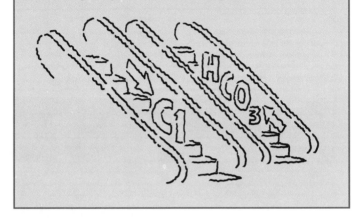

Chloride and bicarbonate

Chloride and bicarbonate have an inverse relationship. When the level of one goes up, the level of the other goes down.

When chloride levels decrease, the kidneys retain bicarbonate and bicarbonate levels increase. When chloride levels rise, the kidneys excrete bicarbonate and bicarbonate levels fall. Therefore, changes in chloride and bicarbonate levels can lead to acidosis or alkalosis. (See *Chloride and bicarbonate.*)

Hypochloremia

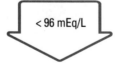

< 96 mEq/L

Hypochloremia is a deficiency of chloride in extracellular fluid reflected by a serum chloride level below 96 mEq/L. When serum chloride levels drop, levels of sodium, potassium, calcium, and other electrolytes may be affected. If much more chloride than sodium is lost, hypochloremic alkalosis may occur.

How it happens

Serum chloride levels drop when chloride intake or absorption decreases or when chloride losses increase. Losses may occur through the skin (chloride is found in sweat), the GI tract, or the kidneys. Changes in sodium levels or acid-base balance also alter chloride levels.

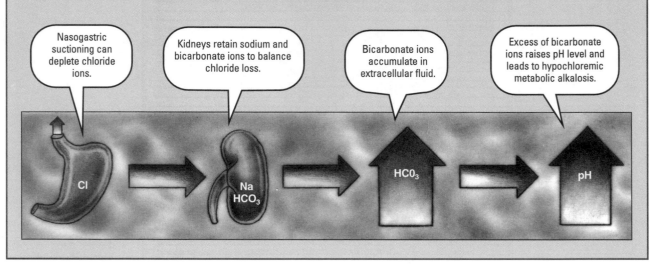

Dangerous development

Here's how hypochloremia can lead to hypochloremic metabolic alkalosis.

Nasogastric suctioning can deplete chloride ions.

Kidneys retain sodium and bicarbonate ions to balance chloride loss.

Bicarbonate ions accumulate in extracellular fluid.

Excess of bicarbonate ions raises pH level and leads to hypochloremic metabolic alkalosis.

Down with intake

Reduced chloride intake may occur in infants being fed chloride-deficient formula and in people on salt-restricted diets. Patients dependent on I.V. fluids are also at risk if the fluids lack chloride (for example, a dextrose solution without electrolytes).

Excessive chloride losses can occur with prolonged vomiting, diarrhea, severe diaphoresis, gastric surgery, nasogastric (NG) suctioning, and other GI tube drainage. Severe vomiting can cause a loss of hydrochloric acid from the stomach, an acid deficit in the body, and subsequent metabolic alkalosis. Patients with cystic fibrosis can also lose more chloride than normal. Any prolonged and untreated hypochloremic state can result in a state of hypochloremic alkalosis. (See *Dangerous development.*)

People at risk for hypochloremia include children with prolonged vomiting from pyloric obstruction and those with draining fistulas and ileostomies that can cause a loss of chloride from the GI tract. Diuretics such as furosemide (Lasix), ethacrynic acid (Edecrin), and hydrochlorothiazide, can also cause an excessive loss of chloride from the kidneys. (See *Drug culprits.*)

Drug culprits

Drugs commonly associated with hypochloremia include these kinds of diuretics:

- loop (such as furosimide)
- osmotic (such as mannitol)
- thiazide (such as hydrochlorothiazide).

Wait, there's more

Other causes of hypochloremia include sodium and potassium deficiency or metabolic alkalosis; conditions that cause alterations in acid-base or electrolyte balance, such as untreated diabetic ketoacidosis and Addison's disease; and rapid removal of ascitic fluid (which contains sodium) during paracentesis. In addition, patients who have congestive heart failure may develop hypochloremia as serum chloride levels are diluted by excess fluid in the body. (See *Key facts about hypochloremia*.)

What to look for

Patients who have hypochloremia may have signs and symptoms of acid-base and electrolyte imbalances. You may notice signs of hyponatremia, hypokalemia, or metabolic alkalosis. Alkalosis results in a high pH and, to compensate, respirations become slow and shallow as the body tries to retain carbon dioxide and restore the pH level to normal.

The nerves also become more excitable, so look for tetany, hyperactive deep-tendon reflexes, and muscle hypertonicity. (See *Signs of hypochloremia*.) The patient may have muscle cramps, twitching, and weakness and be agitated or irritable. If hypochloremia goes unrecognized, it can become life-threatening. As the chloride imbalance worsens (along with other imbalances), the patient may suffer arrhythmias, seizures, coma, or respiratory arrest.

What tests show

The following diagnostic test results are associated with hypochloremia:
- serum chloride level below 96 mEq/L
- serum sodium level below 135 mEq/L (indicates hyponatremia)
- serum pH greater than 7.45 and serum bicarbonate level greater than 26 mEq/L (indicates metabolic alkalosis).

How hypochloremia is treated

The treatment for hypochloremia focuses on correcting the underlying cause, such as low dietary chloride intake, prolonged vomiting, or gastric suctioning. Chloride may

---

Key facts about hypochloremia

☑ When chloride levels are low, potassium, sodium, and ionized calcium levels may also be low.

☑ When chloride levels decrease, bicarbonate levels rise to compensate.

☑ Signs and symptoms of hypochloremic metabolic alkalosis generally reflect metabolic alkalosis.

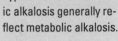
I can't waste time

Signs of hypochloremia

The signs and symptoms of hypochloremia include:

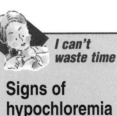

- agitation, irritability
- hyperactive deep-tendon reflexes and tetany
- muscle cramps and hypertonicity
- slow, shallow respirations and weakness
- seizures and coma
- arrhythmias.

be replaced through the administration of fluids or through drug therapy. The patient also may require treatment for associated metabolic alkalosis or electrolyte imbalances such as hypokalemia.

Chloride may be given orally; for example, in a salty broth. If the patient can't take oral supplements, he may receive medications or normal saline solution I.V. To avoid hypernatremia (high sodium level) or to treat hypokalemia, potassium chloride may be administered I.V.

Check out underlying causes

Treatments for associated metabolic alkalosis usually address the underlying causes. The underlying cause of diaphoresis, vomiting or other GI losses, or renal losses should be investigated. Rarely, metabolic alkalosis may be treated by administering ammonium chloride, an acidifying agent used when alkalosis is caused by chloride loss. The dosage of the drug depends on the severity of the alkalosis. The effects of ammonium chloride last for only 3 days. After that, the kidneys begin to excrete the extra acid. (See *When treatment isn't working*.)

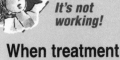

It's not working!

When treatment isn't working

If treatment for hypochloremia doesn't seem to be working, make sure the patient isn't drinking large amounts of free water or bottled water, which can cause him to excrete large amounts of chloride. Review the causes of hypochloremia to identify new or coexisting conditions that might be causing chloride loss.

How you intervene

Make sure to monitor patients at risk for hypochloremia, such as those receiving diuretic therapy or NG suctioning. When caring for a patient with hypochloremia, you'll also want to take these nursing actions.

Monitor

• Monitor level of consciousness, muscle strength, and movement. Notify the doctor if the patient's condition worsens.
• Monitor vital signs, especially respiratory rate and pattern, and observe for worsening respiratory function. Also monitor cardiac rhythm because hypokalemia may be present with hypochloremia. Have emergency equipment handy in case the patient's condition deteriorates.
• Monitor and record serum electrolyte levels, especially chloride, sodium, potassium, and bicarbonate; also assess arterial blood gas (ABG) results for acid-base imbalance.

Administer and maintain

• Offer foods high in chloride, such as tomato juice or salty broth, if the patient is alert and able to swallow with-

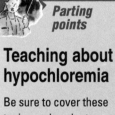

Parting points

Teaching about hypochloremia

Be sure to cover these topics and evaluate your patient's learning:

• signs and symptoms, complications and risk factors for hypochloremia
• warning signs to report to the doctor
• dietary supplements
• medications if prescribed.

out difficulty. Don't let the patient fill up on plain drinking water. (See *Teaching about hypochloremia.*)

• Insert an I.V., as ordered, and keep it patent. Administer chloride and potassium replacements, as ordered.

• If administering ammonium chloride, assess for pain at the infusion site and adjust the rate, if necessary. This drug is metabolized by the liver, so don't give it to patients who have severe hepatic disease.

• Use normal saline solution, not tap water, to flush the patient's NG tube.

• Accurately measure and record intake and output, including the volume of emesis, gastric contents from suction, or other GI drainage tubes.

• Provide a safe environment. Help the patient ambulate, and keep his personal items and call button within reach. Institute seizure precautions, as needed.

• Provide a quiet environment, explain interventions, and reorient the patient, as needed.

• Document all care and the patient's response. (See *Documenting hypochloremia.*)

Hyperchloremia

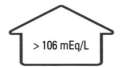

> 106 mEq/L

Hyperchloremia is an excess of chloride in extracellular fluid reflected in a serum chloride level above 106 mEq/L. The condition is associated with other acid-base imbalances and rarely occurs alone.

How it happens

Because chloride regulation and sodium regulation are closely related, hyperchloremia may also be associated with hypernatremia. Chloride and bicarbonate have an inverse relationship, so an excess of chloride ions may be linked to a decrease in bicarbonate. Excess serum chloride results from increased chloride intake or absorption, from acidosis, or from chloride retention by the kidneys.

Up with intake and absorption

Increased intake of chloride as sodium chloride can cause hyperchloremia, especially if water is lost from the body at the same time. That water loss raises the chloride level even further. Increased chloride absorption by the bowel

---

Chart smart

Documenting hypochloremia

If your patient has hypochloremia, make sure your documentation includes:

📄 vital signs, including cardiac rhythm

📄 intake and output

📄 serum electrolyte levels and arterial blood gas results

📄 your assessment, including level of consciousness, seizure activity, and respiratory status

📄 I.V. therapy, along with other interventions, and the patient's response

📄 safety measures implemented

📄 teaching done and the patient's response

📄 time of notification of the doctor.

can occur in patients who have had anastomoses joining the ureter and intestines.

Clinical situations that alter electrolyte and acid-base balance and cause metabolic acidosis include dehydration, renal tubular acidosis, renal failure, respiratory alkalosis, salicylate toxicity, hyperparathyroidism, hyperaldosteronism, and hypernatremia.

Drug-related retention

Several medications can also contribute to hyperchloremia. For example, direct ingestion of ammonium chloride or other drugs that contain chloride or cause chloride retention can lead to hyperchloremia. Ion exchange resins that contain sodium, such as Kayexalate, can cause chloride to be exchanged for potassium in the bowel. When chloride follows sodium into the bloodstream, serum chloride levels rise. Carbonic anhydrase inhibitors, like acetazolamide, also promote chloride retention in the body. (See *Drug offenders*.)

What to look for

Hyperchloremia rarely produces signs and symptoms on its own. Instead, the major signs and symptoms are essentially those of metabolic acidosis, including tachypnea, lethargy, weakness, diminished cognitive ability, and deep, rapid respirations (Kussmaul's respirations). (See *Key facts about hyperchloremia*.)

Left untreated, acidosis can lead to arrhythmias, decreased cardiac output, a further decrease in the patient's level of consciousness, and even coma. Metabolic acidosis related to a high chloride level is called "hyperchloremic metabolic acidosis." (See *Anion gap and metabolic acidosis*.)

If a patient has an increased serum chloride level, his serum sodium level is probably high as well, which can lead to fluid retention. He also may be agitated and have dyspnea, tachycardia, hypertension, or pitting edema — signs of hypernatremia and hypervolemia. (See *Signs of hyperchloremia*.)

Drug offenders

These drugs can lead to excess chloride:

- acetazolamide
- ammonium chloride
- phenylbutazone
- sodium polystyrene sulfonate (Kayexalate)
- salicylates (overdose)
- triamterene.

Key facts about hyperchloremia

☑ An inverse relationship exists between chloride and bicarbonate. When the level of one goes up, the level of the other goes down.

☑ Patients are at risk for hyperchloremic acidosis secondary to bicarbonate ion loss.

☑ Signs and symptoms of hyperchloremia generally reflect metabolic acidosis.

☑ In hyperchloremic metabolic acidosis, the anion gap is normal.

Signs of hyperchloremia

I can't waste time

Here's a list of the chief signs and symptoms of hyperchloremia, in association with metabolic acidosis and with hypernatremia.

Metabolic acidosis

- Decreasing level of consciousness
- Rapid, deep breathing (Kussmaul's respirations)
- Weakness

Hypernatremia

- Agitation
- Tachypnea, dyspnea
- Tachycardia
- Hypertension
- Edema

Anion gap and metabolic acidosis

Hyperchloremia increases the likelihood that a patient will develop hyperchloremic metabolic acidosis. The illustration below shows the relationship between chloride and bicarbonate in the development of that form of acidosis.

How it happens

A normal anion gap in a patient with metabolic acidosis indicates that the acidosis is most likely caused by a loss of bicarbonate ions by the kidneys or the GI tract. In such cases, a corresponding increase in chloride ions also occurs.

Acidosis can also result from an accumulation of chloride ions in the form of acidifying salts. A corresponding decrease in bicarbonate ions occurs at the same time. In the illustration, the chloride level is high (> 106 mEq/L) and the bicarbonate level is low (< 22 mEq/L).

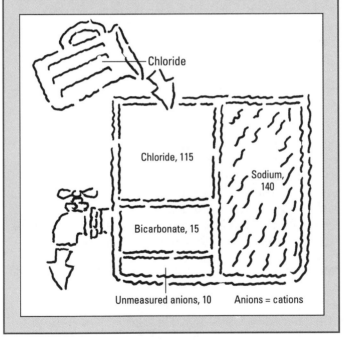

Chloride

Chloride, 115

Sodium, 140

Bicarbonate, 15

Unmeasured anions, 10   Anions = cations

What tests show

The following diagnostic test results typically occur in hyperchloremia:
- serum chloride level greater than 106 mEq/L
- serum sodium level greater than 145 mEq/L

• serum pH level less than 7.35, serum bicarbonate level less than 22 mEq/L, and a normal anion gap (8 to 14 mEq/L). These findings suggest metabolic acidosis.

How hyperchloremia is treated

Treatments for hyperchloremia include correcting the underlying cause as well as restoring fluid, electrolyte, and acid-base balance. (See *Diuretics to the rescue.*) Dehydrated patients may receive fluids to dilute the chloride and speed renal excretion of chloride ions. Sodium and chloride intake also may be restricted.

If the patient's liver function is adequate, he may receive an infusion of lactated Ringer's solution to convert lactate to bicarbonate in the liver and to increase the base bicarbonate level and correct acidosis. In severe hyperchloremia, I.V. sodium bicarbonate may be administered to raise serum bicarbonate levels. Because bicarbonate and chloride compete for sodium, I.V. sodium bicarbonate therapy can lead to renal excretion of chloride ions and correction of acidosis.

How you intervene

Try to prevent hyperchloremia by monitoring high-risk patients. If your patient develops a chloride imbalance:
• Monitor vital signs, including cardiac rhythm.
• Continually assess the patient, paying particular attention to the neurologic, cardiac, and respiratory exam. Report changes to the doctor immediately.
• Look for changes in the respiratory pattern that may indicate a worsening of the acid-base imbalance.
• Insert an I.V. and maintain its patency. Administer I.V. fluids and medications as ordered. Watch for signs of fluid overload.
• Reorient the confused patient as needed and provide a safe, quiet environment to prevent injury. Teach the patient's family to do the same. (See *Teaching about hyperchloremia.*)
• Evaluate muscle strength and adjust activity level accordingly.
• If the patient is receiving high doses of sodium bicarbonate, watch for signs and symptoms of overcompensation, such as metabolic alkalosis, which may cause central

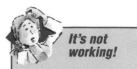

It's not working!

Diuretics to the rescue

If the patient doesn't seem to respond to therapy, the doctor may order diuretics to eliminate chloride. Although other electrolytes will be lost, the chloride level should decrease.

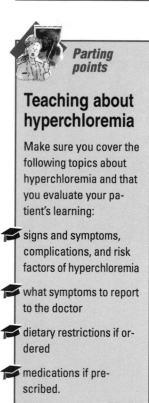

Parting points

Teaching about hyperchloremia

Make sure you cover the following topics about hyperchloremia and that you evaluate your patient's learning:

✒ signs and symptoms, complications, and risk factors of hyperchloremia

✒ what symptoms to report to the doctor

✒ dietary restrictions if ordered

✒ medications if prescribed.

✒ importance of replenishing lost fluids during hot weather.

and peripheral nervous system overexcitation. Also watch for signs of hypokalemia as potassium is forced into the cells.

• Restrict fluids, sodium, and chloride, if ordered.

• Monitor and record serum electrolyte levels and ABG results.

• Monitor and record fluid intake and output. (See *Documenting hyperchloremia*.)

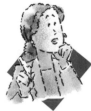

Quick quiz

1. Chloride is largely produced by the:
   A. brain.
   B. kidneys.
   C. stomach.

Answer: C. The chloride ion is largely produced by gastric mucosa and occurs in the form of hydrochloric acid.

2. If the level of bicarbonate ions increases, the level of chloride ions:
   A. increases.
   B. decreases.
   C. stays the same.

Answer: B. The relationship between chloride ions and bicarbonate ions is inversely proportional. If one level rises, the other level drops.

3. If your postoperative patient has a chloride imbalance, you would also expect to see a change in the electrolyte:
   A. calcium.
   B. potassium.
   C. sodium.

Answer: C. Sodium and chloride move together through the body, so an imbalance in one often causes an imbalance in the other.

4. For a patient who has a low serum chloride level, you would expect the patient to have the acid-base imbalance:
   A. respiratory acidosis.
   B. metabolic acidosis.
   C. metabolic alkalosis.

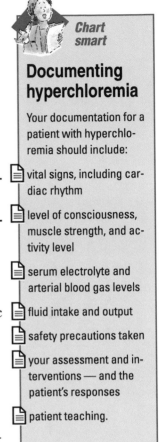

Chart smart

Documenting hyperchloremia

Your documentation for a patient with hyperchloremia should include:

◻ vital signs, including cardiac rhythm

◻ level of consciousness, muscle strength, and activity level

◻ serum electrolyte and arterial blood gas levels

◻ fluid intake and output

◻ safety precautions taken

◻ your assessment and interventions — and the patient's responses

◻ patient teaching.

Answer: C. A drop in chloride ions causes the body to retain bicarbonate, a base, and results in hypochloremic metabolic alkalosis.

5. Deep, rapid breathing may indicate a:
   A. serum chloride level greater than 106 mEq/L.
   B. serum chloride less than 96 mEq/L.
   C. pH greater than 7.45.

Answer: A. Deep, rapid breathing, or Kussmaul's respirations, is the body's attempt to blow off excess acid in the form of carbon dioxide. When this occurs, suspect metabolic acidosis, a condition associated with a serum chloride greater than 106 mEq/L.

Scoring

☆☆☆ If you answered all five items correctly, incredible! You're hereby named Most Exalted Keeper of the Chloride Key!

☆☆ If you answered three or four correctly, super! You're hereby named Royal High Assistant to the Most Exalted Keeper of the Chloride Key!

☆ If you answered fewer than three correctly, that's OK. You're hereby named Notable Grand Associate to the Royal High Assistant to the Most Exalted Keeper of the Chloride Key.

When acids and bases tip the balance

Just the facts

This chapter explains the basics — and more — of acidosis and alkalosis. In this chapter, you'll learn:

♦ how the body compensates for acid-base imbalances

♦ what conditions can trigger those imbalances

♦ how to differentiate among the four major acid-base imbalances — respiratory acidosis and alkalosis, and metabolic acidosis and alkalosis

♦ how to care for a patient with an acid-base imbalance.

A look at acid-base imbalances

The body constantly works to maintain the balance between acids and bases. Without that balance, the cells can't function properly. Acid-base balance depends on the regulation of free hydrogen ions. The concentration of hydrogen ions in body fluids determines the extent of acidity or alkalinity, both of which are measured in pH. (For more information about pH, see Chapter 3.)

When acid-base values stray...

Blood gas measurements remain the major diagnostic tool for evaluating acid-base states. An arterial blood gas (ABG) analysis includes the following tests: pH, $Paco_2$ (reflecting the adequacy of ventilation by the lungs), and

HCO_3 (reflecting the activity of the kidneys in retaining or excreting bicarbonate). (See *An ABG reminder*.)

Normal fix-me-ups

Most of the time, the body's compensatory mechanisms restore acid-base balance or at least prevent the life-threatening consequences of an imbalance. Those compensatory mechanisms include chemical buffers, certain respiratory reactions, and certain kidney reactions.

For example, the body compensates for a primary respiratory disturbance, such as respiratory acidosis, by inducing metabolic alkalosis. Unfortunately, not all attempts to compensate are equal. The respiratory system is efficient and can compensate for metabolic disturbances quickly, whereas the metabolic system, working through the kidneys, can take hours or days to compensate for an imbalance. This chapter takes a closer look at each of the four major acid-base imbalances.

> ### An ABG reminder
>
> Use these three main values when assessing acid-base balance.
>
> pH   7.35 to 7.45
> $Paco_2$ 35 to 45 mm Hg
> HCO_3 22 to 26 mEq/L

Respiratory acidosis

A compromise in any of the three essential parts of breathing — ventilation, perfusion, or diffusion — may result in respiratory acidosis. This acid-base disturbance is characterized by alveolar hypoventilation, meaning that the patient's pulmonary system is unable to rid the body of enough carbon dioxide (CO_2) to maintain a healthy pH balance.

The lack of efficient CO_2 release leads to hypercapnia, in which the partial pressure of carbon dioxide in arterial blood ($Paco_2$) is greater than 45 mm Hg. The condition can be acute, resulting from sudden failure in ventilation, or chronic, resulting from long-term pulmonary disease.

In acute respiratory acidosis, the pH drops below normal (lower than 7.35). In chronic respiratory acidosis, often due to chronic obstructive pulmonary disease (COPD), the pH stays within normal limits (7.35 to 7.45), because the kidneys have had time to compensate for the imbalance. (More on that complex phenomenon later.)

How it happens

When a patient hypoventilates, carbon dioxide builds up in the bloodstream and the pH drops below normal — respiratory acidosis. The body tries to compensate for a drop in pH by retaining more bicarbonate (base) in the kidney, which in turn raises the pH. (See *What happens in respiratory acidosis,* pages 182 and 183.)

Respiratory acidosis can result from neuromuscular problems, from depression of the respiratory center in the brain, from lung disease, or from an airway obstruction.

Respirations lack drive

In certain neuromuscular diseases, such as Guillain-Barré syndrome, myasthenia gravis, and poliomyelitis, the respiratory muscles fail to respond properly to the respiratory drive, resulting in respiratory acidosis. Diaphragmatic paralysis, which often occurs with spinal cord injury, works the same way to cause respiratory acidosis.

Hypoventilation from central nervous system trauma or brain lesions such as tumors, vascular disorders, or infections, may impair the patient's ventilatory drive. In addition, certain drugs, including narcotics, anesthetics, hypnotics, and sedatives, can depress the respiratory center of the brain, leading to hypercapnia. (See *Drugs associated with respiratory acidosis.*) Obesity (as in pickwickian syndrome) or primary hypoventilation (as in Ondine's curse) can also contribute to this imbalance.

Pulmonary problems risky

Lung diseases that decrease the amount of pulmonary surface area available for gas exchange can prompt respiratory acidosis. Less surface area decreases the amount of gas exchange that can occur, thus impeding CO_2 exchange. Examples of those diseases include respiratory infections, COPD, acute asthmatic attacks, chronic bronchitis, late stages of adult respiratory distress syndrome, pulmonary edema, conditions in which there is increased dead space in the lungs (hypoventilation), and physiologic or anatomic shunts.

Chest wall trauma (leading to pneumothorax or flail chest) can also cause respiratory acidosis. The ventilatory drive remains intact, but the chest wall mechanics of the collapsed lung don't allow for sufficient alveolar ventilation to meet the body's needs. Chest wall mechanics can also

Drugs associated with respiratory acidosis

The following drugs are associated with respiratory acidosis:

- anesthetics
- hypnotics
- narcotics
- sedatives.

What happens in respiratory acidosis

This series of illustrations shows at the cellular level how respiratory acidosis develops.

Step 1

When pulmonary ventilation decreases, retained carbon dioxide (CO_2) combines with water (H_2O) to form carbonic acid (H_2CO_3) in larger-than-normal amounts. The carbonic acid dissociates to release free hydrogen ions (H) and bicarbonate ions (HCO_3). The excessive carbonic acid causes a drop in pH. *Look for a $Paco_2$ level above 45 mm Hg and a pH level below 7.35.*

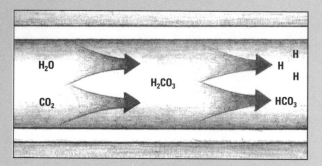

Step 2

As the pH level falls, 2,3-diphosphoglycerate (2,3-DPG) increases in the red blood cells and causes a change in hemoglobin (Hb) that makes the hemoglobin release oxygen (O_2). The altered hemoglobin, now strongly alkaline, picks up hydrogen ions and CO_2, thus eliminating some of the free hydrogen ions and excess CO_2. *Look for decreased arterial oxygen saturation.*

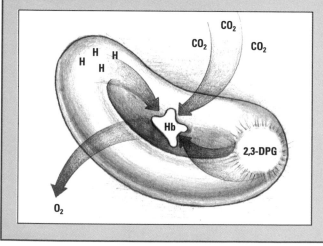

Step 3

Whenever $Paco_2$ increases, CO_2 builds up in all tissues and fluids, including cerebrospinal fluid and the respiratory center in the medulla. The CO_2 reacts with water to form carbonic acid, which then breaks into free hydrogen ions and bicarbonate ions. The increased amount of CO_2 and free hydrogen ions stimulate the respiratory center to increase the respiratory rate. An increased respiratory rate expels more CO_2 and helps to reduce the CO_2 level in the blood and other tissues. *Look for rapid, shallow respirations and a decreasing $Paco_2$.*

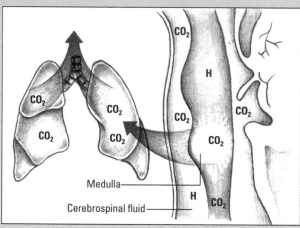

Medulla

Cerebrospinal fluid

Step 4

Eventually, CO_2 and hydrogen ions cause cerebral blood vessels to dilate, which increases blood flow to the brain. That increased flow can cause cerebral edema and depress central nervous system activity. *Look for headache, confusion, lethargy, nausea, or vomiting.*

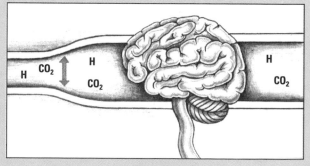

What happens in respiratory acidosis (continued)

Step 5

As respiratory mechanisms fail, the increasing $Paco_2$ stimulates the kidneys to retain bicarbonate and sodium ions and to excrete hydrogen ions, some of which are excreted in the form of ammonium (NH_4). The additional bicarbonate and sodium combine to form extra sodium bicarbonate ($NaHCO_3$), which is then able to buffer more free hydrogen ions. *Look for increased acid content in the urine, increasing serum pH and bicarbonate levels, and shallow, depressed respirations.*

Step 6

As the concentration of hydrogen ions overwhelms the body's compensatory mechanisms, the hydrogen ions move into the cells and potassium ions move out. A concurrent lack of oxygen causes an increase in the anaerobic production of lactic acid, which further skews the acid-base balance and critically depresses neurologic and cardiac functions. *Look for hyperkalemia, arrhythmias, increased $Paco_2$, decreased Pao_2, decreased pH, and decreased level of consciousness.*

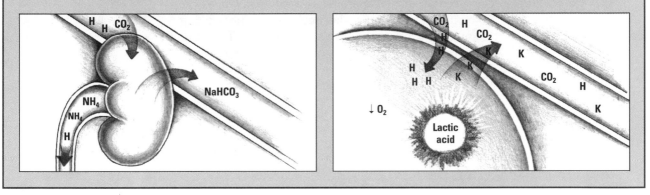

be impeded as a result of the rib cage distortion caused by fibrothorax or kyphoscoliosis.

Danger! Obstruction!

Respiratory acidosis can also be caused by airway obstruction, which leads to carbon dioxide retention in the lungs. Airway obstruction can occur as a result of retained secretions, tumors, anaphylaxis, laryngeal spasm, or lung diseases that interfere with alveolar ventilation. *Keep in mind that children are prone to airway obstruction. So are elderly or debilitated patients who may not be able to clear secretions effectively.*

Who's at risk?

Treatments can induce respiratory acidosis. For instance, mechanical ventilation that underventilates a patient can cause CO_2 retention. A postoperative patient is at risk for respiratory acidosis if fear of pain prevents him from participating in pulmonary hygiene measures. In addition, analgesics or sedatives can depress the medulla, which is responsible for controlling respirations. Depressing the medulla can lead to inadequate ventilation and subsequent respiratory acidosis.

What to look for

Signs and symptoms of respiratory acidosis depend on the cause of the condition. The patient may complain of a headache, since carbon dioxide dilates cerebral blood vessels. (See *Signs of respiratory acidosis.*)

Central nervous system (CNS) depression may result in an altered level of consciousness ranging from restlessness, confusion, and apprehension to somnolence and coma. If the acidosis remains untreated, a fine flapping tremor and depressed reflexes may develop. The patient may also report nausea and vomiting, and the skin may be warm and flushed.

Most patients with respiratory acidosis have rapid, shallow respirations. If acidosis stems from CNS trauma or lesions or drug overdose, however, the respiratory rate will be greatly decreased.

The patient will be dyspneic and possibly diaphoretic. Auscultation will reveal diminished or absent breath sounds over the affected area.

High CO_2 levels affect alveolar gas exchange, causing hypoxemia. In a patient with acidosis coupled with hyperkalemia and hypoxemia, you may note tachycardia and ventricular arrhythmias. Cyanosis is a late sign of the condition. Resulting myocardial depression may lead to shock and ultimately cardiac arrest.

I can't waste time

Signs of respiratory acidosis

The following assessment findings commonly occur in patients with respiratory acidosis:

- apprehension
- confusion
- decreased deep-tendon reflexes
- diaphoresis
- dyspnea, with rapid, shallow respirations
- nausea or vomiting
- restlessness
- tachycardia
- tremors
- warm, flushed skin.

What tests show

The following test results may help confirm the diagnosis and guide the treatment, of respiratory acidosis:
- ABG analysis is the key test for detecting respiratory acidosis. Typically, the pH is below 7.35 and the Pa_{CO_2} is above 45 mm Hg. The bicarbonate level may vary, depending on how long the acidosis has been present. In an acute episode, the bicarbonate may be normal; in a chronic episode, the bicarbonate may be above 26 mEq/L. (See *ABG results in respiratory acidosis.*)
- Chest X-rays often pinpoint causes, such as pulmonary edema, pneumonia, COPD, and pneumothorax.

ABG results in respiratory acidosis

This chart shows typical ABG findings in uncompensated and compensated respiratory acidosis.

	Uncompensated	Compensated
pH	< 7.35	Normal
$Paco_2$ (mm Hg)	> 45	> 45
HCO_3 (mEq/L)	Normal	> 26

• Serum electrolyte studies typically show hyperkalemia, with potassium levels greater than 5 mEq/L. In acidosis, potassium leaves the cell, so expect the serum level to be elevated.
• Drug screening may confirm a suspected overdose.

How respiratory acidosis is treated

Treatment of respiratory acidosis focuses on improving ventilation and lowering the $Paco_2$ level. If respiratory acidosis stems from nonpulmonary conditions, such as neuromuscular disorders or a drug overdose, treatment goals involve correcting the underlying cause.

Treatment for respiratory acidosis with a pulmonary cause includes:
• bronchodilators to open constricted airways
• supplemental oxygen as needed
• drug therapy to treat hyperkalemia
• antibiotics to treat infection
• chest physiotherapy to remove secretions from the lungs
• removal of a foreign body from the patient's airway, if necessary. (See *When hypoventilation can't be corrected*.)

How you intervene

If your patient develops respiratory acidosis, maintain a patent airway. Assist with removing any foreign bodies from the airway and establishing an artificial airway. Pro-

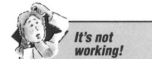

It's not working!

When hypoventilation can't be corrected

If hypoventilation can't be corrected, expect your patient to have an artificial airway inserted and to be placed on mechanical ventilation. Be aware that retained secretions may need to be removed by bronchoscopy.

vide adequate humidification to ensure moist secretions. Additional measures include the following.

Assess and monitor

• Monitor vital signs, and assess cardiac rhythm. Respiratory acidosis can cause tachycardia, alterations in respiratory rate and rhythm, hypotension, and arrhythmias.
• Continue to assess respiratory patterns, and report changes quickly. Prepare for mechanical ventilation, if indicated.
• Monitor the patient's neurologic status, and report significant changes. In addition, monitor the patient's cardiac function, since respiratory acidosis may progress to shock and cardiac arrest.
• Report any variations in ABG, pulse oximetry, or serum electrolyte levels.

Maintain

• Give medications, such as antibiotics and bronchodilators, as prescribed. (See *Teaching about respiratory acidosis*.)
• Administer oxygen as ordered. Generally, lower concentrations of oxygen are given to patients with COPD. The medulla of a patient with COPD is accustomed to high CO_2 levels. A lack of oxygen, called the "hypoxic drive," stimulates those patients to breathe. Too much oxygen diminishes that drive and depresses respiratory efforts.
• Perform tracheal suctioning, incentive spirometry, postural drainage, and coughing and deep breathing, as indicated.
• Maintain adequate hydration through oral or I.V. fluid intake, and maintain accurate intake and output records. (See *Documenting respiratory acidosis*.)
• Provide reassurance to the patient and family.
• Keep in mind that any sedatives you give to the patient can decrease his respiratory rate.
• Institute safety measures as needed to protect a confused patient.

Questions to consider

As you reevaluate your patient's condition, consider the following questions:
• Have the patient's respiratory rate and level of consciousness returned to normal?
• Does auscultation of the patient's chest reveal reduced adventitious breath sounds?

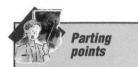

Parting points

Teaching about respiratory acidosis

Be sure to cover these topics with your patient and evaluate his learning:

description of the condition and how to prevent it;

deep-breathing exercises

home oxygen therapy, if indicated

warning signs and symptoms and when to report them

reasons for repeated ABG analyses

prescribed medications

proper technique for using bronchodilators, if appropriate

need for frequent rest

need for increased caloric intake, if appropriate.

• Have all tachycardias or ventricular arrhythmias been stabilized?
• Have the patient's cyanosis and dyspnea diminished?
• Have the patient's ABG results and serum electrolyte levels returned to normal?
• Do chest X-rays show improvement in the condition of the patient's lungs?

Respiratory alkalosis

The opposite of respiratory acidosis, respiratory alkalosis results from alveolar hyperventilation and hypocapnia. In respiratory alkalosis, the pH is greater than 7.45 and the $Paco_2$ falls below 35 mm Hg. The condition may be acute, resulting from a sudden increase in ventilation, or chronic. Chronic respiratory acidosis may be difficult to identify because of renal compensation.

How it happens

Any clinical condition that increases the respiratory rate or depth can cause CO_2 to be eliminated, or "blown off," from the lungs. Because CO_2 is an acid, blowing off CO_2 causes a decrease in the $Paco_2$ and an increase in pH — alkalosis. (See *What happens in respiratory alkalosis,* pages 188 and 189.)

Hyperventilation (gasp!)

The most common cause of acute respiratory alkalosis is hyperventilation associated with anxiety. Pain, which also causes an increased respiratory rate, can have the same effect. Hyperventilation is an early sign of salicylate intoxication and also occurs with the use of nicotine and xanthines, such as aminophylline. (See *Drugs associated with respiratory alkalosis*, page 189.)

Hypermetabolic states, such as fever and sepsis (especially gram-negative sepsis), and liver failure can lead to respiratory alkalosis. Certain drugs can also stimulate an increase in respiratory drive.

Conditions that affect the brain's respiratory control center can also lead to respiratory alkalosis. For example, the respiratory control center in the medulla may be stimulated by the higher progesterone levels of pregnancy or

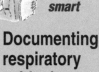

Chart smart

Documenting respiratory acidosis

When providing nursing care for a patient with respiratory acidosis, be sure to document:

vital signs and cardiac rhythm

intake and output

your assessment and interventions, and the patient's response

notification of doctor

patient teaching

medications administered, oxygen therapy, and ventilator settings

character of pulmonary secretions

serum electrolyte levels and ABG results.

What happens in respiratory alkalosis

This series of illustrations shows at the cellular level how respiratory alkalosis develops.

Step 1

When pulmonary ventilation increases above the amount needed to maintain normal carbon dioxide (CO_2) levels, excessive amounts of CO_2 are exhaled. This causes hypocapnia (a fall in $Paco_2$), which leads to a reduction in carbonic acid (H_2CO_3) production, a loss of hydrogen ions (H) and bicarbonate ions (HCO_3), and a subsequent rise in pH. *Look for a pH level above 7.45, a $Paco_2$ level below 35 mm Hg, and a bicarbonate level below 22 mEq/L.*

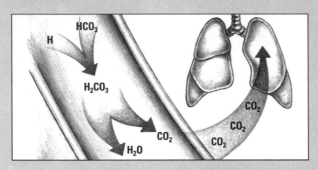

Step 2

In defense against the rising pH, hydrogen ions are pulled out of the cells and into the blood in exchange for potassium ions (K). The hydrogen ions entering the blood combine with bicarbonate ions to form carbonic acid, which lowers the pH. *Look for a further decrease in bicarbonate levels, a fall in pH, and a fall in serum potassium levels (hypokalemia).*

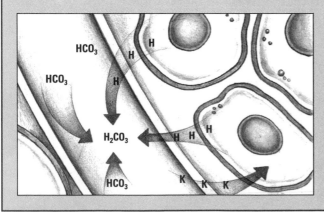

Step 3

Hypocapnia stimulates the carotid and aortic bodies and the medulla, which causes an increase in heart rate without an increase in blood pressure. *Look for angina, electrocardiogram changes, restlessness, and anxiety.*

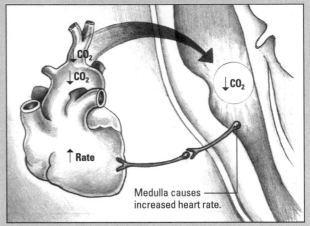

Medulla causes increased heart rate.

Step 4

Simultaneously, hypocapnia produces cerebral vasoconstriction, which prompts a reduction in cerebral blood flow. Hypocapnia also overexcites the medulla, pons, and other parts of the autonomic nervous system. *Look for increasing anxiety, diaphoresis, dyspnea, alternating periods of apnea and hyperventilation, dizziness, and tingling in the fingers or toes.*

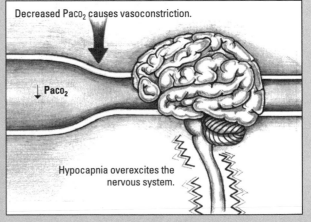

Decreased $Paco_2$ causes vasoconstriction.

Hypocapnia overexcites the nervous system.

What happens in respiratory alkalosis *(continued)*

Step 5

When hypocapnia lasts more than 6 hours, the kidneys increase secretion of bicarbonate and reduce excretion of hydrogen. Periods of apnea may result if the pH remains high and the $Paco_2$ remains low. *Look for slowing of the respiratory rate, hypoventilation, and Cheynes-Stokes respirations.*

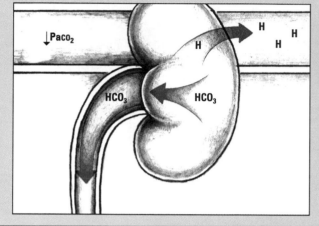

Step 6

Continued low $Paco_2$ increases cerebral and peripheral hypoxia from vasoconstriction. Severe alkalosis inhibits calcium (Ca) ionization, which in turn causes increased nerve excitability and muscle contractions. Eventually, the alkalosis overwhelms the central nervous system and the heart. *Look for decreasing level of consciousness, hyperreflexia, carpopedal spasm, tetany, arrhythmias, seizures, and coma.*

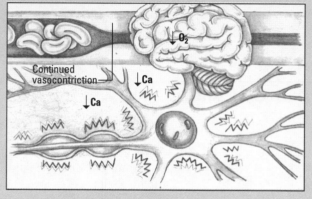

injured by stroke or trauma. Both contitions can result in respiratory alkalosis.

Another offender: Hypoxia

Respiratory alkalosis can be caused by acute hypoxia secondary to high altitude, pulmonary disease, severe anemia, pulmonary embolus, and hypotension. Those conditions may overstimulate the respiratory center and make the patient breathe faster and deeper. Overventilation during mechanical ventilation causes more CO_2 to be "blown off," resulting in respiratory alkalosis.

What to look for

An increase in the rate and depth of respirations is a primary sign of respiratory alkalosis. Tachycardia is often present as well. The patient may appear anxious and restless and may complain of muscle weakness or difficulty breathing.

Drugs associated with respiratory alkalosis

The following drugs are associated with respiratory alkalosis:

• catecholamines
• nicotine
• salicylates
• xanthines such as aminophylline.

In extreme alkalosis, confusion or syncope may occur. Due to the lack of CO_2 in the blood and its effect on cerebral blood flow and the respiratory center, you may see alternating periods of apnea and hyperventilation. The patient may complain of tingling in the fingers and toes.

You may see electrocardiogram (ECG) changes, including a prolonged PR interval, a flattened T wave, a prominent U wave, and a depressed ST segment. (For more information, see Chapter 6.)

Symptoms worsen as calcium levels drop because of vasoconstriction of peripheral and cerebral vessels resulting from hypoxia. You may see hyperreflexia, carpopedal spasm, tetany, arrhythmias, a progressive decrease in the patient's level of consciousness, seizures, or coma. (See *Signs of respiratory alkalosis*.)

What tests show

The following diagnostic test results may be helpful in detecting and treating respiratory alkalosis.
- ABG analysis is the key diagnostic test for identifying respiratory alkalosis. Typically, the pH is above 7.45 and the $Paco_2$ level is below 35 mm Hg. The bicarbonate level may be normal (22 to 26 mEq/L) in the acute stage but usually falls below 22 mEq/L in the chronic stage. (See *ABG results in respiratory alkalosis*.)
- Serum electrolyte studies may detect metabolic disorders that could be causing compensatory respiratory alkalosis. Hypokalemia may be evident. The ionized serum calcium level may be decreased in severe respiratory alkalosis.

I can't waste time

Signs of respiratory alkalosis

The following assessment findings commonly occur in patients with respiratory alkalosis:

- anxiety
- diaphoresis
- dyspnea, increased respiratory rate and depth
- electrocardiogram changes
- hyperreflexia
- paresthesias
- restlessness
- tachycardia
- tetany.

ABG results in respiratory alkalosis

This chart shows typical ABG findings in uncompensated and compensated respiratory alkalosis.

	Uncompensated	Compensated
pH	>7.45	Normal
$Paco_2$ (mm Hg)	< 35	< 35
HCO_3 (mEq/L)	Normal	< 22

- ECG findings may indicate arrhythmias or the changes associated with hypokalemia or hypocalcemia.
- Toxicology screening may reveal salicylate poisoning.

How respiratory alkalosis is treated

Treatment focuses on correcting the underlying disorder, which may require removal of the causative agent, such as a salicylate or other drug, or measures to reduce fever and eliminate the source of sepsis.

If acute hypoxemia is the cause, oxygen therapy is initiated. If anxiety is the cause, the patient may receive sedatives or antianxiety agents.

Hyperventilation can be counteracted by having the patient breathe into a paper bag, which forces the patient to breathe exhaled carbon dioxide, thereby raising the CO_2 level. If a patient's respiratory alkalosis is iatrogenic, mechanical ventilator settings may be adjusted by decreasing the tidal volume or the number of breaths per minute.

How you intervene

- Monitor patients who are at risk for developing respiratory alkalosis. Allay anxiety whenever possible to prevent hyperventilation. Recommend activities that promote relaxation. Assist the patient with breathing into a paper bag, if indicated.
- Monitor vital signs. Report changes in neurologic, neuromuscular, or cardiovascular functioning.
- Monitor ABG and serum electrolyte levels closely, and report any variations immediately. *Remember that twitching and cardiac arrhythmias may be associated with alkalosis and electrolyte imbalances.*
- If the patient is receiving mechanical ventilation, check ventilator settings frequently. Monitor ABG levels after making changes in settings.
- Provide undisturbed rest periods after the patient's respiratory rate returns to normal. Hyperventilation may result in severe fatigue.
- Stay with the patient during periods of extreme stress and anxiety. Offer reassurance, and maintain a calm, quiet environment. (See *Teaching about respiratory alkalosis.*)

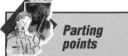

Parting points

Teaching about respiratory alkalosis

Be sure to cover these topics with your patient and evaluate his learning:

- explanation of the condition and its treatment
- warning signs and symptoms and when to report them
- anxiety-reducing techniques, if appropriate
- controlled-breathing exercises, if appropriate
- prescribed medications.

• Institute safety measures and seizure precautions as necessary, and document all care. (See *Documenting respiratory alkalosis.*)

Metabolic acidosis

Metabolic acidosis is characterized by a pH below 7.35 and a serum bicarbonate (HCO_3) level below 22 mEq/L. This disorder depresses the CNS. Left untreated, it may lead to ventricular arrhythmias, coma, and cardiac arrest.

How it happens

The underlying mechanism in metabolic acidosis is a loss of HCO_3 from extracellular fluid, an accumulation of metabolic acids, or a combination. An anion gap greater than 14 mEq/L is associated with acidosis due to an accumulation of metabolic acids (unmeasured anions).

When metabolic acidosis is associated with a normal anion gap (8 to 14 mEq/L), loss of HCO_3 may be the cause. (See *What happens in metabolic acidosis,* pages 194 and 195.)

Gain acids, lose bases

Metabolic acidosis is characterized by a gain in acids or a loss of base from the plasma. The condition may be related to an overproduction of ketone bodies. Fatty acids are converted to ketone bodies when glucose supplies have been used up and the body draws on fat stores for energy. Conditions that cause an overproduction of ketone bodies include diabetes mellitus, chronic alcoholism, severe malnutrition or starvation, poor dietary intake of carbohydrates, hyperthyroidism, and severe infection with accompanying fever.

Other factors may cause or contribute to metabolic acidosis. Lactic acidosis can cause or worsen metabolic acidosis and can occur secondarily to shock, heart failure, pulmonary disease, hepatic disorders, seizures, or strenuous exercise.

Chart smart

Documenting respiratory alkalosis

For a patient with respiratory alkalosis, be sure to document the following:

📄 vital signs

📄 intake and output

📄 I.V. therapy

📄 interventions, including measures taken to alleviate anxiety

📄 patient's response to interventions

📄 patient teaching

📄 serum electrolyte and ABG results

📄 safety measures

📄 notification of doctor.

Lots of other causes

Metabolic acidosis can also stem from a decreased ability of the kidneys to excrete acids, as occurs in renal insufficiency or renal failure with acute tubular necrosis.

Metabolic acidosis also occurs with excessive GI losses from diarrhea, intestinal malabsorption, a draining fistula of the pancreas or liver, or a urinary diversion to the ileum. Other causes include hypoaldosteronism and the use of potassium-sparing diuretics such as acetazolamide, which inhibit the secretion of acid.

At particular risk for metabolic acidosis are patients with poisoning or drug toxicity, which can occur following inhalation of toluene or ingestion of salicylates (aspirin or aspirin-containing medications), methanol, ethylene glycol, paraldehyde, hydrochloric acid, or ammonium chloride.

What to look for

Metabolic acidosis typically produces respiratory, neurologic, and cardiac signs and symptoms. As acid builds up in the bloodstream, the lungs try to compensate by "blowing off" CO_2.

Hyperventilation, especially increased depth of respirations, is the first clue to metabolic acidosis. Called Kussmaul's respirations, the breathing is rapid and deep. A diabetic who experiences Kussmaul's respirations may have a fruity odor to his breath. The odor stems from catabolism of fats and excretion of acetone through the lungs.

Depressed CNS

As the pH drops, the central nervous system is further depressed, as is myocardial function. Cardiac output and blood pressure drop, and arrhythmias may occur if the patient also has hyperkalemia.

Initially, the skin is warm and dry as a result of peripheral vasodilation, but as shock develops, the skin becomes cold and clammy. The patient may complain of weakness and a dull headache as the cerebral vessels dilate.

The patient's level of consciousness may deteriorate from confusion to stupor and coma. A neuromuscular exam may show diminished muscle tone and deep tendon reflexes. Metabolic acidosis also has an effect on the GI

What happens in metabolic acidosis

This series of illustrations shows at the cellular level how metabolic acidosis develops.

Step 1

As hydrogen ions (H) start to accumulate in the body, chemical buffers (plasma bicarbonate and proteins) in the cells and extracellular fluid bind with them. *No signs are detectable at this stage.*

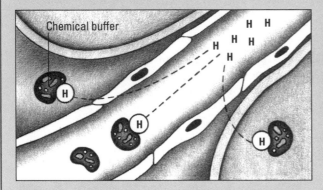

Step 2

Excess hydrogen ions that the buffers can't bind with decrease the pH and stimulate chemoreceptors in the medulla to increase the respiratory rate. The increased respiratory rate lowers the Paco$_2$, which allows more hydrogen ions to bind with bicarbonate ions (HCO$_3$). Respiratory compensation occurs within minutes but isn't sufficient to correct the imbalance. *Look for a pH level below 7.35, a bicarbonate level below 22 mEq/L, a decreasing Paco$_2$ level, and rapid, deeper respirations.*

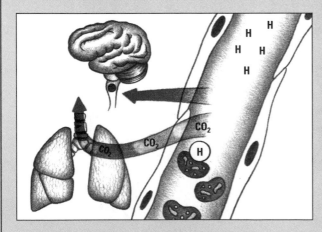

Step 3

Healthy kidneys try to compensate for the acidosis by secreting excess hydrogen ions into the renal tubules. Those ions are buffered by phosphate or ammonia and then are excreted into the urine in the form of a weak acid. *Look for acidic urine.*

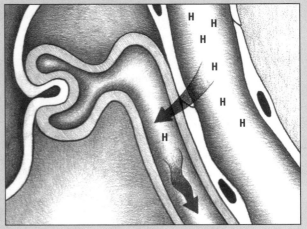

Step 4

Each time a hydrogen ion is secreted into the renal tubules, a sodium ion (Na) and a bicarbonate ion are absorbed from the tubules and returned to the blood. *Look for pH and bicarbonate levels that return slowly to normal.*

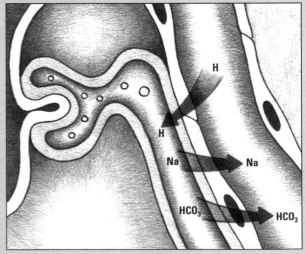

What happens in metabolic acidosis *(continued)*

Step 5

Excess hydrogen ions in the extracellular fluid diffuse into cells. To maintain the balance of the charge across the membrane, the cells release potassium ions into the blood. *Look for signs of hyperkalemia, including colic and diarrhea, weakness or flaccid paralysis, tingling and numbness in the extremities, bradycardia, a tall T wave, a prolonged PR interval, and a wide QRS complex.*

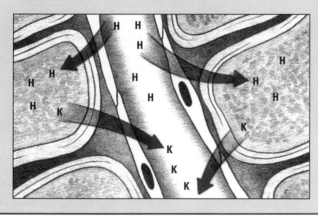

Step 6

Excess hydrogen ions alter the normal balance of potassium, sodium, and calcium ions (Ca), leading to reduced excitability of nerve cells. *Look for signs and symptoms of progressive central nervous system depression, including lethargy, dull headache, confusion, stupor, and coma.*

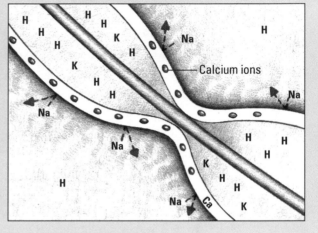

system, causing anorexia, nausea, and vomiting. (See *Signs of metabolic acidosis,* page 196.)

What tests show

The following test results may be helpful in diagnosing and treating metabolic acidosis.

• ABG analysis is the key diagnostic test for detecting metabolic acidosis. Typically, the pH is below 7.35. The $Paco_2$ may be less than 35 mm Hg, indicating compensatory attempts by the lungs to rid the body of excess carbon dioxide. (See *ABG results in metabolic acidosis,* page 196.)

• Serum potassium levels are usually elevated as hydrogen ions move into the cells and potassium moves out to maintain electroneutrality.

• Blood glucose and serum ketone body levels rise in diabetic ketoacidosis.

• Plasma lactate levels rise in lactic acidosis. (See *A look at lactic acidosis,* page 197.)

ABG results in metabolic acidosis

This chart shows typical ABG findings in uncompensated and compensated metabolic acidosis.

	Uncompensated	Compensated
pH	< 7.35	Normal
$Paco_2$ (mm Hg)	Normal	< 35
HCO_3 (mEq/L)	< 22	< 22

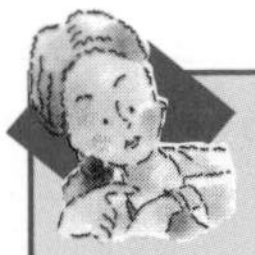

• The anion gap is increased. This measurement is calculated by subtracting the amount of negative ion (chloride plus bicarbonate) from the amount of the positive ion (sodium). Sometimes the amount of potassium ion is added to the amount of positive ion, but the amount of potassium ion is usually so small that the calculation doesn't change. The normal anion gap is 8 to 14 mEq/L.
• ECG changes associated with hyperkalemia, such as tall T waves, prolonged PR intervals, and wide QRS complexes, may be found.

How metabolic acidosis is treated

Treatment aims to correct the acidosis as quickly as possible by addressing both the symptoms and the underlying cause. Respiratory compensation is usually the first line of therapy, including mechanical ventilation if needed.

Adjust the potassium

For diabetics, expect administration of rapid-acting insulin to reverse diabetic ketoacidosis and drive potassium back into the cell. For any patient with metabolic acidosis, monitor serum potassium levels. Even though high serum levels exist initially, serum potassium levels will drop as the acidosis is corrected and may result in hypokalemia. Any other electrolyte imbalances are evaluated and corrected.

Replace the bicarbonate

Sodium bicarbonate is administered I.V. to neutralize blood acidity in patients who have a pH lower than 7.1 and

I can't waste time

Signs of metabolic acidosis

The following assessment findings commonly occur in patients with metabolic acidosis:

• confusion
• decreased deep-tendon reflexes
• dull headache
• hyperkalemic symptoms, including abdominal cramping, diarrhea, muscle weakness, and electrocardiogram changes
• hypotension
• Kussmaul's respirations
• lethargy
• warm, dry skin.

A look at lactic acidosis

Lactate, produced as a result of carbohydrate metabolism, is metabolized by the liver. The normal lactate level is 0.93 to 1.65 mEq/L. With tissue hypoxia, however, cells are forced to switch to anaerobic metabolism and more lactate is produced. When lactate accumulates in the body faster than it can be metabolized, lactic acidosis occurs. It can happen any time the demand for oxygen in the body outstrips its availability.

The causes of lactic acidosis include septic shock, cardiac arrest, pulmonary disease, seizures, and strenuous exercise.

The latter two cause transient lactic acidosis. Hepatic disorders can also cause lactic acidosis, since the liver isn't able to metabolize lactate.

Treatment

Treatment focuses on eliminating the underlying cause. If the pH is under 7.1, sodium bicarbonate may be given. Use caution when administering sodium bicarbonate, however, since it may cause alkalosis.

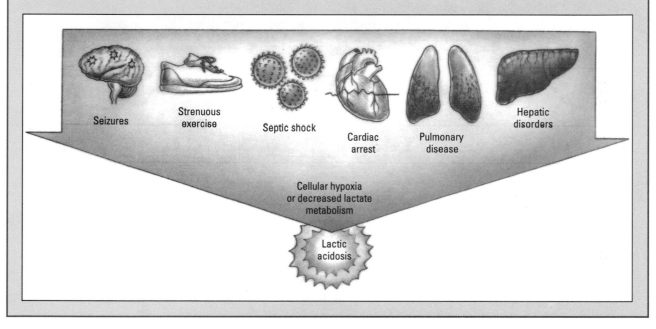

Seizures · Strenuous exercise · Septic shock · Cardiac arrest · Pulmonary disease · Hepatic disorders

Cellular hypoxia or decreased lactate metabolism

Lactic acidosis

who have lost bicarbonate. Fluids are replaced parenterally as required. Dialysis may be initiated in patients with renal failure or certain drug toxicities. The patient may receive antibiotic therapy to treat sources of infection or antidiarrheal agents to treat diarrhea-induced bicarbonate loss.

Get ready for more

Watch for worsening of CNS status or deteriorating laboratory and ABG values. Ventilatory support may be needed, so prepare for intubation. Dialysis may be needed for patients with renal failure, especially when complicated by diabetes. Maintain a patent I.V. line to administer emergency drugs, and flush the line with normal saline solution before and after administering sodium bicarbonate because the bicarbonate may inactivate or cause precipitation of many drugs. (See *Acidosis and dopamine*.)

How you intervene

If your patient is at risk for metabolic acidosis, careful monitoring can help prevent it from developing. If your patient has metabolic acidosis, nursing care includes immediate emergency interventions and long-term treatment of the condition and its underlying causes. Follow these guidelines.

Assess and monitor

- Monitor vital signs, and assess cardiac rhythm.
- Prepare for mechanical ventilation or dialysis as required.
- Monitor the patient's neurologic status closely because changes can occur rapidly. Notify the doctor of any changes in the patient's condition.
- Insert an I.V., as ordered, and maintain patent I.V. access. Have large-bore catheters in place for emergency situations. Administer I.V. fluids, vasopressors, antibiotics, and other medications, as prescribed.
- Administer sodium bicarbonate as ordered. Remember to flush the I.V. line with normal saline solution before and after giving bicarbonate because the chemical can inactivate many drugs or cause them to precipitate. Be aware that too much bicarbonate can cause metabolic alkalosis and pulmonary edema.
- Position the patient to promote chest expansion and facilitate breathing. If he's stuporous, turn him frequently. (See *Teaching about metabolic acidosis*.)
- Take steps to help eliminate the underlying cause. For example, administer insulin and I.V. fluids as prescribed to reverse diabetic ketoacidosis.
- Watch for secondary changes caused by hypovolemia, such as declining blood pressure.
- Monitor the patient's renal function by recording intake and output. (See *Documenting metabolic acidosis*.)
- Watch for serum electrolyte changes and monitor ABG results throughout treatment to check for overcorrection.

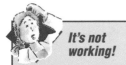

It's not working!

Acidosis and dopamine

If you're administering dopamine hydrochloride to a patient and it doesn't seem to be raising his blood pressure as you expected, investigate your patient's pH. A pH level below 7.1 (as can happen in severe metabolic acidosis) causes resistance to vasopressor therapy. Correct the pH level, and the dopamine may prove more effective.

Parting points

Teaching about metabolic acidosis

Be sure to cover these topics with your patient and evaluate his learning:

- explanation of the condition and its treatment
- blood glucose testing, if indicated
- need for strict adherence to antidiabetic therapy, if appropriate
- avoidance of alcohol
- warning signs and symptoms and when to report them
- prescribed medications
- avoidance of ingestion of toxic substances.

• Orient the patient as needed. If he's confused, take steps to ensure his safety, such as keeping the bed in the lowest position.
• Investigate reasons for the patient's ingestion of toxic substances.

Questions to consider

Physical examination and further diagnostic tests may provide additional information about your patient's metabolic acidosis. As you reevaluate the patient's condition, consider the following questions:
• Has the patient's level of consciousness returned to normal?
• Have his vital signs stabilized?
• Have his ABG results, blood glucose, and serum electrolyte levels improved?
• Is his cardiac output normal?
• Has he regained a normal sinus rhythm (or his previously stable underlying rhythm)?
• Is he ventilating adequately?

Metabolic alkalosis

Metabolic alkalosis is characterized by a blood pH above 7.45 and is accompanied by a serum bicarbonate level above 26 mEq/L. In acute metabolic alkalosis, HCO_3 may be as high as 50 mEq/L. With early diagnosis and prompt treatment, the prognosis for effective treatment is good. Left untreated, metabolic alkalosis can result in coma, arrhythmias, and death.

How it happens

In metabolic alkalosis, the underlying mechanisms include a loss of hydrogen ions (acid), a gain in bicarbonate, or both. $Paco_2$ greater than 45 mm Hg (possibly as high as 60 mm Hg) indicates that the lungs are compensating for the alkalosis. Renal compensation is more effective but is also slower. Metabolic alkalosis is commonly associated with hypokalemia, particularly from the use of thiazides, furosemide, ethacrynic acid, and other diuretics that deplete potassium stores. In hypokalemia, the kidneys conserve potassium. At the same time, the kidneys also in-

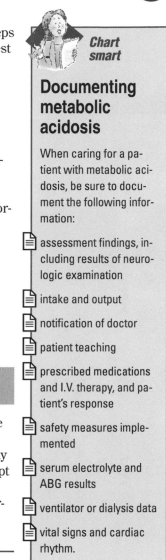

Chart smart

Documenting metabolic acidosis

When caring for a patient with metabolic acidosis, be sure to document the following information:

- assessment findings, including results of neurologic examination
- intake and output
- notification of doctor
- patient teaching
- prescribed medications and I.V. therapy, and patient's response
- safety measures implemented
- serum electrolyte and ABG results
- ventilator or dialysis data
- vital signs and cardiac rhythm.

crease the excretion of hydrogen ions, which prompts alkalosis from the loss of acid. Metabolic alkalosis may also occur with hypochloremia and hypocalcemia. (See *What happens in metabolic alkalosis,* pages 201 and 202.)

GI problems

Metabolic alkalosis can result from many causes, the most common of which is excessive acid loss from the GI tract. Vomiting causes loss of hydrochloric acid from the stomach. Children who have pyloric stenosis can develop this disorder. Alkalosis also results from nasogastric (NG) suctioning, presenting a risk for surgical patients or patients with GI disorders.

Diuretic risks

Diuretic therapy presents another risk of metabolic alkalosis. Thiazide and loop diuretics can lead to hydrogen, potassium, and chloride ion loss from the kidneys. Hypokalemia causes hydrogen ion excretion from the kidneys as they try to conserve potassium. Potassium moves out of the cell as hydrogen moves in, resulting in alkalosis.

With the fluid loss of diuresis, the kidneys attempt to conserve sodium and water. For sodium to be reabsorbed, hydrogen ions must be excreted. In a process known as contraction alkalosis, bicarbonate is reabsorbed and metabolic alkalosis results.

What else?

Cushing's disease can lead to metabolic alkalosis by causing retention of sodium and chloride and urinary loss of potassium and hydrogen. Rebound alkalosis following correction of organic acidosis, such as after cardiac arrest and administration of sodium bicarbonate, can also cause metabolic alkalosis. Post-hypercapnic alkalosis occurs when chronic CO_2 retention is corrected by mechanical ventilation and the kidneys have not yet corrected the chronically high bicarbonate levels.

Metabolic alkalosis can also result from kidney disease, such as renal artery stenosis, or from multiple transfusions. Certain drugs, such as corticosteroids and antacids that contain baking soda, can also lead to metabolic alkalosis. (See *Drugs associated with metabolic alkalosis,* page 202.)

What happens in metabolic alkalosis

This series of illustrations shows at the cellular level how metabolic alkalosis develops.

Step 1

As bicarbonate ions (HCO_3) start to accumulate in the body, chemical buffers (in extracellular fluid and cells) bind with the ions. *No signs are detectable at this stage.*

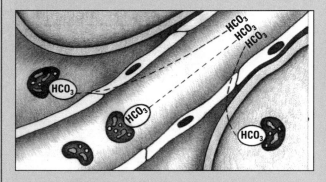

Step 2

Excess bicarbonate ions that don't bind with chemical buffers elevate serum pH levels, which in turn depress chemoreceptors in the medulla. Depression of those chemoreceptors causes a decrease in respiratory rate, which increases the $Paco_2$. The additional CO_2 combines with water to form carbonic acid (H_2CO_3). *Note:* Lowered oxygen levels limit respiratory compensation. *Look for a serum pH level above 7.45, a bicarbonate level above 26 mEq/L, a rising $Paco_2$, and slow, shallow respirations.*

Step 3

When the bicarbonate level exceeds 28 mEq/L, the renal glomeruli can no longer reabsorb excess bicarbonate. That excess bicarbonate is excreted in the urine; hydrogen ions are retained. *Look for alkaline urine and pH and bicarbonate levels that return slowly to normal.*

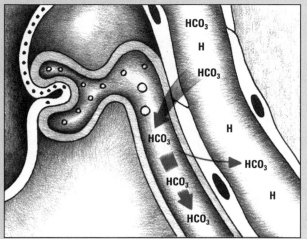

Step 4

To maintain electrochemical balance, the kidneys excrete excess sodium ions (Na), water, and bicarbonate. *Look for polyuria initially, then signs of hypovolemia, including thirst and dry mucous membranes.*

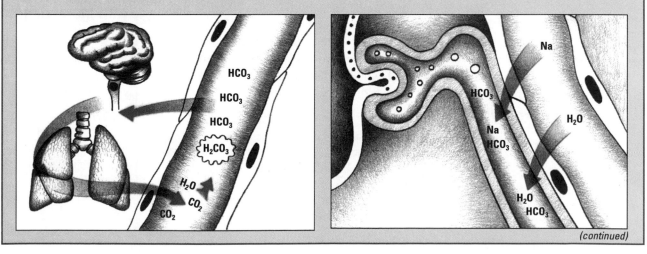

(continued)

What happens in metabolic alkalosis *(continued)*

Step 5

Lowered hydrogen ion levels in the extracellular fluid cause the ions to diffuse out of the cells. To maintain the balance of charge across the cell membrane, extracellular potassium ions (K) move into the cells. *Look for signs of hypokalemia: anorexia, muscle weakness, loss of reflexes, and others.*

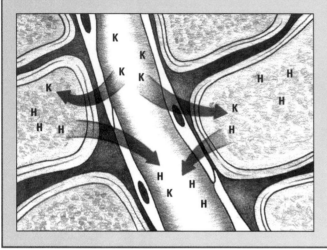

Step 6

As hydrogen ion levels decline, calcium (Ca) ionization decreases. That decrease in ionization makes nerve cells more permeable to sodium ions. Sodium ions moving into nerve cells stimulate neural impulses and produce overexcitability of the peripheral and central nervous systems. *Look for tetany, belligerence, irritability, disorientation, and seizures.*

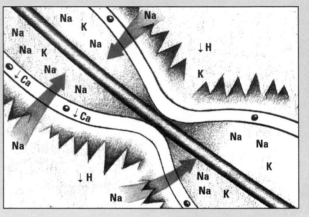

What to look for

Initially, your patient may have slow, shallow respirations as hypoventilation, a compensatory mechanism, occurs. However, this mechanism is limited because hypoxemia soon develops, which stimulates ventilation. The signs and symptoms of metabolic alkalosis are often associated with an underlying condition. The resulting hypokalemic or hypocalcemic ECG changes may be seen, as well as hypotension.

It hits the neuro system

Metabolic alkalosis results in neuromuscular excitability, which causes muscle twitching, weakness, and tetany. Reflexes are hyperactive. The patient may experience numbness and tingling of the fingers, toes, and mouth area. Neurologic symptoms include apathy and confusion. Seizures, stupor, and coma may result.

Drugs associated with metabolic alkalosis

The following drugs are commonly associated with metabolic alkalosis:

• antacids (baking soda, calcium carbonate)
• corticosteroids
• sodium bicarbonate
• thiazide and loop diuretics.

It hits the GI and the GU

If the GI tract is affected by hypokalemia, the patient will probably experience anorexia, nausea, and vomiting. Polyuria may result if the kidneys are affected. If left untreated, metabolic alkalosis can result in arrhythmias and death. (See *Signs of metabolic alkalosis.*)

What tests show

The following tests may be helpful in the diagnosis and treatment of metabolic alkalosis.
• ABG analysis may reveal a blood pH greater than 7.45 and an HCO_3 level greater than 26 mEq/L. If the underlying cause is excessive acid loss, HCO_3 levels may be normal. The $Paco_2$ level may be above 45 mm Hg, indicating respiratory compensation. (See *ABG results in metabolic alkalosis.*)
• Serum electrolyte studies usually show low potassium, calcium, and chloride levels. Bicarbonate levels are elevated.
• ECG changes may occur, such as a low T wave that merges with the P wave.

How metabolic alkalosis is treated

Treatment aims to correct the acid-base imbalance.
• I.V. administration of ammonium chloride is rarely done but may be necessary in severe cases.

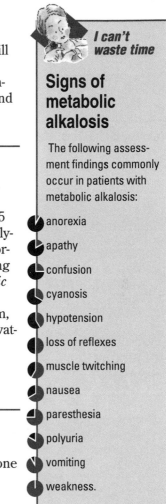

I can't waste time

Signs of metabolic alkalosis

The following assessment findings commonly occur in patients with metabolic alkalosis:

- anorexia
- apathy
- confusion
- cyanosis
- hypotension
- loss of reflexes
- muscle twitching
- nausea
- paresthesia
- polyuria
- vomiting
- weakness.

ABG results in metabolic alkalosis

This chart shows typical ABG findings in uncompensated and compensated metabolic alkalosis.

	Uncompensated	Compensated
pH	> 7.45	Normal
$Paco_2$ (mm Hg)	Normal	> 45
HCO_3 (mEq/L)	> 26	> 26

• Thiazide diuretics and NG suctioning are discontinued. Antiemetics may be administered to treat underlying nausea and vomiting.
• Acetazolamide (Diamox) may be added to increase excretion of bicarbonate by the kidneys.

How you intervene

If your patient is at risk for metabolic alkalosis, careful monitoring can help prevent its development. If your patient has metabolic alkalosis, follow these guidelines:
• Monitor vital signs, including cardiac rhythm and respiratory pattern.
• Assess the patient's level of consciousness during the health history or by talking with him while you're performing the physical examination. For instance, apathy and confusion may be evident in a patient's conversation.
• Administer oxygen, as ordered, to treat hypoxemia.
• Institute seizure precautions when necessary, and explain them to the patient and his family. (See *Teaching about metabolic alkalosis*.)
• Maintain patent I.V. access as ordered.
• Administer diluted potassium solutions with an infusion device.
• Monitor intake and output. (See *Documenting metabolic alkalosis*.)
• Infuse 0.9% ammonium chloride no faster than 1 L over 4 hours. Faster administration may cause hemolysis of red blood cells. Don't administer the drug to a patient who has hepatic or renal disease.
• Irrigate an NG tube with normal saline solution instead of tap water, to prevent loss of gastric electrolytes.
• Assess laboratory values, such as ABG and serum electrolyte results. Notify the doctor of any changes.
• Watch closely for signs of muscle weakness, tetany, or decreased activity.

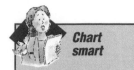

Parting points

Teaching about metabolic alkalosis

Be sure to cover these topics with your patient and evaluate his learning:

☞ explanation of the condition and its treatment

☞ need to avoid overuse of alkaline agents and diuretics

☞ prescribed medications, especially adverse effects of potassium-wasting diuretics or potassium chloride supplements

☞ warning signs and symptoms and when to report them.

Chart smart

Documenting metabolic alkalosis

When providing nursing care to a patient with metabolic alkalosis, be sure to document:

▤ vital signs

▤ I.V. therapy

▤ interventions and the patient's response

▤ medications

▤ intake and output

▤ oxygen therapy

▤ notification of doctor

▤ safety measures

▤ serum electrolyte levels and ABG results.

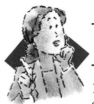

Quick quiz

1. The body compensates for chronic respiratory alkalosis by developing:
   A. metabolic alkalosis.
   B. respiratory acidosis.
   C. metabolic acidosis.

Answer: C. When hypocapnia lasts more than 6 hours, the kidneys compensate by increasing excretion of HCO_3 and reducing excretion of hydrogen ions. Hydrogen ions return to the blood to decrease the pH, causing chemoreceptors in the medulla to decrease the respiratory rate.

2. You are taking care of a patient with obesity-hypoventilation syndrome. You expect to see signs of chronic respiratory acidosis in the patient's ABG results. The compensatory mechanism you'll look for is:
   A. respiratory alkalosis.
   B. metabolic acidosis.
   C. metabolic alkalosis.

Answer: C. As respiratory mechanisms fail, the body compensates by using the increasing $Paco_2$ to excrete hydrogen and to stimulate the kidneys to retain HCO_3 and sodium ions. As a result, more sodium bicarbonate is available to buffer free hydrogen ions (metabolic alkalosis). Ammonium ions are also excreted to remove hydrogen.

3. If your patient's NG tube is attached to suction, you know the patient may develop metabolic alkalosis. The body compensates for metabolic alkalosis by developing:
   A. respiratory alkalosis.
   B. respiratory acidosis.
   C. metabolic acidosis.

Answer: B. Excess unbound HCO_3 elevates the blood pH, which depresses the chemoreceptors in the medulla, decreasing respirations and increasing blood carbon dioxide (respiratory acidosis). CO_2 combines with water to form carbonic acid.

4. In assessing a patient with diabetic ketoacidosis, you detect Kussmaul's respirations. You realize the body is compensating for primary metabolic acidosis with:

A. respiratory alkalosis.
    B. respiratory acidosis.
    C. metabolic alkalosis.

Answer: A. Excess hydrogen that can't be buffered reduces blood pH and stimulates chemoreceptors in the medulla, which in turn increases the respiratory rate (leading to respiratory alkalosis). This mechanism lowers carbon dioxide levels and allows more hydrogen to bind with bicarbonate.

5. In a patient with COPD, you would expect to see the primary imbalance:
    A. respiratory alkalosis.
    B. respiratory acidosis.
    C. metabolic alkalosis.

Answer: B. COPD results in destruction of the alveoli, thereby decreasing the surface area of the lungs available for gas exchange. With alveolar ventilation decreased, the Pa_{CO_2} increases. The CO_2 combines with H_2O to form excessive amounts of carbonic acid. The H_2CO_3 dissociates to release free hydrogen and bicarbonate ions, thereby decreasing the pH (respiratory acidosis).

6. Your bedridden patient has these ABG results: pH, 7.5; Pa_{CO_2}, 26 mm Hg; HCO_3, 24 mEq/L. He is dyspneic and has a swollen right calf. The patient most likely is suffering from:
    A. a pulmonary embolus.
    B. congestive heart failure.
    C. dehydration.

Answer: A. Unexplained respiratory alkalosis may mean a pulmonary embolus (in this case, most likely a thrombus in the leg as a result of immobility).

Scoring

☆☆☆   If you answered all six items correctly, *wow!* Test the pH of the nearest pool, and jump in for a refreshing swim!

☆☆   If you answered four or five correctly, excellent! You're just about ready to do your first solo balancing act!

☆   If you answered fewer than four correctly, take heart. You're still a boffo buffer in our book. *(Buffer,* get it? For chemical buffers? Oh, well, can't win 'em all.)

Part III

Disorders that cause imbalances

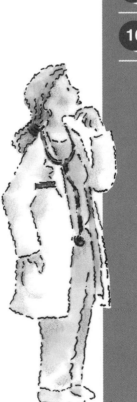

Congestive heart failure

Just the facts

This chapter explains the basics about this disorder and its effects on fluid, electrolyte, and acid-base balance. In this chapter, you'll learn:

♦ what congestive heart failure (CHF) is and how it happens

♦ which imbalances can occur as a result of CHF or its treatment

♦ how to care for patients with CHF effectively

♦ how to chart the care you give to patients with CHF.

A look at CHF

CHF is a syndrome of myocardial dysfunction that causes diminished cardiac output and outright heart failure, or congestion. It occurs when the heart can't pump enough blood to meet the body's metabolic needs. CHF may result from left or right ventricular failure. However, because a properly functioning heart depends on both ventricles, failure of one ventricle almost always leads to failure of the other.

How it happens

Normally, the pumping actions of the right and left sides of the heart complement each other, producing a synchronized and continuous blood flow. With an underlying disorder, though, one side may fail while the other continues to function normally for some time. Because of the prolonged strain, the functioning side eventually fails, resulting in total heart failure.

First, the left side

Usually, the heart's left side fails first. Left ventricular failure typically leads to and is the main cause of right ventricular failure.

Here's what happens: Diminished left ventricular function allows blood to pool in the ventricle and atrium and eventually to back up into the pulmonary veins and capillaries. (See *Left-sided heart failure.*)

As the pulmonary circulation becomes engorged, rising capillary pressure pushes sodium and water into the interstitial space, causing pulmonary edema. The right ventricle becomes stressed because it is pumping against greater pulmonary vascular resistance and left ventricular pressure.

Then, the right side

As the right ventricle starts to fail, symptoms worsen. Blood pools in the right ventricle and the right atrium. The backed-up blood causes pressure and congestion in the vena cava and systemic circulation. (See *Right-sided heart failure,* page 210.)

Blood also distends the visceral veins, especially the hepatic vein. As the liver and spleen become engorged, their function is impaired. Rising capillary pressure forces excess fluid from the capillaries into the interstitial space. This causes tissue edema, especially in the lower extremities and abdomen.

Left-sided heart failure

This illustration shows what happens when left-sided heart failure develops. The left side of the heart normally receives oxygenated blood returning from the lungs and then pumps blood through the aorta to all tissues. Left-sided heart failure causes blood to back up into the lungs, which results into such respiratory symptoms as tachypnea and shortness of breath.

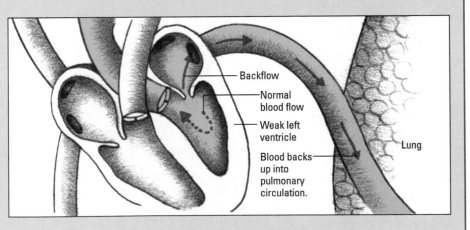

Next, compensation occurs

When the heart begins to fail, the body responds with compensatory mechanisms to maintain blood flow to the periphery. These mechanisms include hypertrophy of the heart wall, dilation of the heart chambers, and sympathetic nervous system activation. In the short term, these mechanisms may help keep the failing heart going. But ultimately, they worsen CHF.

The heart's response

When the heart is under strain, it responds by increasing its muscle mass, a condition called cardiac hypertrophy. As the cardiac wall thickens, the heart's demand for blood and oxygen grows. The patient's heart may be unable to meet this demand, further compromising the condition.

When pressure inside the chambers (usually the left ventricle) rises for a sustained period, the heart compensates by stretching, a condition called cardiac dilation. Eventually, stretched muscle fibers become overstrained, reducing the heart's ability to pump.

Problematic pumping

Diminished cardiac output activates the sympathetic nervous system, causing an increased heart rate and increased myocardial contractility. Blood then shunts away from areas of low priority (such as the skin and kidneys) to areas of high priority (such as the heart and brain).

Right-sided heart failure

This illustration shows what happens when right-sided heart failure develops. The right side of the heart normally receives deoxygenated blood returning from the tissues and then pumps that blood through the pulmonary artery into the lungs. Right-sided heart failure causes blood to back up past the vena cava and into the systemic circulation. This, in turn, causes enlargement of the abdominal organs and tissue edema.

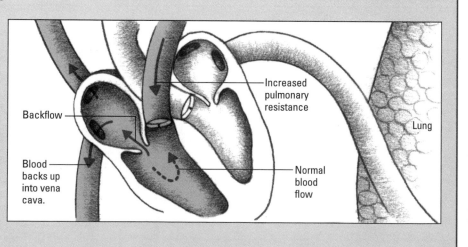

Sensing a reduced renal blood flow, the kidneys activate the renin-angiotensin system, and aldosterone is secreted. Vasoconstriction occurs in the kidneys, along with sodium and water retention. These factors make it more difficult for the heart to pump blood.

Pulmonary congestion, a complication of CHF, can lead to pulmonary edema, a life-threatening condition. Decreased perfusion to major organs, particularly the brain and kidneys, may cause these organs to fail, necessitating dialysis for kidney failure. The patient's level of consciousness may decrease, possibly leading to coma. Myocardial infarction (MI) may occur because myocardial oxygen demands can't be sufficiently met.

Imbalances caused by heart failure

Several imbalances may result from the heart's failure to pump blood and to perfuse tissues adequately. Imbalances may also result from stimulation of the renin-angiotensin system or from certain treatments such as diuretic therapy. Fluid, electrolyte, and acid-base imbalances associated with CHF include hypervolemia, hyponatremia, hypokalemia, hypomagnesemia, hyperkalemia, hypochloremia, hypovolemia, metabolic acidosis, metabolic alkalosis, respiratory acidosis, and respiratory alkalosis.

Volume problems

Extracellular fluid volume excess — the most common fluid imbalance associated with CHF — results from the heart's failure to propel blood forward, consequent vascular pooling, and the sodium and water reabsorption triggered by the renin-angiotensin system. Excess extracellular fluid volume commonly causes peripheral edema. Hypovolemia is usually associated with overly aggressive diuretic therapy and can be especially dangerous in older adult patients because it causes confusion and hypotension.

Hyponatremia

Hyponatremia may result from sodium loss due to diuretic abuse. In some cases, it may result from a dilutional effect that occurs when water reabsorption is greater than sodium reabsorption.

Other electrolyte imbalances

In CHF, hypokalemia is caused by prolonged diuretic use without adequate potassium replacement. Hypomagnesemia may accompany hypokalemia, particularly in patients recieving diuretics. Many diuretics cause the kidneys to excrete magnesium.

Hyperkalemia may occur from the use of potassium-sparing diuretics. Hypochloremia results from excessive diuretic therapy.

Lactic acid on the rise

When cells do not receive enough oxygen, they produce more lactic acid. Poor tissue perfusion in the patient with CHF allows lactic acid to accumulate, which in turn leads to metabolic acidosis. Metabolic alkalosis may be caused by excessive diuretic use, which causes bicarbonate retention.

In early CHF, as the respiratory rate increases, more carbon dioxide (CO_2) is blown off from the lungs, which raises the pH and leads to respiratory alkalosis. As heart failure progresses, gas exchange is further impaired. CO_2 accumulates, resulting in respiratory acidosis.

What causes CHF

A wide range of pathophysiologic processes can cause CHF. The syndrome commonly results from conditions that directly damage the heart. Such conditions include MI, myocarditis, myocardial fibrosis, and ventricular aneurysm. The damage caused by those disorders causes a subsequent decrease in the contractility of the heart.

Ventricular overload can also cause CHF. The condition is caused by an overload of blood volume in the heart (called increased preload) as a result of aortic insufficiency or a ventricular septal defect. Ventricular overload can also be caused by systemic or pulmonary hypertension or by an overload of pressure in the heart (called increased afterload) as a result of aortic or pulmonic stenosis.

CHF may also be caused by restricted ventricular diastolic filling, characterized by the presence of so little blood that the ventricle can't pump it effectively. This disorder is triggered by constrictive pericarditis or cardiomyopathy, tachyarrhythmias, cardiac tamponade, or mitral stenosis.

Increasing the risk

Certain conditions can predispose a person to CHF, especially if he has an underlying disease. Those conditions include:
• anemia, which causes the heart rate to speed up to maintain tissue oxygenation
• pregnancy and thyrotoxicosis, which increase the demand for cardiac output
• infections, which increase metabolic demands and further burden the heart
• increased physical activity, emotional stress, greater sodium or water intake, or failure to comply with the prescribed treatment regimen for underlying heart disease
• pulmonary embolism, which elevates pulmonary arterial pressures and can cause right ventricular failure.

What to look for

Signs and symptoms of CHF vary according to the site of the failure and the stage of the disease. Expect to encounter a combination of the following findings.

Left-sided failure

With left ventricular failure and tissue hypoxia, expect the patient to complain of fatigue, weakness, orthopnea, and exertional dyspnea. The patient may report paroxysmal nocturnal dyspnea.

He may use two or three pillows to elevate his head to sleep, or he may have to sleep sitting up in a chair. Shortness of breath may awaken him shortly after he falls asleep, forcing him to quickly sit upright to catch his breath. He may have dyspnea, coughing, and wheezing even when he sits up. Tachypnea may occur, and you may note crackles on inspiration. Coughing may progress to the point where the patient produces pink, frothy sputum as he develops pulmonary edema.

The patient may be tachycardic. Auscultation of heart sounds may reveal S_3 and S_4 as the myocardium becomes less compliant. Hypoxia and hypercapnia can affect the central nervous system, causing restlessness, confusion, and a progressive worsening of level of consciousness. Later, with continued decrease in cardiac output, oliguria may develop as the kidneys are affected by CHF.

Right ventricular failure

In right ventricular failure, inspection may reveal venous engorgement. When the patient sits upright, his neck veins may appear distended, feel rigid, and exhibit exaggerated pulsations. Edema may develop, and the patient may report a weight gain. Nail beds may appear cyanotic. Anorexia and nausea may occur. The liver may be enlarged and slightly tender. This may progress to congestive hepatomegaly, ascites, and jaundice.

Advanced CHF

In advanced CHF, pulse pressure may be diminished, reflecting reduced stroke volume. Occasionally, diastolic pressure rises from generalized vasoconstriction. The skin feels cool and clammy. Progression of CHF may lead to palpitations, chest tightness, and arrhythmias. Cardiac arrest may occur. (See *Signs of CHF*.)

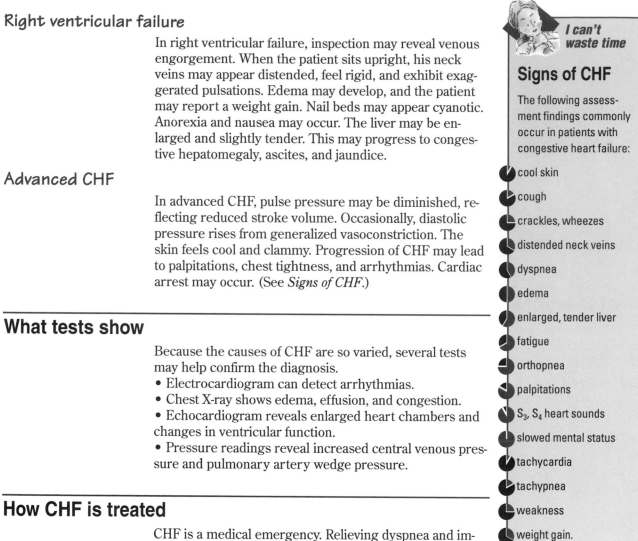

I can't waste time

Signs of CHF

The following assessment findings commonly occur in patients with congestive heart failure:

- cool skin
- cough
- crackles, wheezes
- distended neck veins
- dyspnea
- edema
- enlarged, tender liver
- fatigue
- orthopnea
- palpitations
- S_3, S_4 heart sounds
- slowed mental status
- tachycardia
- tachypnea
- weakness
- weight gain.

What tests show

Because the causes of CHF are so varied, several tests may help confirm the diagnosis.
- Electrocardiogram can detect arrhythmias.
- Chest X-ray shows edema, effusion, and congestion.
- Echocardiogram reveals enlarged heart chambers and changes in ventricular function.
- Pressure readings reveal increased central venous pressure and pulmonary artery wedge pressure.

How CHF is treated

CHF is a medical emergency. Relieving dyspnea and improving arterial oxygenation are the immediate therapeutic goals. Secondary goals include minimizing or eliminating the underlying cause, reducing sodium and water retention, decreasing cardiac preload and afterload, and enhancing myocardial contractility.

Diuretics: First-line treatment

Management of CHF usually requires one or more drugs, such as diuretics, vasodilators, and inotropic agents. Diuretic therapy, the starting point for CHF treatment, increases sodium and water elimination by the kidneys. By reducing fluid overload, diuretics decrease total blood volume and relieve circulatory congestion. *For most diuretics to work effectively, the patient must control his sodium intake.*

Diuretic agents include thiazide diuretics and loop diuretics, such as furosemide or bumetanide. Because thiazide and loop diuretics work at different sites in the nephron, they produce a synergistic effect when given in combination. Potassium-sparing diuretics, such as spironolactone and triamterene, may be used.

Patients on diuretic therapy require careful monitoring because those drugs may disturb the electrolyte balance and lead to metabolic alkalosis, metabolic acidosis, or other complications.

Reducing preload and afterload

Vasodilators can reduce preload or afterload by decreasing arterial and venous vasoconstriction. Reducing preload and afterload helps increase stroke volume and cardiac output.

Angiotensin-converting enzyme (ACE) inhibitors, such as captopril, decrease both afterload and preload. Because ACE inhibitors prevent potassium loss, hyperkalemia may develop in patients receiving concomitant potassium-sparing diuretics. For this reason, those diuretics should be discontinued when ACE inhibitor therapy begins.

Nitrates, primarily vasodilators, also dilate arterial smooth muscle at higher doses. Most CHF patients tolerate nitrates well. Nitrates are available in several forms. In CHF therapy, I.V., oral, and topical ointment or patches are considered the most useful forms.

Inotropic drugs such as digoxin increase contractility in the failing heart muscle. They also slow conduction through the atrioventricular node. Other drugs, such as dopamine, dobutamine, and amrinone, may be indicated in acute CHF to increase myocardial contractility and cardiac output. Hydralazine and nitroprusside may also be used in the treatment of CHF.

Morphine is commonly used in CHF patients with acute pulmonary edema. Besides reducing anxiety, it decreases preload and afterload by dilating veins.

Sometimes, surgery is needed

In severe cases of heart failure, the patient's condition may require a heart transplant or the use of intra-aortic balloon counterpulsation (which helps the ventricles propel blood through the vascular system) or other ventricular assist devices.

How you intervene

To properly care for a patient with CHF, you'll need to perform a number of specific nursing interventions, including the following.

Assess, monitor, and administer

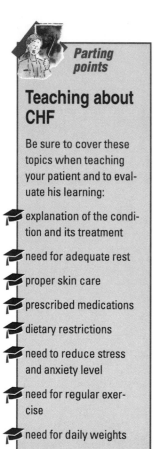

Parting points

Teaching about CHF

Be sure to cover these topics when teaching your patient and to evaluate his learning:

- explanation of the condition and its treatment
- need for adequate rest
- proper skin care
- prescribed medications
- dietary restrictions
- need to reduce stress and anxiety level
- need for regular exercise
- need for daily weights
- warning signs and symptoms and when to report them
- importance of follow-up.

• Assess the patient's mental status, and report changes in vital signs or mental status immediately.

• Assess for signs and symptoms of impending cardiac failure, such as fatigue, restlessness, hypotension, rapid respiratory rate, dyspnea, coughing, decreased urine output, liver enlargement, and a rapid, thready pulse.

• Assess for the presence, amount, and location of edema. Note the degree of pitting, if present. (See *Documenting CHF*.)

• Monitor sodium and fluid intake as prescribed. Hyponatremia and fluid volume deficit can stimulate the renin-angiotensin system and exacerbate CHF. Usually, a mild sodium restriction — such as no added salt — with no water restriction is prescribed.

• Check patient's weight and fluid intake and output daily for significant changes. (See *Teaching about CHF*.)

• Monitor vital signs, including blood pressure, pulse and respirations, and heart and breath sounds, for abnormalities that might indicate a fluid excess or deficit.

• Monitor serum electrolyte levels — especially sodium and potassium — for changes that may indicate an imbalance. Remember that hypokalemia can lead to digitalis toxicity. Monitor arterial blood gas results to assess adequacy of ventilation.

• Maintain continuous cardiac monitoring during acute and advanced stages of disease to identify arrhythmias promptly.

• Administer prescribed medications — such as digitalis glycosides, diuretics, and potassium supplements — to support cardiac function and minimize symptoms.

• Administer oral potassium supplements in orange juice or with meals to promote absorption and prevent gastric irritation.

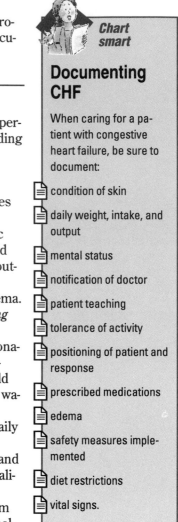

Chart smart

Documenting CHF

When caring for a patient with congestive heart failure, be sure to document:

- condition of skin
- daily weight, intake, and output
- mental status
- notification of doctor
- patient teaching
- tolerance of activity
- positioning of patient and response
- prescribed medications
- edema
- safety measures implemented
- diet restrictions
- vital signs.

Provide comfort measures

• Place the patient in Fowler's position and give supplemental oxygen as ordered to help him breathe more easily.
• Encourage independent activities of daily living as tolerated, though bed rest may be required for some patients. Reposition the patient as needed every 1 to 2 hours. Edematous skin is prone to breakdown.
• Instruct the patient and his family to notify the staff of any changes in his condition, such as increased shortness of breath, chest pain, or dizziness.
• Instruct the patient to call the doctor if his pulse rate is irregular, if it measures fewer than 60 beats/minute, or if he experiences dizziness, blurred vision, shortness of breath, a persistent dry cough, palpitations, increased fatigue, nocturnal dyspnea that comes and goes, swollen ankles, or decreased urine output.

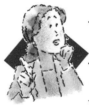

Quick quiz

1. While assessing a patient with left-sided heart failure, you would expect to detect:
    A. distended neck veins.
    B. edema of lower extremities.
    C. dyspnea on exertion.

Answer: C. Diminished left ventricular function allows blood to pool in the ventricle and atrium and eventually to back up into the pulmonary veins and capillaries. As the pulmonary circulation becomes engorged, rising capillary pressure pushes sodium and water into the interstitial space, causing pulmonary edema. Chief complaints include fatigue, exertional dyspnea, orthopnea, weakness, and paroxysmal nocturnal dyspnea.

2. The most common fluid imbalance associated with CHF is:
    A. hypervolemia.
    B. hypovolemia.
    C. hyperkalemia.

Answer: A. Extracellular fluid volume excess results from the heart's failure to propel blood forward, which causes vascular pooling, and from the sodium and water reabsorption triggered by the renin-angiotensin system.

3. Of the following patients admitted to the emergency department, the one *most likely* to develop CHF is:

    A. a 31-year-old woman with pneumonia.

    B. a 52-year-old man suffering a heart attack.

    C. an 82-year-old woman with chronic dehydration.

Answer: B. The man suffering the heart attack has the greatest risk of developing CHF from the myocardial damage, which prevents the heart from pumping as effectively as it needs to.

4. Your assessment of a patient reveals an enlarged liver, distended neck veins, and pitting edema of the lower extremities. You suspect that the patient has:

    A. right-sided heart failure.

    B. left-sided heart failure.

    C. pulmonary hypertension.

Answer: A. These findings indicate that fluid has backed up into the systemic circulation from the right side of the heart.

5. A patient with CHF is more likely to develop drug toxicity if he has concurrent:

    A. hyponatremia.

    B. hyperkalemia.

    C. hypokalemia.

Answer: C. Hypokalemia, which can occur with diuretic therapy, may lead to digitalis toxicity.

Scoring

☆☆☆ If you answered all five items correctly, we salute your heartfelt heroism!

  ☆☆ If you answered three or four correctly, great! We applaud your boisterous bravado!

    ☆ If you answered fewer than three correctly, relax. We still commend your veritable valor!

Respiratory failure

Just the facts

This chapter provides essential information about respiratory failure and its effect on fluid, electrolyte, and acid-base balance. In this chapter, you'll learn:

♦ how respiratory failure occurs

♦ how to recognize the signs and symptoms of respiratory failure

♦ which imbalances occur with respiratory failure and how to manage them.

A look at respiratory failure

When the lungs can't sufficiently maintain arterial oxygenation or eliminate carbon dioxide (CO_2), acute respiratory failure results. Unchecked and untreated, this condition can lead to decreased oxygenation of the body tissues and metabolic acidosis.

In patients with essentially normal lung tissue, respiratory failure usually produces hypercapnia (an above-normal amount of carbon dioxide in the arterial blood) and hypoxemia (a deficiency of oxygen in the arterial blood).

In patients with chronic obstructive pulmonary disease (COPD), however, respiratory failure is signaled only by an acute drop in arterial blood gas (ABG) values and clinical deterioration. The reason? Patients with COPD consistently have high $Paco_2$ and low Pao_2 levels but are able to compensate and maintain a normal, or near-normal, pH level.

How it happens

In acute respiratory failure, gas exchange is diminished by any combination of the following factors:
- alveolar hypoventilation
- ventilation-perfusion ($\dot{V}/\dot{Q}$) mismatch
- intrapulmonary shunting.

Imbalances associated with respiratory failure include hypervolemia, hypovolemia, hypokalemia, hyperkalemia, respiratory acidosis, respiratory alkalosis, and metabolic acidosis. Let's look at each one in turn. (See *What happens in acute respiratory failure.*)

What happens in acute respiratory failure

Three major malfunctions account for impaired gas exchange and subsequent acute respiratory failure. They include alveolar hypoventilation, ventilation-perfusion ($\dot{V}/\dot{Q}$) mismatch, and intrapulmonary (right to left) shunting.

Alveolar hypoventilation

In alveolar hypoventilation (shown below as the result of airway obstruction), the amount of oxygen brought to the alveoli is diminished, which causes a drop in the Pao_2 level and an increase in alveolar carbon dioxide. The accumulation of CO_2 in the alveoli prevents diffusion of adequate amounts of CO_2 from the capillaries, which increases $Paco_2$ levels.

$\dot{V}/\dot{Q}$ mismatch

$\dot{V}/\dot{Q}$ mismatch, the leading cause of hypoxemia, occurs when insufficient ventilation exists with a normal flow of blood or when, as shown below, normal ventilation exists with an insufficient flow of blood.

Intrapulmonary shunting

Intrapulmonary shunting occurs when blood passes from the right side of the heart to the left side without being oxygenated. Shunting can result from untreated ventilation or perfusion imbalances.

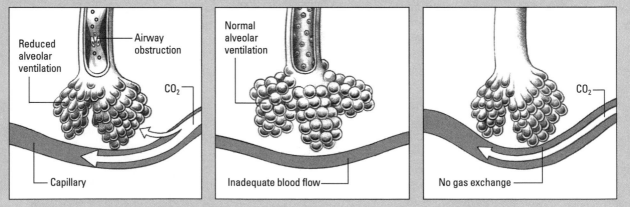

Hypovolemia

Because the lungs remove water daily through exhalation, an increased respiratory rate can promote excessive loss of water. Excessive loss can also occur with fever or any other condition that increases the metabolic rate and thus the respiratory rate. (See *Causes of respiratory failure,* page 222.)

Hypervolemia

Prolonged respiratory treatments, such as nebulizer use, can lead to inhalation and absorption of water vapor. Excessive fluid absorption may also result from increased lung capillary pressure or permeability, which typically occurs in adult respiratory distress syndrome. The excessive fluid absorption may precipitate pulmonary edema.

Hypokalemia

If a patient begins to hyperventilate and alkalosis results, hydrogen ions will move out of the cells and potassium ions will move from the blood into the cells. That shift can cause hypokalemia.

Hyperkalemia

In acidosis, excess hydrogen ions move into the cell. Potassium ions then move out of the cell and into the blood to balance the positive charges between the two fluid compartments. Hyperkalemia may result.

Respiratory acidosis

Respiratory acidosis results from the inability of the lungs to eliminate sufficient quantities of CO_2 and is due to hypoventilation. The excess CO_2 combines with water to form carbonic acid. Increased carbonic acid levels result in decreased pH, which contributes to respiratory acidosis.

Respiratory alkalosis

Respiratory alkalosis develops from an excessively rapid respiratory rate, or hyperventilation, and causes excessive carbon dioxide elimination. Loss of carbon dioxide decreases the blood's acid-forming potential and results in respiratory alkalosis.

Causes of respiratory failure

Problems with the brain, nerves, muscles, chest wall, alveoli, or pulmonary circulation can impair gas exchange and cause respiratory failure. Here's a list of conditions that can cause respiratory failure.

Brain
- Anesthesia
- Cerebral hemorrhage
- Cerebral tumor
- Drug overdose
- Head trauma
- Skull fracture

Muscles and nerves
- Amyotrophic lateral sclerosis
- Guillain-Barré syndrome
- Multiple sclerosis
- Muscular dystrophy
- Myasthenia gravis
- Polio
- Spinal cord trauma

Lungs
- Adult respiratory distress syndrome
- Asthma
- Chronic obstructive pulmonary disease
- Cystic fibrosis
- Flail chest
- Massive bilateral pneumonia
- Sleep apnea
- Tracheal obstruction

Circulation
- Congestive heart failure
- Pulmonary edema
- Pulmonary embolism

Metabolic acidosis

Conditions that cause hypoxia cause cells to use anaerobic metabolism. That metabolism creates an increase in the production of lactic acid, which can lead to metabolic acidosis.

What to look for

The hypoxemia and hypercapnia characteristic of acute respiratory failure stimulate strong compensatory responses from all body systems, especially the respiratory, cardiovascular, and central nervous systems.

Lungs first

When the body senses hypoxemia or hypercapnia, the respiratory center responds by increasing respiratory depth and then respiratory rate. Signs of labored breathing — flared nostrils, pursed-lip exhalation, and the use of accessory breathing muscles, among others — may signify respiratory failure.

As respiratory failure worsens, muscle retractions between the ribs, above the clavicle, and above the sternum may also occur. The patient is dyspneic and may become cyanotic. Auscultation of the chest reveals diminished or absent breath sounds over the affected area. You may also hear wheezes, crackles, or rhonchi. Respiratory arrest may occur.

The heart next

The sympathetic nervous system usually compensates by increasing the heart rate and constricting blood vessels in an effort to improve cardiac output. The patient's skin may become cool, pale, and clammy. Eventually, as myocardial oxygenation diminishes, cardiac output, blood pressure, and heart rate drop. Arrhythmias develop, and cardiac arrest may occur.

CNS next

Even a slight disruption in oxygen supply and carbon dioxide elimination can affect brain function and behavior. Hypoxia initially causes anxiety and restlessness, which can progress to marked confusion, agitation, and lethargy. The primary sign of hypercapnia, headache, occurs as cerebral vessels dilate in an effort to increase the brain's blood supply. If the carbon dioxide level continues to rise, the patient is at risk for seizures and coma. (See *Signs of respiratory failure.*)

What tests show

The following diagnostic tests can help diagnose respiratory failure and guide its treatment.
• ABG changes indicate respiratory failure. Always compare ABG results with your patient's baseline values. For a patient with previously normal lungs, the pH is usually less than 7.35, the Pao_2 less than 50 mm Hg, and the $Paco_2$ greater than 50 mm Hg. In a patient with COPD, respiratory failure is indicated by an acute drop in the Pao_2 level of 10 mm Hg or more. *Keep in mind that patients with chronic COPD have a chronically low Pao_2, increased $Paco_2$, increased bicarbonate, and normal pH.*
• Chest X-rays may identify an underlying pulmonary condition.
• Electrocardiogram (ECG) changes may show arrhythmias.
• Changes in serum potassium levels may be related to acid-base balance.

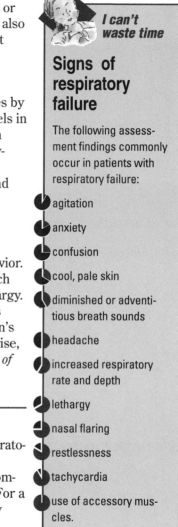

I can't waste time

Signs of respiratory failure

The following assessment findings commonly occur in patients with respiratory failure:

• agitation
• anxiety
• confusion
• cool, pale skin
• diminished or adventitious breath sounds
• headache
• increased respiratory rate and depth
• lethargy
• nasal flaring
• restlessness
• tachycardia
• use of accessory muscles.

How respiratory failure is treated

The underlying cause of respiratory failure must be addressed and the oxygen and carbon dioxide levels improved.

Increase O_2 saturation

Oxygen is given in controlled concentrations, often using a Venturi rebreathing mask. The goal of oxygen therapy is to prevent oxygen toxicity by administering the lowest dose of oxygen for the shortest period of time, while achieving an oxygen saturation of 90% or more or a Pao_2 level of at least 60 mm Hg.

Intubate and ventilate

Intubation and mechanical ventilation are indicated if conservative treatment fails to raise oxygen saturation above 90%. The patient may also be intubated and ventilated if acidemia continues, if he becomes exhausted, or if respiratory arrest occurs. Intubation provides a patent airway. Mechanical ventilation decreases the work of breathing, ventilates the lungs, and improves oxygenation.

Positive end-expiratory pressure (PEEP) therapy may be ordered during mechanical ventilation to improve gas exchange. PEEP maintains positive pressure at the end of expiration, thus preventing the airways and alveoli from collapsing between breaths.

Open the airways

Bronchodilators, especially inhalants, are used to open the airways. If the patient can't inhale effectively or is on a mechanical ventilator, he may receive a bronchodilator by nebulizer. Corticosteroids, theophylline, and antibiotics may also be ordered, as may be chest physiotherapy, including postural drainage, chest percussion, and chest vibration. Suctioning may be required to clear the airways. I.V. fluids may be ordered to correct dehydration and to help thin secretions. Diuretics may be used in cases of fluid overload.

How you intervene

To care effectively for a patient with respiratory failure, follow these guidelines.

Assess and monitor

• Assess respiratory status; monitor rate, depth, and character of respirations, making sure to check breath sounds for abnormalities.
• Monitor vital signs frequently.
• Monitor the patient's neurologic status; it may become depressed as respiratory failure worsens.
• Ongoing respiratory assessment should include level of consciousness, accessory muscle use, changes in breath sounds, ABG test analysis, secretion production and clearance, and respiratory rate, depth, and pattern. Notify the doctor if interventions don't improve the patient's condition.
• Monitor fluid status by maintaining accurate fluid intake and output records. Obtain daily weights.
• Evaluate serum electrolyte levels for abnormalities that can occur with acid-base imbalances.
• Evaluate ECG for arrhythmias.
• Monitor oxygen saturation values with a pulse oximeter.
• Monitor ABG levels to assess ventilation.

Maintain and administer

• Intervene as necessary to correct underlying respiratory problems and associated alterations in acid-base status.
• Keep a handheld resuscitation bag at the bedside.
• Maintain patent I.V. access as ordered for medication and I.V. fluid administration.
• Administer oxygen as ordered to help maintain adequate oxygenation and to restore the normal respiratory rate.
• Use caution when administering oxygen to a patient with COPD. Increased serum oxygen levels can depress the breathing stimulus.
• Make sure the ventilator settings are at the ordered parameters.
• Perform chest physiotherapy and postural drainage as needed to promote adequate ventilation.
• If the patient is retaining carbon dioxide, encourage slow deep breaths with pursed lips. Urge him to cough up secretions. If he can't mobilize secretions, suction him when necessary. (See *Teaching about respiratory failure*.)
• Unless the patient is retaining fluid or has heart failure, increase his fluid intake to 2 L/day, to help liquefy secretions.

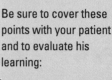

Parting points

Teaching about respiratory failure

Be sure to cover these points with your patient and to evaluate his learning:

▰ explanation of the condition and its treatment

▰ proper pulmonary hygiene and coughing techniques

▰ need for proper rest

▰ need to quit smoking, if appropriate

▰ prescribed medications

▰ warning signs and symptoms and when to report them

▰ importance of follow-up appointments

▰ diet restrictions, if appropriate.

Provide comfort measures

• Reposition the immobilized patient every 1 to 2 hours.
• Sit the conscious patient upright as tolerated in a supported, forward-leaning position to promote diaphragm movement. Supply an overbed table and pillows for support.
• If the patient isn't on a ventilator, avoid giving him narcotics and other central nervous system depressants, because they can further suppress respirations.

Provide nutritional support

• Limit carbohydrate intake and increase protein intake, because carbohydrate metabolism causes more carbon dioxide production than protein.
• Calm and reassure the patient while giving care. Anxiety can raise oxygen demands.
• Pace care activities to maximize the patient's energy level and to provide needed rest. Limit his need to respond verbally. Talking may cause shortness of breath.
• Implement safety measures as needed to protect the patient. Reorient the confused patient.

Follow up

• Stress the importance of returning for routine follow-up appointments with the doctor.
• Explain how to recognize signs and symptoms of overexertion, fluid retention, and heart failure. These may include a weight gain of 2 to 3 lb (0.9 to 1.4 kg)/day, edema of the feet or ankles, nausea, loss of appetite, or abdominal tenderness.
• Help the patient develop the knowledge and skills he needs to perform pulmonary hygiene. Encourage adequate hydration to thin secretions — but instruct the patient to notify the doctor of any signs of fluid retention or heart failure.
• Chart all instructions given and care provided. (See *Documenting respiratory failure*.)

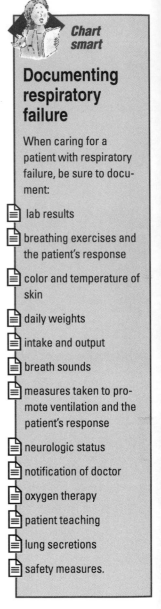

Chart smart

Documenting respiratory failure

When caring for a patient with respiratory failure, be sure to document:

📄 lab results

📄 breathing exercises and the patient's response

📄 color and temperature of skin

📄 daily weights

📄 intake and output

📄 breath sounds

📄 measures taken to promote ventilation and the patient's response

📄 neurologic status

📄 notification of doctor

📄 oxygen therapy

📄 patient teaching

📄 lung secretions

📄 safety measures.

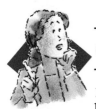

Quick quiz

1. When the body senses hypoxemia or hypercapnia, the brain's respiratory center responds by:
   A. slowing down the respiratory rate.
   B. decreasing the heart rate.
   C. increasing the depth and rate of respirations.

Answer: C. The brain's respiratory center initially causes an increase in respiratory rate. It then causes an increase in respiratory depth in an effort to blow off excess carbon dioxide.

2. Respiratory alkalosis can develop from:
   A. hyperventilation.
   B. excessive vomiting.
   C. prolonged use of antacids.

Answer: A. Respiratory alkalosis develops from an excessively rapid respiratory rate — hyperventilation — which causes excessive carbon dioxide elimination.

3. Prolonged respiratory treatment, such as nebulizer use, can lead to:
   A. hypovolemia.
   B. hypervolemia.
   C. respiratory acidosis.

Answer: B. Prolonged respiratory treatments, such as nebulizer use, can lead to the inhalation and absorption of water vapor, which can lead to hypervolemia.

4. The leading cause of hypoxemia is:
   A. alveolar hypoventilation.
   B. intrapulmonary shunting.
   C. ventilation-perfusion mismatch.

Answer: C. Ventilation-perfusion mismatch is the leading cause of hypoxemia and stems from an imbalance in the lungs between ventilation and blood flow.

5. You notice paradoxical chest-wall movement in a patient in the emergency department. You're concerned about respiratory failure because the patient could have:
   A. amyotrophic lateral sclerosis.
   B. flail chest.
   C. a tracheal obstruction.

Answer: B. Paradoxical chest-wall movement indicates flail chest, which interferes with normal lung mechanics and prevents alveolar expansion and adequate gas exchange; together this can lead to respiratory failure.

6. You're concerned about possible respiratory failure in your newly admitted patient. When administering drugs, you should avoid giving him:

    A. anticholinergics.
    B. corticosteroids.
    C. narcotics.

Answer: C. Narcotics depress the respiratory center of the brain and may hasten the development of respiratory failure.

Scoring

☆☆☆ If you answered all six items correctly, outstanding! You're ready to run the marathon!

☆☆ If you answered four or five correctly, great! You're the new pivot person for the 400-meter relay.

☆ If you answered fewer than four correctly, cool. You're first in line for the 100-meter hurdles!

Excessive GI fluid loss

Just the facts

This chapter will guide you through the processes of GI fluid loss and its effect on the patient. In this chapter you'll learn:

♦ what can cause GI fluid loss

♦ which fluid, electrolyte, and acid-base imbalances occur with excessive GI fluid loss and how to treat them

♦ what the signs and symptoms related to excessive GI fluid loss are

♦ what to teach your patients about excessive GI fluid loss.

A look at GI fluid loss

Normally, very little fluid is lost from the GI system. Most of the fluid is reabsorbed in the intestines. However, the potential for significant fluid loss through this system exists because large amounts of fluids — isotonic and hypotonic — pass through the GI system in the course of a day.

Isotonic fluids that may be lost from the GI tract include gastric juices, bile, pancreatic juices, and intestinal secretions. The only hypotonic fluid that may be lost is saliva, which has a lower solute concentration than other GI fluids.

How it happens

Excessive GI fluid loss may come from physical removal of secretions as a result of vomiting, suctioning, or increased or decreased GI tract motility. Excessive fluids can be excreted as waste products or secreted from the intestinal wall into the intestinal lumen, both of which lead to fluid and electrolyte imbalances.

Osmotic diarrhea may occur in the intestines when a high solute load in the intestinal lumen attracts water into the cavity. Both acids and bases can be lost from the GI tract.

Losing it

Vomiting or mechanical suctioning of stomach contents, as with a nasogastric tube, causes the loss of hydrogen ions and electrolytes, such as chloride, potassium, and sodium. Vomiting also depletes the body's fluid volume supply and causes hypovolemia. Dehydration occurs when there is more water lost than electrolytes. *When assessing acid-base balance, remember that the pH of the upper GI tract is low and that vomiting causes the loss of those acids and raises the subsequent possibility of alkalosis.*

Running on empty

An increase in the frequency and amount of bowel movements and a change in the stool toward a watery consistency can cause excessive fluid loss, resulting in hypovolemia and dehydration. Besides fluid loss, diarrhea can cause a loss of potassium, magnesium, and sodium. Fluids lost from the lower GI tract carry a large amount of bicarbonate with them, which lowers the amount of bicarbonate available to counter the effects of acids in the body.

Bowel cleansers

Laxatives and enemas may be used by patients for constipation or given to patients before abdominal surgery or diagnostic studies to clean the bowel. Excessive use of laxatives, such as magnesium sulfate, milk of magnesia, and Fleet Phospho-Soda, can cause high magnesium and phosphorus levels.

Excessive use of commercially prepared enemas containing sodium and phosphate — such as Fleet enemas — can cause high phosphorus and sodium levels if the enemas are absorbed before they can be eliminated. Excessive use of tap-water enemas can cause a decrease in sodium levels because water absorbed by the colon can have a dilutional effect on sodium.

Who's at risk?

Excessive GI fluid loss can be caused by numerous conditions, including:
- bacterial infections of the GI tract, which are usually accompanied by vomiting or diarrhea
- antibiotic administration, which removes normal flora and promotes diarrhea
- young age, which makes the person vulnerable to diarrhea, a frequent cause of GI fluid loss in children
- pregnancy, which may be accompanied by vomiting
- pancreatitis or hepatitis, which may be accompanied by vomiting
- pyloric stenosis in young children, which may be accompanied by vomiting. (See *Characteristics and causes of vomiting*.)

That ain't all, folks

Imbalances can also result from fecal impaction, poor absorption of foods, poor digestion, anorexia nervosa, or bulimia. (See *Imbalances caused by GI fluid loss,* page 232.) Disorders such as anorexia nervosa and bulimia, which primarily affect young women, often involve the use of laxatives and vomiting as a means of controlling weight. This can lead to numerous fluid, electrolyte, and acid-base imbalances. Other disorders that may cause disturbances in fluid, electrolyte, or acid-base balance include the pres-

---

Characteristics and causes of vomiting

Vomiting may lead to serious fluid, electrolyte, and acid-base disturbances and can occur for a variety of reasons. By carefully observing the characteristics of the vomitus, you may gain clues as to the underlying disorder. Here's what the vomitus may indicate.

Bile-stained (greenish)
Obstruction below the pylorus, as from a duodenal lesion

Bloody
Upper GI bleeding, as from gastritis or peptic ulcer if bright or from gastric or esophageal varices if dark red

Brown with a fecal odor
Intestinal obstruction or infarction

Burning, bitter-tasting
Excessive hydrochloric acid in gastric contents

Coffee-ground
Digested blood from slowly bleeding gastric or duodenal lesions

Undigested food
Gastric outlet obstruction, as from gastric tumor or ulcer

Imbalances caused by GI fluid loss

Excessive GI fluid loss can lead to a number of fluid, electrolyte, and acid-base imbalances. Here's a breakdown of those imbalances.

Fluid imbalances

• *Hypovolemia and dehydration.* Large amounts of fluid can be lost during prolonged, uncorrected vomiting and diarrhea. Hypovolemia can also result if gastric and intestinal suctioning occur without proper monitoring of intake and output to make sure lost fluid and electrolytes are adequately replaced.

Electrolyte imbalances

• *Hypokalemia.* The excessive loss of gastric fluids rich in potassium can lead to hypokalemia.

• *Hypomagnesemia.* Although gastric secretions contain little magnesium, several weeks of vomiting, diarrhea, or gastric suctioning can result in hypomagnesemia. Because hypomagnesemia itself can cause vomiting, the patient's condition may be self-perpetuating.

• *Hyponatremia.* Prolonged vomiting, diarrhea, or gastric or intestinal suctioning can deplete the body's supply of sodium and lead to hyponatremia.

• *Hypochloremia.* Any loss of gastric contents causes the loss of chloride. Prolonged gastric fluid loss can lead to hypochloremia.

Acid-base imbalances

• *Metabolic acidosis.* Anything that promotes intestinal fluid loss can result in metabolic acidosis. Intestinal fluid contains large amounts of bicarbonate. With the loss of bicarbonate, pH falls, creating an acidic condition.

• *Metabolic alkalosis.* Loss of gastric fluids from vomiting or the use of drainage tubes in the upper GI tract can lead to metabolic alkalosis. Gastric fluids contain large amounts of acids that, when lost, lead to an increase in pH and alkalosis. Excessive use of antacids can also worsen the imbalance by adding to the alkalotic state.

ence of fistulas involving the GI tract, GI bleeding, intestinal obstruction, and paralytic ileus.

The use of enteral tube feedings and ostomies (especially ileostomies) may also lead to imbalances. Enteral tube feedings may cause diarrhea or vomiting, depending on their composition and the patient's condition. Suctioning of gastric secretions through tubes may deplete the body of vital fluids, electrolytes, and acids. Saliva may be lost from the body when it cannot be swallowed, as with dysphagia related to extensive head and neck cancer.

What to look for

With excessive fluid loss, the patient may show signs of hypovolemia. Look for these signs and symptoms:
• The body tries to compensate for hypovolemia by increasing the heart rate. Along with tachycardia, blood pressure falls as intravascular volume is lost.
• The patient's skin may be cool and dry as the body shunts blood flow to major organs. There may also be a decrease in skin turgor or sunken eyeballs, as occurs with dehydration. Urine output decreases as kidneys try to conserve fluid and electrolytes.
• Cardiac arrhythmias may occur from electrolyte imbalances, such as those related to potassium and magnesium. The patient may become weak and confused. Mental status may deteriorate as fluid, electrolyte, and acid-base imbalances progress.
• Respirations may change according to the type of acid-base imbalance the patient develops. For instance, acidosis will cause respirations to be deeper as the patient tries to blow off acid from the lungs.
• The patient will also have signs and symptoms related to the underlying disorder — for instance, pancreatitis. (See *Signs of excessive GI fluid loss.*)

What tests show

Diagnostic test results related to the fluid, electrolyte, and acid-base imbalances associated with excessive GI fluid loss can help to direct nursing interventions. Those results include:
• changes in arterial blood gas levels, related to metabolic acidosis and metabolic alkalosis
• alterations in the levels of certain electrolytes, such as potassium, magnesium, and sodium. (See appropriate chapter for specific imbalances.)
• hematocrit levels that may be falsely elevated in a volume-depleted patient
• cultures of body fluid samples that may help to identify bacteria responsible for the underlying disorder.

I can't waste time

Signs of excessive GI fluid loss

In addition to the signs and symptoms related to underlying disorders, the patient with excessive GI fluid loss may show these signs of hypovolemia:

▸ tachycardia

▸ falling blood pressure

▸ cool, dry skin

▸ decreased skin turgor or sunken eyeballs

▸ decreased urine output

▸ possible cardiac arrhythmias

▸ weakness

▸ confusion or deteriorated mental status

▸ changes in respirations.

How GI fluid losses are treated

Treatment is aimed at the underlying cause of the imbalance to prevent further fluid and electrolyte loss. For instance, antiemetics or antidiarrheal drugs may be given for vomiting and diarrhea, respectively. GI drainage tubes or the suction applied to them are discontinued as soon as possible.

The patient is also supported by administering I.V. or oral fluid replacements, depending on the patient's tolerance and the cause of the fluid loss. Electrolytes should also be replaced if serum levels are decreased. Long-term parenteral nutrition may be needed. Antibiotics may be administered if infection is the underlying cause of fluid loss.

How you intervene

Patients who have conditions that alter fluid and electrolyte balance through GI losses need to be closely monitored. An increase in the amount of drainage from GI tubes or an increase in the frequency of vomiting or diarrhea should be taken seriously and reported. Follow these recommendations when caring for a patient with GI fluid losses.

Assess

- Measure and record the amount of fluid lost through vomiting, diarrhea, or gastric or intestinal suctioning. Remember to include GI losses as part of the patient's total output.
- Assess the patient's fluid status by monitoring intake and output, daily weight, and skin turgor.
- Assess vital signs and report any changes that may indicate fluid deficits, such as a decreased blood pressure or increased heart rate.
- Report vomiting so that imbalances do not become severe and treatment can be started early.

Administer and maintain

- Administer oral fluids containing water and electrolytes, such as Gatorade or Pedialyte, if the patient can tolerate fluids. (See *Teaching about GI fluid loss.*)
- Maintain patent I.V. access, as ordered. Administer I.V. replacement fluids as prescribed. Monitor the infusion rate and volume to prevent hypervolemia.

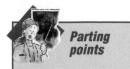

Parting points

Teaching about GI fluid loss

Be sure to cover these points with your patient and to evaluate his learning:

- explanation of the condition and its treatment
- need to report prolonged vomiting or diarrhea
- importance of avoiding repeated use of enemas and laxatives
- proper technique for irrigating a gastric tube, if appropriate
- proper technique for monitoring I.V. infusion, if appropriate.

• Check GI tube placement often if the patient is undergoing gastric suctioning, to prevent fluid aspiration.
• Irrigate the suction tube with isotonic normal saline solution as ordered. *Remember never to use plain water for irrigation. It draws more gastric secretions into the stomach in an attempt to make the fluid isotonic for absorption.* In addition, the fluid is suctioned out of the stomach, causing further depletion of fluids and electrolytes.
• When the patient is connected to gastric suction, restrict the amount of ice chips given by mouth and explain the reason for the restriction. Gastric suctioning of ice chips can deplete fluid and electrolytes from the stomach. (See *Documenting GI fluid loss.*)
• Administer such medications as antiemetics or antidiarrheals, as prescribed, to control the patient's underlying condition.
• Evaluate serum electrolyte and pH levels to detect abnormalities and to monitor the effectiveness of therapy.

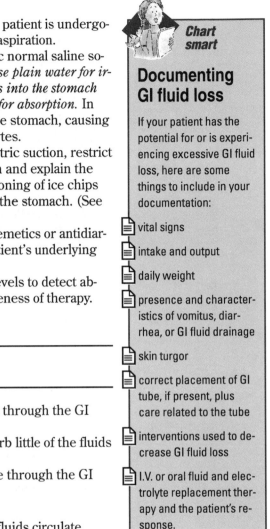

Chart smart

Documenting GI fluid loss

If your patient has the potential for or is experiencing excessive GI fluid loss, here are some things to include in your documentation:

📄 vital signs

📄 intake and output

📄 daily weight

📄 presence and characteristics of vomitus, diarrhea, or GI fluid drainage

📄 skin turgor

📄 correct placement of GI tube, if present, plus care related to the tube

📄 interventions used to decrease GI fluid loss

📄 I.V. or oral fluid and electrolyte replacement therapy and the patient's response.

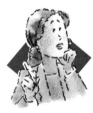

Quick quiz

1. Large amounts of fluid may be lost through the GI system because:
   A. the intestines normally reabsorb little of the fluids contained in food.
   B. large amounts of fluid circulate through the GI system each day.
   C. GI fluids are isotonic.

Answer: B. Because large amounts of fluids circulate through the GI system, anything that disrupts the system can promote excessive fluid loss.

2. The excessive use of Fleet enemas can cause:
   A. hypophosphatemia.
   B. hyponatremia.
   C. hypernatremia.

Answer: C. Hypernatremia can result from the excessive use of Fleet enemas because they contain sodium. If the enema is retained for a long time before it is expelled, excess sodium is absorbed by the bowel, resulting in hypernatremia.

3. Fluid and electrolyte imbalances that can occur with excessive GI fluid loss include:
  A. hypomagnesemia, hypermagnesemia, and hyponatremia.
  B. hypomagnesemia, hypernatremia, and hyperchloremia.
  C. hypervolemia, hyponatremia, and hypernatremia.

Answer: A. These imbalances, in addition to others, may occur with varying types of GI fluid loss.

4. A patient with fluid losses from the upper GI tract is likely to suffer:
  A. metabolic alkalosis.
  B. metabolic acidosis.
  C. respiratory acidosis.

Answer: A. GI fluid losses from the upper GI tract can result in metabolic alkalosis; losses from the lower GI tract can result in metabolic acidosis.

5. Warning signs of hypovolemia associated with GI losses include:
  A. tachycardia, decreased blood pressure, decreased urine output.
  B. tachycardia, increased blood pressure, increased urine output.
  C. decreased blood pressure, increased urine output, and warm, flushed skin.

Answer: A. Tachycardia, decreased blood pressure, and decreased urine output indicate that the patient is experiencing hypovolemia from GI losses.

Scoring

☆☆☆ If you answered all five items correctly, here's a high five! You're a GI genius!

☆☆ If you answered three or four correctly, we want to shake your hand! We're going to renew your membership in the Association of GI Prodigies!

☆ If you answered fewer than three correctly, slap us some skin! You're on your way to GI greatness!

Renal failure

Just the facts

This chapter will help you understand the effects of fluid imbalances associated with renal failure. It will also provide guidelines for treatment and preventive care. In this chapter you'll learn:

♦ how to tell the difference between acute and chronic renal failure

♦ which fluid, electrolyte, and acid-base imbalances occur in renal failure and why

♦ what the signs and symptoms of renal failure are

♦ what nursing interventions are appropriate for patients with renal failure.

A look at renal failure

Renal failure involves a disruption of normal kidney function. The kidneys play a major role in regulating fluids, electrolytes, and acids and bases. Acute renal failure occurs suddenly and is usually reversible. In contrast, chronic renal failure occurs slowly and is irreversible.

Both acute and chronic renal failure affect the kidneys' functional unit, the nephron, which forms urine. Imbalances occur as the kidneys lose the ability to excrete water, electrolytes, wastes, and acid-base products through the urine. Patients may also develop hypertension, anemia, uremia and renal osteodystrophy, the latter of which includes softening of bones and a reduction of bone mass. The following discussion examines how acute and chronic renal failure develop.

How acute renal failure happens

Acute renal failure can stem from intrarenal conditions, which damage the kidneys themselves; from prerenal conditions such as congestive heart failure, which causes a diminished blood flow to the kidneys; or from obstructive postrenal conditions such as prostatitis, which can cause urine to back up into the kidneys. (See *Causes of acute renal failure.*)

About 5% of hospitalized patients develop acute renal failure at some point during their hospitalizations. A multitude of conditions reduce blood flow or otherwise damage the kidney's nephrons. Acute renal failure normally passes through three distinct phases: oliguric-anuric, diuretic, and recovery.

Urine output drops off

A decrease in urine output is the first clinical sign of acute renal failure during the first phase, called the oliguric-anuric phase. Typically, as the glomerular filtration rate decreases, the patient's urine output decreases to less than 400 ml during a 24-hour period.

When the kidneys fail, nitrogenous waste products accumulate, which causes an elevation in the blood urea nitrogen (BUN) and the serum creatinine levels. This in turn results in uremia. Electrolyte imbalances, metabolic acidosis, and other effects follow as the patient becomes increasingly uremic and renal dysfunction disrupts other body systems. Left untreated, the condition is fatal.

The oliguric-anuric phase generally lasts 1 to 2 weeks but may last for several more. The longer the patient remains in this phase, the poorer the prognosis for a return to normal renal function.

Room for improvement

The second phase, the diuretic phase, starts with a gradual increase in daily urine output from 400 ml/24 hours to 1 to 2 L/24 hours. The BUN level stops rising. Although urine output is beginning to increase in this phase, a potential for fluid and electrolyte imbalances still exists as glomerular filtration recovers. The diuretic phase lasts approximately 10 days.

Causes of acute renal failure

The causes of acute renal failure can be broken down into three categories (illustrated here) — prerenal, intrarenal, and postrenal. Prerenal causes include conditions that diminish blood flow to the kidneys. Intrarenal causes include conditions that damage the kidneys themselves. Postrenal causes include conditions that obstruct urine outflow, which causes urine to back up into the kidneys.

Prerenal causes
- Serious cardiovascular disorders
- Hypovolemia
- Peripheral vasodilation
- Severe vasoconstriction
- Renal vascular obstruction

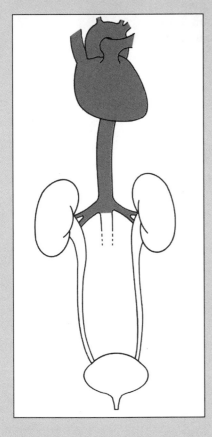

Intrarenal causes
- Acute tubular necrosis
- Nephrotoxins
- Heavy metals
- Aminoglycosides or nonsteroidal anti-inflammatory drugs
- Ischemic damage from poorly treated renal failure
- Eclampsia, postpartum renal failure, or uterine hemorrhage
- Crush injury, myopathy, sepsis, or transfusion reaction

Postrenal causes
- Bladder obstruction
- Ureteral obstruction
- Urethral obstruction

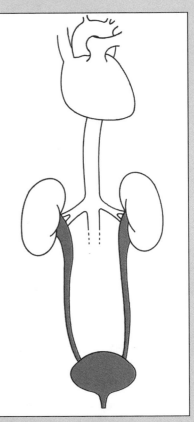

Gettin' better every day

The third phase, the convalescent or recovery phase, begins when fluid and electrolyte values start to stabilize, indicating a return to normal kidney function. The patient may experience a slight reduction in kidney function for the rest of his life, so he will still be at risk for fluid and electrolyte imbalances. The recovery phase generally lasts a few months.

How chronic renal failure happens

Chronic renal failure has a more insidious onset than acute renal failure. Chronic renal failure may result from:
• chronic glomerular disease such as glomerulonephritis
• chronic infections, such as chronic pyelonephritis or tuberculosis
• congenital anomalies such as polycystic kidney disease
• vascular diseases, such as renal nephrosclerosis or hypertension
• obstructions such as from calculi
• collagen diseases such as systemic lupus erythematosus
• nephrotoxic agents such as long-term aminoglycoside therapy
• endocrine diseases such as diabetes mellitus.

Stages of failure

Because chronic renal failure has a slow onset, identifying specific time frames for its stages may be difficult. In addition, the rate at which kidney function deteriorates depends on the specific disease causing the deterioration. It is possible, however, to stage progression of the disease by the degree of kidney function.

Chronic renal failure can be divided into four basic stages:
1. reduced renal reserve (glomerular filtration rate 35% to 50% of normal)
2. renal insufficiency (glomerular filtration rate 20% to 35% of normal)
3. renal failure (glomerular filtration rate 20% to 25% of normal)
4. end-stage renal disease (glomerular filtration rate less than 20% of normal).

In reserve

The kidneys have great functional reserve. Few symptoms develop until more than 75% of glomerular filtration is lost. The remaining functional nephrons then deteriorate progressively; symptoms worsen as renal function diminishes. Failing kidneys cannot regulate fluid balance, filter solutes, or participate effectively in acid-base balance. If chronic renal failure continues unchecked, uremic toxins accumulate and produce potentially fatal physiologic changes in all major organ systems.

Imbalances caused by renal failure

Renal failure — acute or chronic — may cause a number of fluid, electrolyte, and acid-base imbalances, including hypervolemia, hypovolemia, hyperkalemia, hyperphosphatemia, hypocalcemia, hyponatremia, hypernatremia, hypermagnesemia, metabolic acidosis, and metabolic alkalosis.

Water, water, everywhere...or not

When urinary output decreases, especially with the more sudden onset of acute renal failure, the body retains fluid, which can lead to hypervolemia. That condition may also occur if fluid intake exceeds urine output. The resulting fluid retention may lead to hypertension, peripheral edema, congestive heart failure, and pulmonary edema.

Hypovolemic water losses usually occur during the diuretic phase of acute renal failure and can result in hypotension and circulatory collapse.

Potassium to the max

As the kidneys' ability to excrete potassium is impaired, serum potassium levels increase, resulting in hyperkalemia. In chronic renal failure, a patient tends to tolerate high potassium levels more than a patient with acute renal failure, in which the onset is more sudden.

Metabolic acidosis, which occurs in renal failure, causes potassium to move from inside the cells into the extracellular fluid. The release of potassium from any necrotic or injured cells worsens hyperkalemia. Additional stressors — such as infection, GI bleeding, trauma, or surgery — can also lead to a high serum potassium level.

Bad influences

Serum calcium and phosphorus have an inverse relationship, so when one goes out of balance, the other follows suit. Secondary imbalances can occur as a result.

Hyperphosphatemia develops when the kidneys lose the ability to excrete phosphorus. High serum phosphorus levels cause a decrease in calcium levels because calcium and phosphorus have an inverse relationship.

Decreased activation of vitamin D by the kidneys results in decreased GI absorption of calcium — another cause for low serum calcium levels.

The salt mines

Sodium levels may be either abnormally high or unusually low during renal failure.

Hyponatremia can occur in acute renal failure because a decreased glomerular filtration rate and damaged tubules increase water and sodium retention. This dilutional hyponatremic state can also be caused by the intracellular-extracellular exchange between sodium and potassium during metabolic acidosis.

Hypernatremia can occur during chronic renal failure. A progression in the degree of kidney failure causes less sodium to be excreted and makes hypernatremia worse.

Easy on the laxatives

The patient with renal failure may retain magnesium as a result of a decreased glomerular filtration rate and destruction of the tubules. However, a high serum magnesium level is usually not recognized unless the patient receives external sources of magnesium, such as laxatives, antacids, I.V. solutions, or hyperalimentation solutions.

Can't hold the bicarb

Metabolic acidosis is the most common acid-base imbalance occuring in renal failure. It develops as the kidneys lose the ability to secrete hydrogen ions — an acid — in the urine. The imbalance is also exacerbated as the kidneys fail to hold onto bicarbonate — a base.

Patients with chronic renal failure have more time to compensate for this acid-base imbalance than patients with acute renal failure. The lungs try to compensate for the excess acid by increasing the depth and rate of respirations in an attempt to blow off carbon dioxide.

Metabolic alkalosis rarely occurs in renal failure. When it does, it usually results from excessive administration of bicarbonate, given in an effort to correct metabolic acidosis.

What to look for

The patient's history may reveal a disorder that can cause renal failure; it may also include a recent episode of fever, chills, GI problems (such as anorexia, nausea, vomiting, diarrhea, or constipation), and central nervous system problems such as headache.

Signs and symptoms vary, depending on the length of time in which renal failure develops. (See *Lab results in renal failure.*) Fewer signs may appear in acute renal failure due to the condition's shorter clinical course. In chronic renal failure, however, almost all body systems are affected. Your assessment findings may involve several body systems. (See *Effects of renal failure, page 244.*)

Salt shortage

In renal failure, the kidneys may not be able to retain salt and hyponatremia occurs. The patient may complain of dry mouth, fatigue, and nausea. You may note hypotension, loss of skin turgor, and listlessness that progresses to somnolence and confusion.

Later, as the number of functioning nephrons decreases, so does the kidney's capacity to excrete sodium and potassium. Urine output decreases. The urine may be dilute, with casts or crystals present. Accumulation of potassium causes muscle irritability and then muscle weakness, irregular pulse, and life-threatening cardiac arrhythmias. Sodium retention causes fluid overload, and edema becomes palpable. The patient gains weight from fluid retention. Metabolic acidosis can also occur.

Rubs and crackles

When the cardiovascular system is involved, you'll find hypertension and an irregular pulse. Tachycardia may occur. Signs of a pericardial rub, related to pericarditis, may be heard, especially in chronic renal failure. Crackles at the bases of the lungs may be heard, and peripheral edema may be palpated if congestive heart failure occurs.

Lab results in renal failure

Keep alert for these early signs of acute renal failure:

• urine output below 400 ml over 24 hours
• increased blood urea nitrogen level.
• increased serum creatinine level

I can't waste time

Effects of renal failure

Here are signs and symptoms associated with renal failure. Your patient may develop some or all of them.

Neurologic
- Fatigue
- Listlessness and somnolence
- Shortened memory and attention span
- Irritability
- Confusion
- Coma
- Seizures
- Hiccups
- Muscle irritability and twitching
- Pain, burning, and itching in the legs and feet

Cardiovascular
- Hypotension
- Hypertension
- Cardiac arrhythmias
- Weight gain with fluid retention
- Irregular pulse
- Tachycardia
- Pericardial rub
- Heart failure
- Anemia

Pulmonary
- Decreased breath sounds, if pneumonia is present
- Dyspnea
- Crackles
- Kussmaul's respirations

GI
- Dry mouth
- Inflammation and ulceration of GI mucosa
- Bleeding
- Metallic taste in the mouth
- Ammonia smell to the breath
- Anorexia
- Nausea and vomiting
- Pain on abdominal palpation and percussion
- Constipation or diarrhea

Integumentary
- Yellow-bronze skin color
- Dry, scaly skin with purpura, ecchymoses, and petechiae
- Uremic frost (in later stages)

- Thin, brittle fingernails with lines
- Dry mucous membranes
- Dry, brittle hair that may change color or fall out easily
- Severe itching
- Loss of skin turgor

Genitourinary
- Changes in urinary patterns or appearance
- Dilute urine with casts and crystals
- Oliguria or anuria
- Infertility
- Decreased libido
- Amenorrhea in women
- Impotence in men

Musculoskeletal
- Pathologic fractures
- Bone and muscle pain
- Gait abnormalities or loss of ambulation
- Muscle cramps
- Muscle weakness

Rapid respirations

Pulmonary changes include reduced pulmonary macrophage activity with increased susceptibility to infection. If pneumonia is present, breath sounds may decrease over areas of consolidation. Crackles at the lung bases occur with pulmonary edema. Kussmaul's respirations occur with metabolic acidosis.

Metallic hiccups

With inflammation and ulceration of GI mucosa, inspection of the mouth may reveal gum ulceration and bleeding.

The patient may complain of hiccups, a metallic taste in the mouth, anorexia, nausea, and vomiting (caused by esophageal, stomach, or bowel involvement). You may note an ammonia smell to the breath. Abdominal palpation and percussion may cause pain.

Dry, scaly skin

Inspection of the skin typically reveals a yellow-bronze color. The skin is dry and scaly with purpura, ecchymoses, and petechiae that form as a result of thrombocytopenia and platelet dysfunction caused by uremia. In later stages, the patient may experience uremic frost (powdery deposits on the skin as a result of urea and uric acid being excreted in sweat) and thin, brittle fingernails with characteristic lines. Mucous membranes are dry. Hair is dry and brittle and may change color and fall out easily. The patient usually complains of severe itching.

Sexual effects

With chronic renal failure, the patient may have a history of infertility and decreased libido. Women may have amenorrhea, and men may be impotent.

Bone and muscle pain

The patient may have a history of pathologic fractures and complain of bone and muscle pain, which may be caused by an imbalance in calcium and phosphorus or in the amount of parathyroid hormone produced. You may note gait abnormalities or, possibly, that the patient is no longer able to ambulate.

More problems

You may note that the patient has changes in his level of consciousness that may progress from mild behavior changes, shortened memory and attention span, apathy, drowsiness, and irritability to confusion, coma, and seizures. The patient may complain of muscle cramps and twitching caused by muscle irritability. The patient may also complain of pain, burning, and itching in the legs and feet that may be relieved by voluntarily shaking, moving, or rocking them. Those symptoms may eventually progress to paresthesia and motor nerve dysfunction.

What tests show

Diagnostic test results related to renal failure include:
• elevated serum BUN, creatinine, potassium, and phosphorus levels
• arterial blood gas (ABG) results that show metabolic acidosis, indicated by a low pH and a low bicarbonate
• low hematocrit, low hemoglobin, and mild thrombocytopenia
• urinalysis showing casts, cellular debris, decreased specific gravity, and proteinuria
• electrocardiogram (ECG) showing tall, peaked T waves; a widened QRS complex; and disappearing P waves if hyperkalemia is present
• other studies, such as kidney-ureter-bladder radiography and kidney ultrasonography, to find cause of renal failure.

Emergency treatment for hyperkalemia

Emergency treatment for hyperkalemia includes dialysis and administration of 50% hypertonic glucose I.V., regular insulin, calcium gluconate I.V., and sodium bicarbonate I.V. Kayexalate may also be administered.

How renal failure is treated

Treatment for renal failure aims to correct specific symptoms and different aspects of the disease process.

Go low pro

Dietary changes should be made. A low protein diet reduces the production of end-products of protein metabolism that the kidneys can't excrete. Protein consumed should contain all essential amino acids. Such foods include eggs, milk, poultry, and meat.

Consuming those foods will help to prevent the breakdown of body protein. In addition, a high-calorie diet needs to be provided to meet daily requirements and to prevent the breakdown of body protein. The diet also should restrict sodium and potassium.

Balance those fluids

Maintaining fluid balance requires careful monitoring of vital signs, weight changes, and urine output. Fluid retention can be reduced with the use of loop diuretics such as Lasix (if some renal function remains) and with fluid restriction. Careful monitoring of serum potassium levels is necessary to detect hyperkalemia. If hyperkalemia is discovered, emergency treatment should be initiated. (See *Emergency treatment for hyperkalemia.*) Phosphate-binding antacids may be given to lower serum phosphorus levels.

A kick to the marrow

In chronic renal failure, kidney production of erythropoietin is diminished. This hormone controls the rate of red cell production in bone marrow and functions as a growth factor and differentiating factor. Treatment includes the administration of synthetic erythropoietin to stimulate bone marrow to produce red blood cells.

Scrub those fluids

Hemodialysis or peritoneal dialysis are used in both acute and chronic renal failure. By assuming the function of the kidneys, those measures help correct fluid and electrolyte disturbances and relieve some of the symptoms of renal failure.

How you intervene

Caring for a patient with renal failure requires careful monitoring, administration of various medicines and therapeutic regimens, and empathic ministering to the patient and the family.

Assess and monitor

- Assess the patient carefully to determine the type and severity of fluid, electrolyte, and acid-base imbalances.
- Maintain accurate fluid intake and output records.
- Weigh the patient daily, and compare the results with the 24-hour intake and output record. (See *Teaching about renal failure.*)
- Monitor vital signs, including breath sounds and central venous pressure when available, to detect changes in fluid volume. Report hypertension, which may occur as a result of fluid and sodium retention.
- Observe the patient for signs and symptoms of fluid overload, such as edema, bounding pulse, and shortness of breath.
- Monitor serum electrolyte and ABG levels for abnormalities. Report significant changes to the doctor.
- Observe for signs and symptoms that may indicate an electrolyte or acid-base imbalance, such as tetany, paresthesia, muscle weakness, tachypnea, or confusion.
- Monitor electrocardiographic readings to detect electrolyte imbalances.
- Monitor hemoglobin and hematocrit levels.

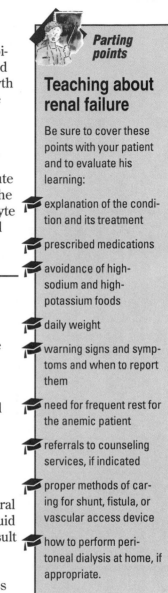

Parting points

Teaching about renal failure

Be sure to cover these points with your patient and to evaluate his learning:

- explanation of the condition and its treatment
- prescribed medications
- avoidance of high-sodium and high-potassium foods
- daily weight
- warning signs and symptoms and when to report them
- need for frequent rest for the anemic patient
- referrals to counseling services, if indicated
- proper methods of caring for shunt, fistula, or vascular access device
- how to perform peritoneal dialysis at home, if appropriate.

• If the patient requires dialysis, check the vascular access site every 2 hours for patency and signs of clotting. Check the site for bleeding after dialysis.

Administer

• Restrict fluids as prescribed.
• Administer prescribed diuretics to patients whose kidneys can still excrete excess fluid.
• Administer other prescribed medications, such as oral or I.V. electrolyte replacement to correct electrolyte imbalances, and vitamin supplements to correct nutritional deficiencies.
• Know the route of excretion for medications being given. Drugs excreted through the kidney or removed during dialysis will need their dosage adjusted.
• Expect to administer sodium bicarbonate I.V. to control acute acidosis and orally to control chronic acidosis. Be aware of the high sodium content of sodium bicarbonate. Multiple doses of the drug may result in hypernatremia, which could contribute to the onset of heart failure and pulmonary edema.
• As necessary, restrict electrolyte intake, especially potassium and phosphorus, to prevent imbalances. Monitor and document the patient's response. (See *Documenting renal failure*.)
• Be prepared to initiate dialysis for electrolyte or acid-base imbalances that don't respond to drugs or when fluid removal isn't possible.

Maintain

• Maintain nutritional status. Provide a diet high in calories and low in protein, sodium, and potassium. Initiate a nutritional consult, as needed.
• If a shunt or fistula for dialysis has been placed in the patient's arm, don't use that extremity for measuring blood pressure, drawing blood, or inserting I.V. catheters.
• Provide emotional support to the patient and his family.
• Teach the patient and his family about renal failure and its treatment.

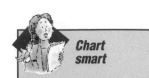

Chart smart

Documenting renal failure

If your patient is in renal failure, here are some things to include in your documentation:

▤ assessment findings, such as those related to fluid, electrolyte, or acid-base imbalances

▤ vital signs, including breath sounds and central venous pressure readings (if available)

▤ daily weight

▤ laboratory test results

▤ intake and output

▤ administration of I.V. or oral electrolyte replacement therapy

▤ dialysis and care of the vascular access site

▤ patient teaching and patient's response

▤ notification of the doctor.

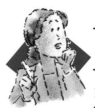

Quick quiz

1. Symptoms may not show up in chronic renal failure until later stages of the disease because:
   A. liver hormones mask the symptoms.
   B. the kidneys have great functional reserve.
   C. other body systems take over some of the kidneys' functions.

Answer: B. Because of the great functional reserve of the kidneys, chronic renal failure develops more slowly than acute renal failure and without apparent signs and symptoms until later stages of the disease.

2. Metabolic acidosis worsens the electrolyte imbalance known as:
   A. hyperkalemia.
   B. hypervolemia.
   C. hypokalemia.

Answer: A. Metabolic acidosis causes the movement of potassium from intracellular to extracellular fluid, causing high blood potassium levels.

3. Low serum calcium levels in renal failure can be due to:
   A. decreased amounts of parathyroid hormone.
   B. decreased activation of vitamin D.
   C. demineralization of bone.

Answer: B. Decreased activation of vitamin D in renal failure causes a decreased GI absorption of calcium. Although demineralization of bone can happen with renal failure, the condition is due to repeated episodes of hypocalcemia.

4. In the oliguric phase of acute renal failure, urine output drops to less than:
   A. 800 ml/24 hours.
   B. 400 ml/24 hours.
   C. 100 ml/24 hours.

Answer: B. The oliguric phase involves a urine output below 400 ml/24 hours.

5. A patient with hyperkalemia may experience several ECG changes, including:
    A. flat T waves, a small QRS, and normal P waves.
    B. tall, peaked T waves; a widened QRS; and disappearing P waves.
    C. no T waves, a normal QRS, and flattened or misshapened P waves.

Answer: B. High potassium levels may result in disappearing P waves, a widened QRS complex, and tall, peaked T waves because of the effect on cardiac cells.

6. The optimal diet for the patient in renal failure is:
    A. high-calorie, low-protein, low-sodium, low-potassium.
    B. high-calorie, high-protein, high-sodium, high-potassium.
    C. low-calorie, high-protein, low-sodium, low-potassium.

Answer: A. A high-calorie, low-protein, low-sodium, and low-potassium diet is the optimal diet for meeting the metabolic and nutritional requirements of a patient with renal failure.

Scoring

☆☆☆   If you answered all six items correctly, great job! You're the Royal Renal Ruler!

☆☆   If you answered four or five correctly, way to go! You're a true Renal Renegade!

☆   If you answered fewer than four correctly, cool, you Renal Recluse, you!

Burns

Just the facts

This chapter explains how burn injuries affect the entire body system. In this chapter, you'll learn:

♦ what physiologic changes occur with a severe burn injury

♦ what fluid, electrolyte, and acid-base imbalances occur as a result of a severe burn injury

♦ what signs and symptoms occur with a burn injury

♦ how treatment methods vary for burn injuries

♦ how to provide appropriate nursing care for a burn patient.

A look at burns

A major burn is a horrifying injury, requiring painful treatment and a long period of rehabilitation. The destruction of the epidermis, dermis, or subcutaneous layers of the skin can affect the entire body and frequently is life-threatening. If not fatal, it is often permanently disfiguring and incapacitating, both emotionally and physically.

A burn, like any injury to the skin, interferes with the skin's ability to help keep out infectious organisms, maintain fluid balance, and regulate body temperature. Burn injuries cause major changes in the body's fluid and electrolyte balance. Many of those imbalances change over time as the initial injury progresses.

The extreme heat from a burn can be severe enough to completely destroy cells. Even with a lesser injury, normal cell activity is disrupted. With minimal injury, the cell may recover its function. The burn patient's prognosis depends on the size and severity of the burn.

Several factors determine the severity of a burn, including the cause, degree, and extent of the burn, as well as the part of the body involved. The outcome for the burned patient is also affected by the presence of preexisting medical conditions and the patient's age.

Types of burns

Burns may be caused by chemicals or radiation, or as a result of thermal, mechanical, or electrical injuries. Thermal burns, the most common type of burn injury, frequently result from residential fires, motor vehicle accidents, childhood accidents, exposure to improperly stored gasoline, exposure to space heaters or electrical malfunctions, and arson. Other causes include improper handling of firecrackers, scalding liquids, and kitchen accidents. Because its effects are similar to the effects of a burn, frostbite is included in the thermal burn category.

Chemical burns result from the contact, ingestion, inhalation, or injection of acids, alkalies, or vesicants. Mechanical burns, such as those caused by friction or abrasion, happen when the skin is rubbed harshly against a coarse surface.

Radiation burns may be caused by excessive exposure to sunlight. Electrical burns commonly occur after contact with faulty electrical wiring, high-voltage power lines, or immersion in water that has been electrified. Those injuries may also be caused by lightning strikes.

When caring for a patient with an electrical burn, keep in mind that there may be more damage internally than meets the eye. Tissue damage from an electrical burn is difficult to assess because internal destruction along the conduction pathway usually is greater than the surface burn would indicate. An electrical burn that ignites the patient's clothing may cause thermal burns as well.

Classification of burns

Classifying the degree of burn helps to determine the type of intervention needed, since burn thickness is associated with the cells' ability to function.

First-degree

Partial-thickness (first-degree) burns affect the superficial layer of the epidermis. Those burns are usually pink or red, and dry and painful. No blistering occurs with a partial-thickness burn; however, some edema may be present. Partial-thickness burns are not classified as severe since the epidermis remains intact and continues to prevent water loss from the skin, so fluid and electrolyte balances are not affected. Regrowth of the epidermis occurs and healing is generally rapid without scarring.

Second-degree

Deep partial-thickness (second-degree) burns affect both the epidermis and dermis. Those burns are caused by prolonged exposure — usually longer than 10 seconds — to intense heat or by prolonged contact with hot liquids or objects.

To identify a deep partial-thickness burn, look for the area to be painful, swollen, and red, with blister formation. When pressure is applied to the burn, it blanches and refills.

Regeneration of the epithelial layer may occur. The amount of scarring varies with this type of burn. Fluid and electrolyte imbalances are associated with second-degree burns that cover significant areas of the body.

Third-degree

Full-thickness (third-degree) burns affect the epidermis, the dermis, and tissues below the dermis. This burn will look dry and leathery, be painless (because nerve endings are destroyed), and will not blanch when pressure is applied. The color of the burned area can vary from white to black or charred.

Third-degree burn injuries require skin grafting. Full-thickness burns carry the greatest risk of fluid and electrolyte imbalance.

Extent of a burn

Assessment tools, such as the Rule of Nines or the Lund and Browder chart, are used to estimate the percentage of body surface area involved in a burn injury. (See *Estimating the extent of a burn.*)

The severity of a burn can be estimated by correlating its depth and size. Burns are categorized as major, moderate, and minor.

Major burn

Major burns include:
• second-degree burns covering more than 25% of an adult body surface
• third-degree burns covering more than 10% of the body surface area
• burns of the hands, face, eyes, ears, feet, or genitalia
• all inhalation injuries
• all electrical burns
• burn injuries complicated by fractures or other major trauma
• all burns in poor-risk patients, such as children younger than age 2, adults older than age 60, and patients who have preexisting medical conditions such as heart disease.

Moderate burn

Moderate burns include:
• third-degree burns on 2% to 10% of the body surface area, regardless of body size
• second-degree burns on 15% to 25% of an adult's body surface area (10% to 20% of a child's).

Minor burn

Minor burns include:
• third-degree burns that appear on less than 2% of the body surface area, regardless of body size
• second-degree burns on less than 15% of an adult's body surface area (10% of a child's).

Phases of a burn

Burn phases describe the physiologic changes that occur after a burn and include the fluid accumulation, fluid remobilization, and convalescent phases. Burns affect many

Estimating the extent of a burn

You can quickly estimate the extent of an *adult* patient's burns by using the Rule of Nines (below, left). This method divides an adult's body surface into percentages.

 To use this method, mentally transfer your adult patient's burns to the body chart shown here. Then add up the corresponding percentages for each burned section. The total — a rough estimate of the extent of your patient's burns — enters into the formula to determine his initial fluid replacement needs.

 An infant or a child's body-section percentages differ from those of an adult. For instance, an infant's head accounts for a greater percentage of his total body surface when compared with an adult's. For an *infant* or *child,* use the Lund and Browder chart (below, right).

Rule of nines

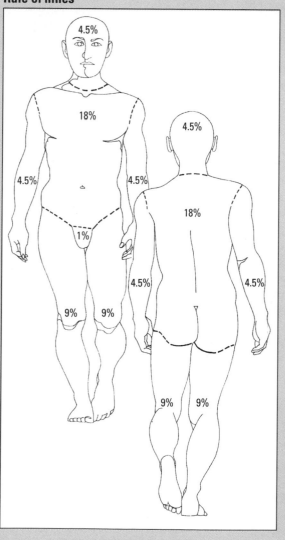

Lund and Browder

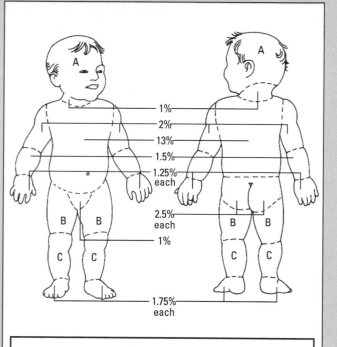

Relative percentages of areas affected by growth

	At birth	1–4 yr.	5–9 yr.	10–14 yr.	15 yr.	Adult
A: *Half of head*	9.5%	8.5%	6.5%	5.5%	4.5%	3.5%
B: *Half of thigh*	2.75%	3.25%	4%	4.25%	4.5%	4.75%
C: *Half of leg*	2.5%	2.5%	2.75%	3%	3.25%	3.5%

body systems and can lead to several serious fluid and electrolyte imbalances, which vary depending on the phase of the burn.

Fluid accumulation phase

The fluid accumulation phase lasts for 36 to 48 hours after a burn injury. During that phase, fluid shifts from the vascular compartment to the interstitial space, a process known as third-space shift. That shift of fluids causes edema. Typically, the edema reaches its maximum extent within 8 hours after the injury. Severe edema may compromise circulation and diminish pulses. Other conditions occur during this phase.

Plasma, proteins, and permeability

Because of the burn injury, capillary damage alters the permeability of the vessels. Plasma — the liquid and protein part of blood — also escapes from the vascular compartment into the interstitium. Because less fluid is available to dilute the blood, the blood becomes hemoconcentrated and the patient's hemoglobin and hematocrit rise.

Because of the third-space shift (fluids moving out of the vascular compartment), hypovolemia occurs. Hypovolemia causes a decreased cardiac output, tachycardia, and hypotension. Shock, cardiac arrhythmias, and a decreased mental status may develop.

With the burn's damage to the skin surface, the skin's ability to prevent water loss is also decreased. As a result, the patient can lose up to 8 L of fluid per day, or 400 ml/hour.

Back in the kidneys...

Diminished kidney perfusion causes decreased urine output. In response to a burn, the body produces and releases stress hormones — aldosterone and antidiuretic hormone — which cause the kidneys to retain sodium and water.

Uneasy breathing

Depending on the type of burn, a patient may have a compromised, edematous airway. Look for burns of the head or neck, singed nasal hairs, soot in the mouth or nose, coughing, voice changes, mucosal burns, and stridor. You may hear crackles or wheezes over the lung fields. The patient may breathe rapidly or pant. Circumferential burns and edema of the neck or chest can restrict respirations and cause shortness of breath.

Acid test

Injured tissue causes the release of acids that can cause a drop in the pH level of the blood and subsequent metabolic acidosis. Damage to muscle tissue in full-thickness burns causes a release of myoglobin, which can cause renal damage and acute tubular necrosis. Myoglobin gives urine a darkened appearance.

Paralyzed GI system

Hypovolemia can cause a decrease in circulation to the GI system, resulting in a paralytic ileus. The development of gastric ulceration is also common among severe burn patients. Due to tissue destruction, protein loss, and the body's stress response, a negative nitrogen balance can occur after a burn injury. In those instances, protein loss exceeds intake and leads to a negative nitrogen balance.

In addition, the body's metabolic needs are increased due to the burn injury. The increase in metabolic need is usually proportional to the size of the burn wound.

Unbalanced!

Many electrolyte imbalances can occur during the fluid accumulation phase because of the hypermetabolic needs and the priority that fluid replacement takes over nutritional needs during the emergent phase.

Potassium and fluid

Hyperkalemia can result from massive cellular trauma, metabolic acidosis, or renal failure. The condition develops as potassium is released into the extracellular fluid in the initial days following the injury.

Hypovolemia can occur as a result of fluid losses and fluids moving from the vascular space to the interstitial space. Lost fluid resembles intravascular fluid in composition and contains proteins and electrolytes.

Sodium

Hyponatremia can result from the increased loss of sodium and water from the cells. Large amounts of sodium become trapped in edematous fluid during the fluid accumulation phase. Aqueous silver nitrate dressings may also contribute to this electrolyte imbalance.

Other imbalances

Hypernatremia can occur as a result of the aggressive use of hypertonic sodium solutions during fluid replacement therapy.

Hypocalcemia can develop in burn patients, because calcium travels to the damaged tissue and becomes immobilized at the burn site. That movement can occur 12 to 24 hours after the burn injury. Hypocalcemia may also occur due to an inadequate dietary intake of calcium or inadequate supplementation during treatment.

Metabolic acidosis can develop as a result of the accumulation of acids released from the burned tissue. It can also occur due to decreased tissue perfusion from hypovolemia. Respiratory acidosis can result from inadequate ventilation, as happens in inhalation burns.

Fluid remobilization phase

The fluid remobilization phase, also known as the diuresis stage, starts approximately 48 hours after the initial burn injury. Here, the fluid shifts back to the vascular compartment. Edema at the burn site decreases and blood flow to the kidneys increases, which increases urine output. Sodium is lost through the increase in diuresis, and potassium is lost through the urine or moves back into the cells.

Fluid and electrolyte imbalances present during the initial phase after a burn can change during the diuretic phase. Here's a rundown of those imbalances.

• Hypokalemia can develop as potassium shifts from the extracellular fluid back into the cells. The condition usually occurs 4 or 5 days after a major burn.

• Hypervolemia can occur during the fluid remobilization phase because fluid shifts back to the vascular compartment. The condition may be exacerbated by the excessive administration of I.V. fluids.

• Hyponatremia may occur when sodium is lost during diuresis.

Convalescent phase

This phase begins after the first two phases have been resolved and is characterized by the need to focus on the healing or reconstruction of the burn wound. Although the major fluid shifts have been resolved, further fluid and electrolyte imbalances can continue to occur as a result of inadequate dietary intake. Anemia often develops at this time because of the destruction of red blood cells typical of severe burns.

What tests show

Diagnostic test results you may see when caring for a burn patient include:
• increased hemoglobin and hematocrit
• increased serum potassium
• decreased serum sodium
• increased blood urea nitrogen and creatinine with renal failure
• low pH and bicarbonate levels shown in arterial blood gas (ABG) analyses, indicating metabolic acidosis
• increased carboxyhemoglobin level, which indicates smoke inhalation
• electrocardiogram (ECG) changes reflective of electrolyte imbalances or myocardial damage
• myoglobin in the urine.

Be alert!

Be alert for signs and symptoms of pulmonary edema, which can occur because of the fluid shift back to the vascular compartment as well as because of fluid replacement therapy. Check for a decrease in hemoglobin and hematocrit due to hemodilution from the shift of fluids back to the vascular compartment.

Skin impairment leads not only to body temperature alterations and chills but also to infection. Blisters, charring, and scarring may appear, depending on the type and age of the burn. With infected wounds, there may be a foul odor and purulent drainage.

How burns are treated

Priorities in treating a burn patient reflect the ABCs — airway, breathing, and circulation. For a patient with severe facial burns or suspected inhalation injury, treatment to prevent hypoxia includes endotracheal intubation, administration of high concentrations of oxygen, and positive-pressure ventilation. Be aware that adult respiratory distress syndrome may develop from the combination of the body's immune response to injury and fluid leakage across the alveolar-capillary membrane.

Rehydrate

Fluid resuscitation is a vital part of treatment. Several formulas have been created to guide initial treatment for the burn victim. The Parkland formula is one of the more commonly used formulas. (See *Fluid replacement formula*.)

Initial treatment includes administration of lactated Ringer's solution through a large-bore I.V. line to expand vascular volume. This balanced isotonic solution supplies water, sodium, and other electrolytes and can help correct metabolic acidosis because lactate in the solution is quickly metabolized into bicarbonate.

Colloid controversy and insensible losses

Hypertonic solutions called colloids may be used to increase blood volume. Colloids draw water from the interstitial space into the vasculature. However, the use of colloids in the immediate postburn period is controversial; those fluids increase colloid osmotic pressure in the interstitial space, which may worsen edema at the burn site. Examples of colloid solutions are plasma, albumin, and dextran.

A solution of dextrose 5% in water may be used to replace normal insensible water loss as well as the loss of water associated with damage to the skin barrier. Central and peripheral I.V. lines are inserted as necessary. Potassium may be added to I.V. fluids 48 to 72 hours after the burn injury.

More help

An indwelling urinary catheter permits accurate monitoring of urine output. I.V. morphine (2 to 4 mg) alleviates

---

Fluid replacement formula

Here's a commonly used formula, the Parkland formula, for calculating fluid replacement. Vary volumes of infusions depending on the patient's response, especially the urine output.

Formula

4 ml of lactated Ringer's solution per kilogram of body weight per percentage of body surface area over 24 hours.

Example for a 68 kg person with 27% body surface area burns: 4 ml x 68 kg x 27 = 7,344 ml over 24 hours. Give one half of the total over the first 8 hours after the burn and the remainder over the next 16 hours.

pain and anxiety. The patient may need an NG tube to prevent gastric distention from paralytic ileus.

All burn patients need a booster of 0.5 ml of tetanus toxoid given I.M. Most burn centers don't recommend administering prophylactic antibiotics because overuse of antibiotics fosters the development of resistant bacteria.

Caring for the wound

Treatment of the wound includes:
• initial debridement by washing the surface of the wound area with mild soap
• sharp debridement of loose tissue and blisters because blister fluid contains vasospastic agents that can worsen tissue ischemia
• coverage of the wound with an antibacterial agent, such as silver sulfadiazine, and an occlusive cotton gauze dressing
• removal of eschar (escharotomy) if the patient is at risk for vascular, circulatory, or respiratory compromise, as occur with circumferential burns that circle around an extremity, the chest cavity, or the abdomen. Skin grafts may be required.

How you intervene

In a burn patient, good nursing care can mean the difference between life and death. The priority during the emergent phase is to provide immediate, aggressive burn treatment to increase the patient's chance for survival. Later, the priority shifts to providing supportive measures and using strict aseptic technique to minimize the risk of infection. (For tips on how to handle burns outside the health care system, see *Emergency burn care*.)

First steps

• Maintain head and spinal alignment until head and spinal cord injuries have been ruled out.
• Give emergency treatment for electric shock if needed. If an electric shock caused ventricular fibrillation and subsequent cardiac and respiratory arrest, begin cardiopulmonary resuscitation at once. Try to obtain an estimate of the voltage that caused the injury.

Emergency burn care

Here's what you should do if you come upon a person who has just been burned.

• Extinguish any remaining flames on clothing.
• Do not directly touch a patient still connected to live electricity. Unplug or disconnect the electrical source if possible.
• Assess the ABCs (airway, breathing, circulation), and initiate cardiopulmonary resuscitation if necessary.
• Assess the scope of the burns and other injuries.
• Remove clothing but don't pull at clothing that sticks to the skin.
• Irrigate areas of chemical burns with copious amounts of water.
• Remove jewelry or other metal objects that retain heat.
• Cover the person with a blanket.
• Send for emergency medical assistance.

• Ensure that the patient has an adequate airway and effective breathing and circulation. If needed, assist with endotracheal intubation. The patient may have a tracheostomy tube inserted if endotracheal intubation is not possible. Administer 100% oxygen as ordered, and adjust the flow to maintain adequate gas exchange. Draw blood for ABG analyses as ordered.

• Assess vital signs every 15 minutes. Assess breath sounds, and watch for signs of hypoxia and pulmonary edema.

• Take steps to control bleeding, and remove clothing that's still smoldering. If clothing is stuck to the patient's skin, soak it in saline solution. Remove rings and other constricting items.

• Assess the skin for the location, depth, and extent of the burn.

• Assist with the insertion of a central venous line and additional arterial and I.V. lines.

• Start I.V. therapy at once to prevent hypovolemic shock and maintain cardiac output. Follow the Parkland formula or another fluid resuscitation formula, as ordered by the doctor.

• Insert an indwelling urinary catheter as ordered, and monitor intake and output every 15 to 30 minutes.

• Maintain adequate pulmonary hygiene by turning the patient and performing postural drainage regularly.

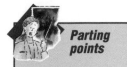

Parting points

Teaching about burns

Teach the patient and his family about his burns and make sure to evaluate his learning. Include the following:

▰ what a burn is and how to prevent it

▰ the patient's particular treatment plan and wound management

▰ signs and symptoms to report to the doctor

▰ long-term care issues such as home care follow-up and rehabilitation.

Assess and monitor

• Watch for signs of decreased tissue perfusion, increased confusion, and agitation. Assess peripheral pulses for adequacy.

• Assess the patient's heart and hemodynamic status for changes that might indicate fluid imbalances, such as hypervolemia or hypovolemia.

• Observe the pattern of third-space shifting (generalized edema, ascites, and pulmonary or intracranial edema) and document the evidence you find.

• Monitor potassium levels, and watch for signs of hyperkalemia (slowed, irregular heart rate; cardiac rhythm strip changes; weakness; and diarrhea).

• Monitor sodium levels, and watch for signs of hyponatremia (increasing confusion, twitching, seizures, abdominal pain, nausea, and vomiting). (See *Teaching about burns*.)

• Watch for signs of metabolic acidosis (headache, disorientation, drowsiness, nausea, vomiting, and rapid, shallow breathing).
• Monitor ABG results.
• Monitor other laboratory results.
• Monitor ECG for arrhythmias.

Maintain

• Anticipate administering maintenance I.V. replacement fluids based on daily assessment of fluid, electrolyte, acid-base, and nutritional needs.
• Maintain core body temperature by covering the patient with a sterile blanket and exposing only small areas of his body at a time.
• Insert an NG tube, if ordered, to decompress the stomach. Avoid aspiration of stomach contents during the procedure.

Weigh and measure

• Obtain a preburn weight from the patient or from a family member or friend.
• If bowel sounds are present, provide a diet high in potassium, protein, vitamins, fats, nitrogen, and calories to maintain the patient's preburn weight. If necessary, feed the patient enterally until he can tolerate oral feedings.
• Weigh the patient every day at the same time. If he can't tolerate oral or enteral feedings, administer hyperalimentation as ordered.

Care for the wounds

• Use strict aseptic technique for all patient care, including routine hand washing and the use of protective isolation clothing.
• Observe the patient for signs and symptoms of infection, such as fever, tachycardia, and purulent wound drainage. Burn patients have an increased risk of infection because of destruction of the skin barrier and the loss of nutrients.
• Administer analgesics 30 minutes before wound care.
• Culture wounds before applying a topical antibiotic for the first time.
• Cover burns with a dry, sterile dressing. Never cover large burns with saline-soaked dressings because they can drastically lower body temperature. Topical ointments

and antibiotic agents may be applied as appropriate. Silver nitrate and mafenide acetate (Sulfamylon) can cause electrolyte imbalances and metabolic alterations.
• Maintain joint function with physical therapy and use of support garments and splints.
• Notify the doctor of significant changes in the patient's condition or pertinent laboratory test results.

Communicate with the patient

• Explain all procedures to the patient before performing them. Speak calmly and clearly to help alleviate anxiety. Encourage the patient to participate in self-care as much as possible.
• Give opportunities for the patient to voice concerns, especially about altered body image. If appropriate, arrange a meeting with another patient with similar injuries. When possible, show the patient how bodily functions are improving. If necessary, refer the patient for mental health counseling.
• Prepare the patient to go home.
• Document all care given, all teaching done, and the patient's reaction to each. (See *Documenting burn care.*)

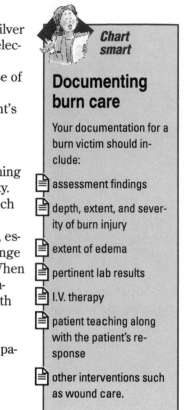

Chart smart

Documenting burn care

Your documentation for a burn victim should include:

- assessment findings
- depth, extent, and severity of burn injury
- extent of edema
- pertinent lab results
- I.V. therapy
- patient teaching along with the patient's response
- other interventions such as wound care.

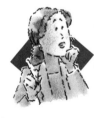

Quick quiz

1. During the fluid accumulation phase of a major burn injury, fluids shift from the:
   A.   intravascular space to the interstitial space.
   B.   interstitial space to the intravascular space.
   C.   intracellular space to the interstitial space.

Answer: A. During the fluid accumulation phase, fluids shift from the intravascular space to the interstitial space.

2. Hypovolemia usually occurs during the:
   A.   fluid remobilization phase of a major burn.
   B.   fluid accumulation phase of a major burn.
   C.   convalescent phase of a major burn.

Answer: B. Hypovolemia usually occurs during the fluid accumulation phase as fluid moves from the intravascular space to the interstitial spaces, a process known as third-spacing.

3. Hypervolemia can occur during the fluid remobilization phase of a major burn as a result of:
    A. fluids shifting back into the intracellular space.
    B. fluids shifting back into the interstitial space.
    C. giving too much I.V. fluids.

Answer: C. Hypervolemia can be exacerbated by administering excessive I.V. fluids.

4. Your patient has second and third degree burn injuries to his anterior chest, anterior abdomen, and entire right arm. Using the Rule of Nines, the percent of total body surface area involved can be estimated at:
    A. 18%.
    B. 27%.
    C. 45%.

Answer: B. The anterior chest and abdomen constitute 18% of the body surface area, and the entire right arm is 9%, for a total of 27%.

5. You insert I.V. lines and begin fluid resuscitation. The doctor wants you to use the Parkland formula. The patient is a 155 lb (70 kg) male and is estimated at having 50% of his total body surface area burned. The amount of lactated Ringer's solution to be administered over the first 8 hours is:
    A. 700 ml.
    B. 7,000 ml.
    C. 1,400 ml.

Answer: B. The Parkland formula is 4 ml $\times$ the percent of total body surface area burned $\times$ weight in kg. So, 4 ml $\times$ 50% $\times$ 70 kg = 14,000 ml or 14 L of lactated Ringer's solution in the first 24 hours. Give 7,000 ml (or half) in the first 8 hours.

6. During the fluid accumulation phase of a patient with burn injuries, the nurse would expect to see signs of the electrolyte imbalance:
    A. hypokalemia.
    B. hyperkalemia.
    C. hyponatremia.

Answer: A. Hypokalemia occurs in the fluid mobilization stage as the potassium shifts from extracellular fluid back into the cells.

Scoring

★★★   If you answered all six items correctly, outstanding! You're simply a burn care superstar!

★★   If you answered four or five correctly, way to go! You're clearly a burn care expert!

★   If you answered fewer than four correctly, that's OK. You're surely a burn care expert-in-training!

Part IV

Treating imbalances

I.V. fluid replacement

Just the facts

This chapter focuses on I.V. fluid replacement therapy. In this chapter, you'll learn:

♦ what the types of I.V. fluids are and how they're used

♦ what methods are used to administer I.V. fluids

♦ what complications are associated with I.V. therapy

♦ how to provide nursing care for a patient receiving I.V. therapy.

A look at I.V. therapy

To maintain health, the balance of fluids and electrolytes in the intracellular and extracellular spaces needs to remain relatively constant. Whenever a person experiences an illness or a condition that prevents normal fluid intake or causes excessive fluid loss, I.V. fluid replacement may be necessary.

I.V. therapy that provides the patient with life-sustaining fluids, electrolytes and medications offers the advantages of immediate and predictable therapeutic effects. The I.V. route is, therefore, the preferred route, especially for fluid, electrolyte, and drug administration in emergencies.

This route also allows for fluid intake when a patient has GI malabsorption. I.V. therapy permits accurate dosage titration for analgesics and other medications. Potential disadvantages associated with I.V. therapy include drug and solution incompatibility, adverse reactions, infection, and other complications.

Types of solutions

Solutions used for I.V. fluid replacement fall into the broad categories of crystalloids (which may be isotonic, hypotonic, or hypertonic) and colloids (which are always hypertonic). The following closely examines each category.

Crystalloids

Crystalloids are solutions with small molecules that flow easily from the bloodstream into cells and tissues. Isotonic crystalloids contain about the same concentration of osmotically active particles as extracellular fluid, so fluid doesn't shift between the extracellular and intracellular areas.

Hypotonic crystalloids are less concentrated than extracellular fluid, so they move from the bloodstream into the cell, causing the cell to swell. In contrast, hypertonic crystalloids are more highly concentrated than extracellular fluid, so fluid is pulled into the bloodstream from the cell, causing the cell to shrink. (See *Comparing fluid tonicity,* page 270.)

Sugar and saline

Isotonic solutions, such as dextrose 5% in water (D_5W), have an osmolality (or concentration) of about 275 to 295 mOsm/L. The dextrose metabolizes quickly, though, leaving water behind and acting like a hypotonic solution. Large amounts of the solution may cause hyperglycemia.

Normal saline solution, another isotonic solution, contains only the electrolytes sodium and chloride. Other isotonic fluids are more similar to extracellular fluid. For instance, Ringer's solution contains sodium, potassium, calcium, and chloride. Lactated Ringer's solution contains those electrolytes plus lactate, which the liver converts to bicarbonate.

Swelled cells

Hypotonic fluids are those fluids that have an osmolality less than 275 mOsm/L. Examples of hypotonic fluids include:
• 0.45% sodium chloride or half-normal saline solution
• 0.33% sodium chloride solution
• dextrose 2.5% in water.

Comparing fluid tonicity

The illustrations below show the effects of different types of I.V. fluids on fluid movement and cell size.

Isotonic

Isotonic fluids such as normal saline solution have a concentration of dissolved particles, or tonicity, equal to that of the intracellular fluid. Osmotic pressure is therefore the same inside and outside the cells, so they neither shrink nor swell with fluid movement.

Hypertonic

Hypertonic fluid has a tonicity greater than that of intracellular fluid, so osmotic pressure is unequal inside and outside the cells. Dehydration or rapidly infused hypertonic fluids, such as 3% saline or 50% dextrose, draw water out of the cells into the more highly concentrated extracellular fluid.

Hypotonic

Hypotonic fluids such as half-normal saline solution have a tonicity less than that of intracellular fluid, so osmotic pressure draws water into the cells from the extracellular fluid. Severe electrolyte losses or inappropriate use of I.V. fluids can make body fluids hypotonic.

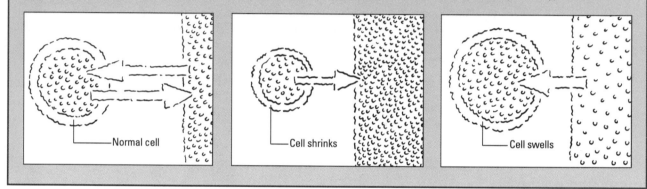

Normal cell   Cell shrinks   Cell swells

Hypotonic solutions should be given cautiously since fluid moves from the extracellular space into cells, causing them to swell. That fluid shift can cause cardiovascular collapse from vascular fluid depletion. It can also cause increased intracranial pressure (ICP) from fluid shifting into brain cells.

Hypotonic solutions should not be given to a patient at risk for increased ICP—for example, those who have had a stroke, head trauma, or neurosurgery. Signs of increased ICP include a change in the patient's level of consciousness, motor or sensory deficits, and changes in the size, shape, or response to light in the pupils. Hypotonic solutions also shouldn't be used in patients who suffer from abnormal fluid shifts into the interstitial space or the body cavities, such as those that occur in liver disease, after a burn, or as a result of trauma.

Dry cells

Hypertonic solutions are those that have an osmolality greater than 295 mOsm/L. Examples include:
• dextrose 5% in half-normal saline solution
• dextrose 5% in normal saline solution
• dextrose 5% in lactated Ringer's solution
• dextrose 10% in water.

A hypertonic solution draws fluids from the intracellular space, causing cells to shrink and the extracellular space to expand. Patients with cardiac or renal disease may be unable to tolerate extra fluid. Be alert for fluid overload and possibly pulmonary edema.

Since hypertonic solutions draw fluids from cells, patients at risk for cellular dehydration (diabetics in ketoacidosis, for example) should not receive them. (See *A look at I.V. solutions,* page 272.)

Colloids

The use of colloids over crystalloids is controversial. Still, the doctor may prescribe a colloid — or plasma expander — if your patient's blood volume doesn't improve with crystalloids. Examples of colloids that may be given include:
• albumin (available in 5% solutions, which are osmotically equal to plasma, and 25% solutions, which draw about four times their volume in interstitial fluid into the circulation within 15 minutes of administration)
• plasma protein fraction
• dextran
• hetastarch.

Colloids pull fluid into the bloodstream. The effects of colloids last several days if the lining of the capillaries is normal. The patient needs to be closely monitored during a colloid infusion for increased blood pressure, dyspnea, and bounding pulse, which are all signs of hypervolemia.

If neither crystalloids nor colloids are effective in treating the imbalance, the patient may require blood transfusions or other treatment.

A look at I.V. solutions

This chart shows examples of some commonly used I.V. fluids, including some of their clinical uses and special considerations associated with their use.

Solution	Uses	Special considerations
Isotonic		
Dextrose 5% in water	• Fluid loss and dehydration • Hypernatremia	• Solution is isotonic initially; becomes hypotonic when dextrose is metabolized. • Don't use for resuscitation; can cause hyperglycemia. • Use cautiously in renal and cardiac disease; can cause fluid overload. • Does not provide enough daily calories for prolonged use; may cause eventual breakdown of protein.
0.9% sodium chloride (normal saline)	• Shock • Hyponatremia • Blood transfusions • Resuscitation • Fluid challenges • Metabolic alkalosis • Hypercalcemia • Fluid replacement in diabetic ketoacidosis	• Since this replaces extracellular fluid, don't use in patients with CHF, edema, or hypernatremia; can lead to overload.
Lactated Ringer's	• Dehydration • Burns • Lower GI tract fluid loss • Acute blood loss • Hypovolemia due to third spacing	• Electrolyte content is similar to serum but doesn't contain magnesium. • Contains potassium; don't use with renal failure; can cause hyperkalemia. • Don't use in liver disease because the patient can't metabolize lactate; functional liver converts it to bicarbonate; don't give if pH > 7.5.
Hypotonic		
0.45% sodium chloride (half-normal saline)	• Water replacement • Diabetic ketoacidosis after initial normal saline solution and before dextrose infusion • Hypertonic dehydration • Sodium and chloride depletion • Gastric fluid loss from nasogastric suctioning or vomiting	• Use cautiously; may cause cardiovascular collapse or increased intracranial pressure. • Don't use in patients with liver disease, trauma, or burns.

A look at I.V. solutions *(continued)*

Solution	Uses	Special considerations
Hypertonic Dextrose 5% in half-normal saline solution	• Diabetic ketoacidosis after initial treatment with normal saline solution and half-normal saline solution — prevents hypoglycemia and cerebral edema (occurs when serum osmolality is reduced too rapidly)	• In diabetic ketoacidosis, use only when glucose falls < 250 mg/dl.
Dextrose 5% in normal saline solution	• Hypotonic dehydration • Temporary treatment of circulatory insufficiency and shock if plasma expanders not available • Syndrome of inappropriate antidiuretic hormone (or use 3% sodium chloride) • Addisonian crisis	• Don't use in cardiac or renal patients because of danger of CHF and pulmonary edema.
Dextrose 10% in water	• Water replacement • Conditions in which some nutrition with glucose is required	• Monitor serum glucose levels.

Delivery methods

The choice of I.V. delivery is based on the purpose of the therapy and its duration; the patient's diagnosis, age, and health history; and the condition of the patient's veins. I.V. solutions can be delivered through a peripheral or a central vein. Catheters and tubing are chosen depending on the therapy and the site to be used. Here's a look at how to choose a site — peripheral or central — and what equipment you'll need for each.

Peripheral lines

Peripheral I.V. therapy is administered for short-term or intermittent therapy through a vein in the arm, hand, leg, or foot. Potential I.V. sites include the metacarpal, cephalic, basilic, median cubital, and greater saphenous veins.

Using veins in the leg or foot is unusual due to the risk of thrombophlebitis.

Choose the right site

Choose a site that meets the patient's need for fluids while trying to keep the patient as comfortable as possible. Place I.V. catheters in the hand or the lower arm so sites can be moved upward as needed. Use the patient's non-dominant hand, if possible.

For a trauma patient or when a patient has suffered cardiac arrest, use a large vein in the antecubital area to gain rapid access. Avoid the antecubital site in a mobile patient because the catheter may kink with movement or cause other discomfort. Avoid using veins over joints. Catheters in those veins are uncomfortable and awkward and can be displaced easily.

Pick a cath, not just any cath

Three main types of catheters are used for insertion into a peripheral vein.
• Steel scalp-vein (winged-infusion) needles are inserted easily, but infiltration is common. These catheters are small, nonflexible, and used when access with another device proves unsuccessful. The catheters are also used for short-term therapy in adults, especially for giving medications by I.V. push (through a syringe over a short period of time).
• Indwelling catheters inserted over a steel needle are easy to use and less likely to infiltrate. Once in place, these catheters are more comfortable for the patient. They're also more difficult to insert than a scalp-vein needle.
• Plastic catheters inserted through a hollow needle are longer and are used more often for central-vein infusions. The catheter must be threaded through the vein for a greater distance, which makes these catheters more difficult to use.

Needle size

Choosing the right diameter (or gauge) needle or catheter is important for ensuring adequate flow and for patient comfort. The higher the gauge, the smaller the diameter of the needle.

If you want to give a lot of fluid over a short period of time, use a catheter with a lower gauge (such as 14, 16, or 18 gauge) and a shorter length, which offers less resistance to fluid flow. For routine I.V. fluid administration, use higher gauge catheters, such as a 20 or a 22 gauge. *French catheters are the exception to the needle-gauge rule. The higher the number in a French catheter, the greater the diameter.*

Central lines

Central venous therapy involves administering solutions through a catheter placed in a central vein, typically the subclavian or internal jugular vein, less often the femoral vein. Central venous therapy is used for patients who have inadequate peripheral veins, need access for blood sampling, require a large volume of fluid, need a hypertonic solution to be diluted by rapid blood flow in a larger vein, or need a high-calorie nutritional supplement.

One lumen, two lumens, more

Three main types of catheters are used for short- and long-term central venous therapy. The traditional central venous catheter is a multilumen catheter used most often for short-term therapy. Although the lumen size may vary, a multilumen catheter provides multiple I.V. access using one insertion site.

A peripherally inserted central catheter is now commonly used in hospitals and in home care. This catheter can be inserted at the bedside by a certified nurse, through a vein in the antecubital area. Fewer and less severe adverse effects occur with these catheters than with traditional central venous catheters. In addition, the catheters can be left in place for several months, making them ideal for long-term therapy.

For extended long-term therapy, the patient may receive a vascular access port implanted in a pocket surgically constructed in the subcutaneous tissue or a tunneled catheter, such as a Hickman, Broviac, or Groshong. Some of these catheters have multiple lumens and are used in the health care facility and at home.

Tubing systems

The mechanics of infusing a solution require a tubing system that can deliver a drug at the correct infusion rate. I.V. tubing is available principally in microdrip sets, which are designed so that 60 drops equal 1 ml. Microdrip sets are useful for infusion rates lower than 100 ml/hour — for instance, when using a solution to keep a vein open.

A macrodrip set, on the other hand, is designed so that 10 to 15 drops equal 1 ml, depending on the manufacturer. Macrodrip sets are preferred for infusion rates greater than 100 ml/hour — for instance, in the treatment of shock.

Infusion pumps

Electronic infusion pumps and controllers require their own types of tubing. Be sure to check the directions prior to using the machines. Infusion pumps and controllers deliver fluids at precisely controlled infusion rates.

Most tubings contain back-check valves to prevent drugs from mixing inside piggyback systems (one I.V. line plugged into another at a piggyback port). Filters on some tubing eliminate particulate matter, bacteria, and air bubbles. Other types of tubing are available specifically for administering drugs or for use as a piggyback.

Complications of I.V. therapy

Caring for a patient with an I.V. line requires careful monitoring, a clear understanding of the possible complications, what to do when a complication arises, and how to deal with flow issues.

Infiltration, infection, phlebitis, and thrombophlebitis are the most frequent complications of I.V. therapy. Other complications include extravasation, a severed catheter, an allergic reaction, an air embolism, speed shock, and fluid overload. Here's an examination of those complications, one at a time.

Infiltration

During infiltration, fluid may leak from the vein into surrounding tissue. Look for coolness at the site, pain, swelling, leaking, and lack of blood return. Also look for a sluggish flow that continues even if a tourniquet is applied above the site. If you see infiltration, stop the infusion, elevate the extremity, and apply warm soaks.

Infection

I.V. therapy involves puncturing the skin, the body's barrier to infection. Infection may result. Look for purulent drainage at the site, tenderness, erythema, warmth, or hardness on palpation. If the infection becomes systemic, look for fever, chills, and an elevated white blood cell count. Nursing actions for an infected I.V. site include monitoring vital signs and notifying the doctor. Swab the site for culture, and remove the catheter as ordered. Always maintain aseptic technique to prevent this complication.

Phlebitis and thrombophlebitis

Phlebitis is an inflammation of the vein; thrombophlebitis is an irritation of the vein with the formation of a clot and is usually more painful than phlebitis. Look for pain, redness, swelling, or induration at the site; a red line streaking along the vein; fever; or a sluggish flow of the solution. When phlebitis or thrombophlebitis occurs, remove the I.V., monitor the patient's vital signs, notify the doctor, and apply warm soaks to the site.

Extravasation

Extravasation, similar to infiltration, is the leakage of fluid into surrounding tissues. It's caused by the tendency of medications, such as dopamine, calcium solutions, and chemotherapeutic agents, to seep through veins and produce blistering and, eventually, necrosis. Initially, the patient may experience discomfort, burning, or pain at the site. Look also for skin tightness, blanching, and lack of blood return. Delayed effects include inflammation and pain within 3 to 5 days and ulcers or necrosis within 2 weeks.

When administering medications that may extravasate, know the policy of your facility. Nursing actions include stopping the infusion, notifying the doctor, infiltrating the site with an antidote as ordered, applying ice early and warm soaks later, and elevating the extremity. Assess the circulation and nerve function of the limb.

Severed catheter

A severed catheter can occur when a piece of catheter becomes dislodged and is set free in the vein. Look for pain at the fragment site, decreased blood pressure, cyanosis, loss of consciousness, and a weak, rapid pulse. Apply a tourniquet above the site of pain, notify the doctor immediately, monitor the patient, and provide support as needed. This serious complication can be avoided by never reinserting a needle through its plastic catheter once the needle has been withdrawn.

Allergic reaction

A patient may suffer an allergic reaction to the fluid, medication, I.V. catheter, or even the latex port in the I.V. tubing. In any case, the source of the reaction may not be known. Look for a red streak extending up the arm, rash, itching, watery eyes and nose, and wheezing. Left untreated, the condition may progress rapidly to anaphylaxis. Nursing measures for allergic reaction include stopping the I.V. immediately, notifying the doctor, monitoring the patient, and giving oxygen and medications as ordered.

Air embolism

An air embolism occurs when air enters the vein and can cause a decrease in blood pressure, increased pulse, respiratory distress, increased intracranial pressure, and loss of consciousness. You should notify the doctor and clamp off the I.V. Place the patient on his left side, and lower his head to allow the air to enter the right atrium, where it can disperse more safely by way of the pulmonary artery. Monitor the patient and administer oxygen. To avoid this serious complication, prime all tubing completely, tighten all connections securely, and use an air detection device on an I.V. pump.

Speed shock

Speed shock occurs when I.V. solutions or medications are given too rapidly. Almost immediately, the patient will have facial flushing, an irregular pulse, a severe headache, and decreased blood pressure. Loss of consciousness and cardiac arrest may also occur. Clamp off the I.V., and notify the doctor immediately. Provide oxygen, obtain frequent vital signs, and administer medications as ordered.

Fluid overload

Fluid overload can happen gradually or suddenly, depending on the ability of the patient's circulatory system to accommodate the fluid. Look for neck-vein distention, increased blood pressure, increased respirations, shortness of breath, cough, and crackles in the lungs on auscultation. Slow the I.V. rate, notify the doctor, and monitor vital signs. Keep the patient warm, keep the head of the bed elevated, and give oxygen and other medications (such as diuretics) as ordered.

How you intervene

Nursing care for the patient with an I.V. includes the following actions.

Check, measure, monitor

• Check the I.V. order for completeness and accuracy. Most I.V. orders expire after 24 hours. A complete order should specify the amount and type of solution, specific additives and their concentrations, and the rate and duration of the infusion.

• Measure intake and output carefully at scheduled intervals. Notify the doctor if your patient's urine output falls below 30 ml/hour.

• Keep in mind the size, age, and history of your patient when giving I.V. fluids to prevent fluid overload. In pediatric patients, use a Buretrol or other I.V. infusion device to limit the amount of fluid the patient receives hourly and prevent the accidental administration of excessive amounts of fluid. (See *Teaching about I.V. therapy.*)

• Always carefully monitor the infusion of solutions that contain medication, because rapid infusion and circulation of the drug can be dangerous.

• Note the pH of the I.V. solution. The pH can alter the effect and stability of drugs mixed in the I.V. bag. Consult medication literature or the doctor if you have questions.

• Change the site, dressing, and tubing as often as your institution's policy requires. Solutions should be changed at least every 24 hours. (See *Documenting an I.V. infusion.*)

• When changing I.V. tubing, be careful not to move or dislodge the I.V. device. If you have trouble disconnecting the used tubing, use a hemostat to hold the I.V. hub while twisting the tubing to remove it. Don't clamp the hemostat shut because this may crack the hub.

• Always report needle-stick injuries. Exposure to a patient's blood risks infection with these blood-borne viruses: human immunodeficiency virus (HIV), hepatitis B virus, hepatitis C virus, and cytomegalovirus. About 1 out of 300 people with occupational needle-stick injuries become HIV-seropositive.

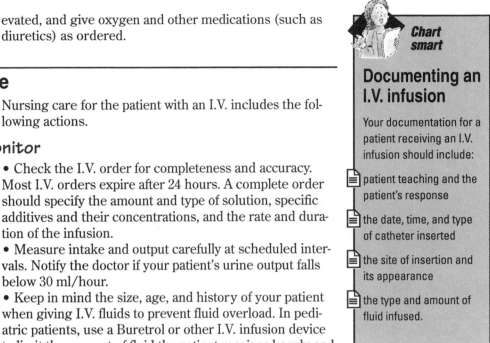

Parting points

Teaching about I.V. therapy

Be sure to cover these points with your patient and evaluate his learning.

✎ what to expect before, during, and after the I.V. procedure

✎ signs and symptoms of complications and when to report them

✎ activity or diet restrictions

✎ how to care for an I.V. line at home.

Chart smart

Documenting an I.V. infusion

Your documentation for a patient receiving an I.V. infusion should include:

📄 patient teaching and the patient's response

📄 the date, time, and type of catheter inserted

📄 the site of insertion and its appearance

📄 the type and amount of fluid infused.

Focus on the patient

• Always listen to your patient carefully. Subtle statements such as "I just don't feel right" may be your clue to the beginning of an allergic reaction.

• Keep in mind that a candidate for home I.V. therapy must have a family member or friend who can safely and competently administer the I.V. fluids, a backup helper, a suitable home environment, a telephone, available transportation, adequate reading skills, and the ability to prepare, handle, store, and dispose of equipment properly. Procedures for caring for the I.V. are the same at home as in a health care facility except that at home, the patient uses clean technique instead of sterile technique.

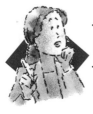

Quick quiz

1. Extravasation of I.V. fluid is associated with:
   A.   administration of hypertonic fluids.
   B.   administration of D_5W.
   C.   administration of neoplastic drugs.

Answer: C. Neoplastic drugs are highly irritating to the veins and are often administered using steel needles. Extravasation is common in those situations.

2. Hypertonic solutions cause fluids to move from the:
   A.   interstitial space to the intracellular space.
   B.   intracellular space to the extracellular space.
   C.   extracellular space to the intracellular space.

Answer: B. Hypertonic solutions, because of their increased osmolality, draw fluids out of the cells and into the extracellular space.

3. The initial solution to be used in treating patients with diabetic ketoacidosis is:
   A. D_5W.
   B.   dextrose 5% in half-normal saline solution.
   C.   normal saline solution.

Answer: C. Normal saline is the optimal choice for patients with diabetic ketoacidosis because the fluid is isotonic and helps to replenish the intravascular volume.

4. Hypotonic fluids should *not* be used for a patient with:
  A. increased intracranial pressure (ICP).
  B. diabetic ketoacidosis whose blood sugar is 200 mg/dl or more.
  C. blood loss as a result of trauma.

Answer: A. Hypotonic fluids cause swelling of the cells and can further increase ICP.

5. Symptoms of an allergy to I.V. tubing include:
  A. shortness of breath.
  B. dry throat.
  C. slow, bounding pulse.

Answer: A. Symptoms of an allergic reaction include shortness of breath, rash, and itching.

6. Your patient is a 90-year-old male with a history of congestive heart failure. When you make rounds, you notice that an I.V. of normal saline solution was mistakenly hung an hour before and has infused 600 ml since then. You should observe this patient for signs of:
  A. septic shock.
  B. decreased intracranial pressure.
  C. circulatory overload.

Answer: C. Because of his advanced age and cardiac condition, the type of fluid infused, and the infusion rate, the patient is at risk for circulatory overload.

7. When a hypotonic crystalloid solution is infused into the bloodstream, it causes the cells to:
  A. shrink.
  B. swell.
  C. release chloride.

Answer: B. Hypotonic crystalloids are less concentrated than extracellular fluids, so they move from the bloodstream into the cell and cause the cell to expand with fluid.

8. Hypertonic solutions should be used cautiously in patients with:
  A. cancer or burns.
  B. cardiac or renal disease.
  C. respiratory or GI disease.

Answer: B. A hypertonic solution draws fluids from the intracellular space into the bloodstream. Patients with cardiac or renal disease may be unable to tolerate that extra fluid volume.

Scoring

☆☆☆ If you answered all eight items correctly, bravo! Here's my arm; plug me in with an I.V., you ace!

☆☆ If you answered five to seven correctly, excellent, you infusion hot shot, you!

☆ If you answered fewer than five correctly, no biggie. A little more I.V. training and you'll be whipping in 18-gaugers in no time!

Total parenteral nutrition

Just the facts

This chapter will help you understand and deal with total parenteral nutrition (TPN). In this chapter, you'll learn:

♦ how to identify patients who would benefit from TPN

♦ what each TPN component is and how TPN is delivered

♦ how to recognize complications associated with TPN

♦ how to care for a patient receiving TPN.

A look at TPN

TPN is a highly concentrated, hypertonic nutrient solution administered by way of an infusion pump through a large central vein. For patients with high caloric and nutritional needs due to illness or injury, TPN provides crucial calories, restores nitrogen balance, and replaces essential fluids, vitamins, electrolytes, minerals, and trace elements. (See *Understanding common TPN additives,* page 284.) It also promotes tissue and wound healing and normal metabolic function. TPN gives the bowel a chance to heal; reduces activity in the gallbladder, pancreas, and small intestine; and is used to improve a patient's response to surgery.

Who needs TPN?

Patients who can't meet their nutritional needs by oral or enteral feedings may require I.V. nutritional supplement

Understanding common TPN additives

Common components of TPN solutions include dextrose 50% in water ($D_{50}W$), amino acids, and other additives and are used for specific purposes. For instance, $D_{50}W$ provides calories for metabolism. Here's a list of other common additives and what purposes each serves. (Lipids may be infused separately.)

Electrolytes
• *Calcium* promotes development of bones and teeth and aids in blood clotting.
• *Chloride* regulates acid-base balance and maintains osmotic pressure.
• *Magnesium* helps absorb carbohydrates and protein.
• *Phosphorus* is essential for cell energy and calcium balance.
• *Potassium* is needed for cellular activity and cardiac function.
• *Sodium* helps control water distribution and maintains normal fluid balance.

Vitamins
• *Folic acid* is needed for DNA formation and promotes growth and development.
• *Vitamin B complex* helps the final absorption of carbohydrates and protein.
• *Vitamin C* helps in wound healing.
• *Vitamin D* is essential for bone metabolism and maintenance of serum calcium levels.
• *Vitamin K* helps prevent bleeding disorders.

Other additives
• *Acetate* prevents metabolic acidosis.
• *Micronutrients* (such as zinc, cobalt, manganese) help in wound healing and red blood cell synthesis.
• *Amino acids* provide the proteins necessary for tissue repair.

or TPN. Generally, this treatment is prescribed for any patient who can't absorb nutrients from the GI tract for more than 10 days. More specific indications include:
• debilitating illnesses lasting longer than 2 weeks
• loss of 10% or more of pre-illness weight
• serum albumin level below 3.5 g/dl

• excessive nitrogen loss from wound infection, fistulas, or abscesses
• renal or hepatic failure
• nonfunction of the GI tract lasting for 5 to 7 days.

TPN triggers

Common illnesses or treatments that can trigger the need for TPN include inflammatory bowel disease, ulcerative colitis, bowel obstruction or resection, radiation enteritis, severe diarrhea or vomiting, AIDS, chemotherapy, and severe pancreatitis, all of which hinder a patient's ability to absorb nutrients. In addition, patients may benefit from TPN after major surgery or if they have a high metabolic rate due to sepsis, trauma, or burns of more than 40% of total body surface area. Infants with congenital or acquired disorders may need TPN to promote proper growth and development.

TPN has limited value for well-nourished patients whose GI tracts are healthy or will most likely resume normal function within 10 days. The treatment also may be inappropriate for a patient with a poor prognosis or when the risks of TPN outweigh its benefits.

Today's TPN trends

The trend of today's nutritional supplementation is to individualize TPN formulas depending on the patient's specific needs. As a result, standard TPN mixtures are becoming less popular. Nutritional support teams consisting of nurses, doctors, pharmacists, and dietitians assess, prescribe for, and monitor patients receiving TPN. The solutions may consist of:
• protein (amino acids in a 2.5% to 8.5% solution), with varying types available for renal or liver failure patients
• dextrose (15% to 50% solution)
• fat emulsions (10% to 20% solution)
• electrolytes
• vitamins
• trace element mixtures
• medications.

Lipid emulsions

Lipid emulsions are thick emulsions of several essential fatty acids and typically supply calories besides the fatty acids. Lipid emulsions assist in wound healing, in the production of red blood cells, and in prostaglandin synthesis. They're given in conjunction with TPN or may be given alone through a peripheral or central venous line.

Lipid emulsions should be given cautiously in patients with liver disease, pulmonary disease, anemia, coagulation disorders, or any patient at risk for developing a fat embolism. These emulsions should be avoided in patients who have conditions that disrupt normal fat metabolism, such as pathologic hyperlipidemia, lipid nephrosis, and acute pancreatitis. Make sure to report adverse reactions to the doctor so the TPN regimen may be changed as needed. (See *Adverse reactions to lipid emulsions*.)

How to infuse TPN

TPN, a hypertonic solution, may be up to six times the concentration of blood, which makes the solution too irritating for a peripheral vein. TPN must be infused through a central vein.

TPN may be infused around the clock or for part of the day — for instance, as the patient sleeps at night. A sterile catheter made of polyurethane, polyvinyl chloride, or silicone rubber (silastic) is inserted into the subclavian or jugular vein. A polyurethane catheter is used for short-term use only because it stiffens within a reasonably short period of time and can cause thrombophlebitis. Silastic catheters offer a better alternative for long-term therapy — months or years — because they're more flexible and durable and are compatible with many medications and solutions.

Why *go peripheral?*

A peripherally inserted central catheter, a variation of central venous therapy, can be used for therapy lasting 3 months or more. The catheter is inserted through the basilic or cephalic vein and threaded so that the tip lies in the superior vena cava.

The patient generally experiences less discomfort with a peripheral catheter, especially if he can move around easily. Movement stimulates blood flow and decreases the risk of phlebitis. Peripherally inserted central catheters are fast becoming the preferred choice for intermediate-term therapy, both at home and in the hospital.

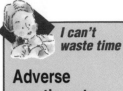

I can't waste time

Adverse reactions to lipid emulsions

Immediate or early adverse reactions to lipid emulsions include:

- dyspnea
- cyanosis
- nausea or vomiting
- headache
- flushing or diaphoresis
- lethargy or syncope
- chest and back pain
- slight pressure over the eyes
- irritation at the site
- hypercoagulability
- thrombocytopenia.

Delayed complications associated with prolonged administration include:

- hepatomegaly
- splenomegaly
- jaundice
- blood dyscrasias
- fatty liver syndrome.

Complications

Signs and symptoms of electrolyte imbalances caused by TPN administration include abdominal cramps, lethargy, confusion, malaise, muscle weakness, tetany, convulsions, and cardiac arrhythmias. Acid-base imbalances can also occur due to the patient's condition or the TPN content. Look for these other complications:

• congestive heart failure (CHF) or pulmonary edema, both of which may occur from fluid and electrolyte administration and can lead to tachycardia, lethargy, confusion, weakness, and labored breathing

• hyperglycemia as a result of dextrose infusing too quickly, a condition that may require an adjustment in the patient's insulin dosage

• adverse reactions to medications added to TPN — for example, added insulin can cause hypoglycemia, which can result in confusion, restlessness, lethargy, pallor, and tachycardia.

Interventions

Constant assessment and rapid intervention are critical for patients receiving TPN. When caring for a patient on TPN, you'll want to take these actions.

Assess and monitor

• Carefully monitor patients receiving TPN to detect early signs of complications, such as metabolic problems, CHF, pulmonary edema, or allergic reactions. Adjust the TPN regimen as needed.

• Assess the patient's nutritional status, and weigh the patient at the same time each morning after he voids, in similar clothing, and on the same scale. Weight gain may indicate fluid overload. A patient shouldn't gain more than 3 lb (1.4 kg) a week.

• Assess for peripheral and pulmonary edema.

• Monitor serum glucose levels every 6 hours initially, then once a day. Stay alert for signs of thirst and polyuria, symptoms of hyperglycemia. Periodically confirm serum glucose meter readings with laboratory tests.

• Monitor for signs and symptoms of glucose metabolism disturbance, fluid and electrolyte imbalances, and nutritional problems. Some patients may require insulin added directly to the TPN for the duration of treatment.

• Monitor electrolyte and protein levels daily at first, and then twice a week for serum albumin. Albumin levels may drop initially as treatment restores hydration.

• Check renal function by monitoring BUN and creatinine levels; increases may indicate excess amino acid intake.

• Assess nitrogen balance with 24-hour urine collection.

• Assess liver function with liver function tests, bilirubin, triglyceride, and cholesterol levels. Abnormal values may indicate intolerance.

• In most institutions, central lines and peripherally inserted central catheters require an order and a patient-consent form. Only an RN specializing in inserting those lines should obtain the form. (See *Teaching about TPN.*)

• Obtain a chest X-ray to check catheter placement after insertion.

Infuse properly

• Review the patient's serum chemistry and nutritional studies, and alert the doctor of abnormal results, which may indicate that the TPN fluid concentration or ingredients may need to be adjusted to meet the patient's specific needs.

• Avoid an adverse reaction by starting TPN slowly — about 1,000 calories over 24 hours — and increasing gradually. Continually monitor the patient's cardiac and respiratory status.

• When a patient is severely malnourished, starting TPN may spark refeeding syndrome, which includes a rapid drop in potassium, magnesium, and phosphorus levels. To avoid compromising cardiac function, initiate feeding slowly and monitor the patient's electrolyte levels closely until they stablize.

• Because the TPN solution is high in glucose, start the infusion slowly. Doing so will allow the patient's pancreatic beta cells to adapt to the glucose by increasing insulin output. Within the first 3 to 5 days of TPN, the typical adult can tolerate about 3 L of solution a day without suffering an adverse reaction.

Parting points

Teaching about TPN

Be sure to cover these topics with your patient and to evaluate his learning:

☛ explanation of TPN and its specific use for the patient

☛ adverse reactions or catheter complications and when to report them

☛ basic care of a TPN line

☛ maintenance of equipment.

• Occasionally a patient may react adversely to specific ingredients in the TPN solution. Protein may need to be reduced if BUN and creatinine levels are elevated.

• Alert the doctor if TPN needs to be stopped and glucose given orally or I.V. The patient's diagnosis and pre-existing physical condition need to be considered when determining the composition and amount of electrolytes used for the TPN solution.

Set up

• Use an infusion pump for rate control.

• Flush central lines according to protocol.

• If using a single-lumen central venous line, don't use the line for blood or blood products, or give a bolus injection, administer simultaneous I.V. solutions, measure the central venous pressure, or draw blood for lab tests.

• Never add medications to a TPN solution container. Don't use a three-way stopcock unless absolutely necessary; add-on devices increase the risk of infection.

• Explain the insertion procedure to the patient.

Monitor during the infusion

• Record vital signs at least every 4 hours. Temperature elevation is one of the earliest signs of catheter-related sepsis.

• Assess the patient daily. Measure arm circumference and skinfold thickness over the triceps, if ordered.

• Perform site care and dressing changes at least three times a week (once a week for transparent semipermeable dressings), or whenever the dressing becomes wet, soiled, or nonocclusive. Use strict aseptic technique.

• Monitor for and document signs of inflammation and infection. (See *Documenting TPN.*)

• Change the I.V. administration set according to your facility's policy, and always use aseptic technique. Changes of I.V. administration sets are usually done every 24 hours for TPN.

• Do not allow TPN solutions to hang for more than 24 hours.

• The TPN solution should be clear. If you see particulate matter, cloudiness, or an oily layer in the bag when preparing to hang a TPN solution, return the bag to the pharmacy.

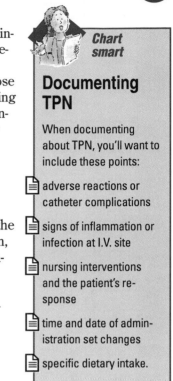

Chart smart

Documenting TPN

When documenting about TPN, you'll want to include these points:

▤ adverse reactions or catheter complications

▤ signs of inflammation or infection at I.V. site

▤ nursing interventions and the patient's response

▤ time and date of administration set changes

▤ specific dietary intake.

Follow up

• Provide emotional support, especially if eating is restricted due to the patient's condition.

• Provide frequent mouth care.

• While weaning the patient from TPN, document his dietary intake and total calorie and protein intake. Use percentages when recording food intake. For instance, chart that "The patient ate 50% of a baked potato," rather than "The patient had a good appetite."

• When discontinuing TPN, decrease the infusion slowly, depending on current glucose intake. Slowly decreasing the infusion minimizes the risk of hyperinsulinemia and resulting hypoglycemia. Weaning usually takes place over 24 to 48 hours but can be completed in 4 to 6 hours if the patient receives sufficient oral or I.V. carbohydrates.

• Report any adverse reactions to the doctor promptly.

• Prepare your patient for home care.

• Accurately document all aspects of care, according to your facility's policy.

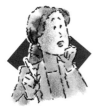

Quick quiz

1. The patient most likely to benefit from TPN is:
   A. a well-nourished patient whose GI tract will resume normal function within 10 days.
   B. a patient with a chronic, intractable condition.
   C. a patient with a nonfunctioning GI tract lasting 5 to 7 days.

Answer: C. A patient whose GI tract is nonfunctioning for 5 to 7 days is a good candidate for TPN; however, TPN has only limited value if the patient is well nourished and normal function is expected to resume within 10 days of function loss. TPN may be inappropriate for a patient with a poor prognosis.

2. When a severely malnourished patient starts receiving TPN, his lab tests show a rapid drop in potassium, magnesium, and phosphorus levels. The findings indicate:
   A. fluid shock.
   B. refeeding syndrome.
   C. hypovolemia.

Answer: B. These findings are signs and symptoms of refeeding syndrome.

3. The type of I.V. catheter recommended for TPN expected to last months or years is the:
    A. silastic catheter.
    B. polyvinyl chloride catheter.
    C. metal-winged catheter.

Answer: A. Silastic catheters are hardy catheters and may be used for months or years.

4. When preparing to hang a TPN solution, you see an oily layer in the bag. You should:
    A. gently agitate the solution to disperse the contents.
    B. hang the solution; the oily layer will disperse in time.
    C. return the solution to the pharmacy.

Answer: C. The solution should be clear. An oily layer indicates that the fluid might be contaminated or have been improperly prepared.

5. Site care and dressing changes for a patient with TPN should be performed at least:
    A. once a week.
    B. three times a week.
    C. every day.

Answer: A. Three times a week is the recommended frequency of site care and dressing changes, though more may be required due to the patient's condition or to institutional policy.

6. Infusions of lipid emulsions are useful for promoting:
    A. wound healing.
    B. coagulation in bleeding disorders.
    C. a reduction in inflammation from pancreatitis.

Answer: A. Lipid emulsions assist in wound healing in the production of red blood cells and in prostaglandin synthesis. Their use should be avoided in patients with acute pancreatitis and coagulation disorders.

7. The tip of a peripherally inserted central catheter is usually placed in the:
    A. right atrium.
    B. internal jugular vein.
    C. superior vena cava.

Answer: C. Periphally inserted central catheters are generally inserted through the basilic or cephalic vein and threaded so that the tip lies in the superior vena cava.

Scoring

☆☆☆ If you answered all seven items correctly, take yourself out for a hearty high-protein meal! You deserve it!

☆☆ If you answered four to six correctly, have a protein-packed peanut butter sandwich and a milkshake. Yummy!

☆ If you anwered fewer than four correctly, don't worry. Have a triple-decker sundae, a fudge brownie, or a luscious cinnamon roll. It won't help you learn about TPN but it will sure taste great!

Blood products

Just the facts

This chapter discusses blood products and their uses. In this chapter, you'll learn:

♦ how blood is typed

♦ what types of blood products are available and when each is used

♦ what complications can occur with transfusions

♦ how to care for a patient receiving a transfusion.

A look at blood transfusions

Transfusion therapy can restore blood volume or correct deficiencies in the blood's oxygen-carrying capacity or coagulation components. Nursing responsibilities in blood transfusion include administering blood products as well as monitoring patients receiving the therapy. Nurses need to be knowledgeable about the various blood products available in order to safely transfuse blood to their patients.

Compatibility

Blood contains various antigens that affect how compatible one person's blood is with another's. The antigens include the Rh factor, the ABO blood group, and the human leukocyte antigen (HLA) blood group. Laboratory technologists cross-match those characteristics — especially the Rh factor and the ABO blood type — to ensure compatibility between the donor's and recipient's blood prior to transfusion.

The ABOs of typing blood

The ABO method of typing blood identifies two antigens on red blood cells (RBCs), A and B. A person has both A and B antigens (type AB), only one antigen (type A or type B), or neither (type O). In the United States, 85% of the population has either type A or type O (with type O being the most common), 10% has type B, and 5% has type AB.

If a patient has A antigens, he has anti-B antibodies floating freely in his plasma. If a patient has B antigens, he has anti-A antibodies in his plasma. A patient may suffer a transfusion reaction if he receives a blood type for which he has antibodies.

Patients who have type AB blood are called universal recipients. They don't have antibodies and so may receive blood type O, A, B, or AB without having an ABO reaction. Patients with type O blood, by contrast, are universal donors. Their blood may be transfused into a person with any blood type, but since type O people have both anti-A and anti-B antibodies, they may receive only type O blood safely.

Ideally, transfusions should be done using the same type of blood as the patient's. If that's not possible, patients should receive blood that's compatible with their own blood type to keep transfusion reactions to a minimum. (See *Identifying compatible blood types.*)

In an emergency, when waiting for a crossmatch would be inadvisable, universal donor blood or plasma solution may be given. (See *Transfusing in a crisis.*)

Rh positives and negatives

About 85% of the U.S. population is Rh-positive, which means that they possess the Rh antigen, an antigen found on the membrane of RBCs. People who don't have the Rh antigen are said to be Rh-negative.

No natural antibodies to Rh exist. However, Rh-negative people may develop an Rh antibody if exposed to Rh-positive blood. The first exposure usually causes sensitization, but the second exposure may result in a fatal hemolytic reaction. Those reactions can occur during transfusions or pregnancy. (See *Fixing an Rh problem.*)

HLA story

HLA is located on the surface of circulating platelets, white blood cells (WBCs), and most tissue cells. HLA is

---

Transfusing in a crisis

In a crisis situation, where it may not be possible to wait for blood cross-matching, the following can be given until tested blood is available:

• type O Rh-negative blood ("universal donor")
• plasma protein solution
• artificial plasma substitute.

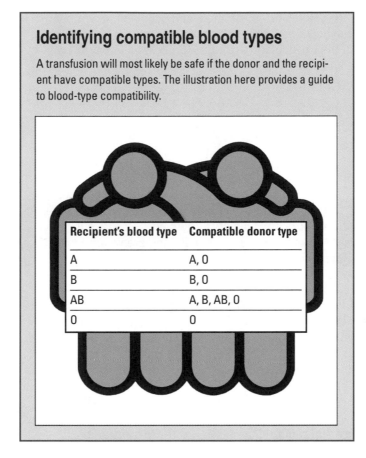

Identifying compatible blood types

A transfusion will most likely be safe if the donor and the recipient have compatible types. The illustration here provides a guide to blood-type compatibility.

Recipient's blood type	Compatible donor type
A	A, O
B	B, O
AB	A, B, AB, O
O	O

Fixing an Rh problem

If an Rh-negative person is exposed to Rh-positive blood, an injection of Rh_o (D) immune globulin can be given within 72 hours of exposure. Rh_o (D) immune globulin inhibits antibody formation. Names of common preparations include Gamulin Rh, HypRho-D, and RhoGAM.

responsible for febrile reactions in patients receiving a transfusion that contains platelets from several donors.

In that instance, an antigen-antibody reaction occurs that causes platelet destruction. As a result, the patient becomes less responsive to platelet transfusions. Giving HLA-matched platelets greatly decreases the risk of such antigen-antibody reactions. Generally, HLA tests benefit patients who receive multiple transfusions over a long period of time or frequent transfusions during a limited illness.

Types of blood products

Many blood products are available for transfusion, including whole blood, RBCs, fresh frozen plasma, cryoprecipi-

tate, granulocytes, albumin, and platelets. In addition to receiving donated blood, patients may receive transfusions
of their own blood through a process called autologous
transfusion. Here's a rundown on the various blood products, one at a time.

It's whole-some

Whole blood is rarely used unless the patient has lost
more than 25% of the total blood volume. It's generally
available in bags of 500 ml and may be used to treat hemorrhage, trauma, or major burns.

Whole blood should be avoided if fluid overload is a
concern. Stored whole blood is also high in potassium. After 24 hours, the viability and function of RBCs decreases.
ABO compatibility and Rh matching are required before
administration.

The cells have it

RBCs are prepared by removing approximately 90% of the
plasma surrounding the cells and adding an anticoagu-
lant preservative. A 250-ml bag of RBCs can help restore
or maintain the oxygen-carrying capacity of the blood in
anemic conditions or correct blood losses during or after
surgery. About 70% of the leukocytes in packed cells have
been removed, which reduces the risk of febrile, nonhemolytic reactions. ABO compatibility and Rh matching
are still required, however, for these transfusions.

Grand ol' granulocytes

Granulocyte transfusion, or WBC transfusion, is used to
treat antimicrobial-resistant neutropenia and congenital
WBC dysfunction. It's also used to treat sepsis that proves
unresponsive to antimicrobials and in granulocytopenia.
HLA compatibility tests are preferable, and Rh matching is
required. One unit of WBCs is given each day up to 5 days
or until the infection resolves.

The big thaw

Fresh frozen plasma is prepared by separating the plasma
from the RBCs and freezing it within 6 hours of collection.
The resulting solution contains plasma proteins, water, fib-
rinogen, some clotting factors, electrolytes, sugar, vitamins, minerals, hormones, and antibodies.

Fresh frozen plasma is used to treat hemorrhage, expand plasma volume, correct undetermined coagulation

factor deficiencies, replace specific clotting factors, and correct factor deficiencies resulting from liver disease. ABO compatibility testing is unnecessary; Rh matching is preferred. Large-volume transfusions of fresh frozen plasma may require correction for hypocalcemia because citric acid in the transfusion binds with calcium.

The even bigger thaw

Cryoprecipitate (also called Factor VIII) is the insoluble portion of plasma recovered from fresh frozen plasma. It's used for the treatment of von Willebrand disease, hypofibrinogenemia, Factor VIII deficiency (antihemophilic factor), hemophilia A, and disseminated intravascular coagulation. ABO compatibility testing is unnecessary.

What an extract!

Albumin is extracted from plasma and contains albumin, globulin, and other proteins. It comes in an isotonic 5% solution or in a hypertonic 25% solution and is used for patients who have acute liver failure, burns, trauma, or surgery and for hemolytic diseases of the newborn when crystalloids prove ineffective. Albumin also assists in replacing volume, preventing marked hemoconcentration, and treating hypoproteinemia with or without edema. ABO matching is unnecessary.

People, people who need platelets

Platelets are used for patients who have platelet dysfunctions or thrombocytopenia. They're also used for patients who have had multiple transfusions of stored blood, acute leukemia, or bone marrow abnormalities. Patients may have febrile or mild allergic reactions to platelet transfusions. Rh matching is preferred.

Banking on your own blood

The term autologous transfusion, also called autotransfusion, refers to the reinfusion of a patient's own blood or blood components. Indications for autologous transfusion include:
• elective surgery in which blood has been donated during a period of time leading up to before the procedure
• nonelective surgery in which blood is withdrawn immediately before surgery

• preoperative emergency where blood lost during a procedure or traumatic injury is collected, filtered, and reinfused.

Examples of operations using autologous transfusions include cardiovascular surgery, hip or knee operations, liver resection, ruptured ectopic pregnancy, and hemothorax.

Possible complications of autologous transfusions include hemolysis, embolus, coagulation disorders, and thrombocytopenia. Autologous transfusions are advantageous, however, because they avoid the risk of transfusion reaction, prevent the transmission of disease-causing organisms such as human immunodeficiency virus (HIV), and avoid depleting the local blood supply.

Disadvantages include the facts that autologous blood donors need more counseling than people who aren't donating their own blood, that blood is often wasted, and storage, preparation, and testing are expensive. In addition, some patients — such as those with malignant neoplasms, coagulopathies, excessive hemolysis, and active infections — aren't candidates for autologous transfusions.

Complications and risks

Transfusions of blood and blood products are not without risk. Concerns have surfaced over the years about the risk of transmitting disease-causing organisms — particularly HIV — through transfusions. With HIV-antibody testing being done on all donated blood and stringent criteria used to exclude high-risk blood donors, studies now show that HIV transmission through infusion is a highly rare occurrence. Testing for hepatitis B and hepatitis C viruses has become more specific, which has also helped to make the blood supply as safe as possible.

No matter how safe the blood supply is, though, transfusion reactions can still occur. (See *Guide to transfusion reactions.*) Be alert for signs of transfusion complications, including endogenous reactions caused by antigen-antibody reaction in the recipient and exogenous reactions caused by external factors related to blood administration.

Guide to transfusion reactions

This chart describes endogenous reactions (those caused by antigen-antibody reactions) and exogenous reactions (those caused by external factors in administered blood).

ENDOGENOUS

What causes it	What to look for	What to do
Allergic • Allergen in donated blood • Donor blood hypersensitive to certain drugs	Anaphylaxis (chills, facial swelling, laryngeal edema, pruritus, urticaria, wheezing), fever, nausea, vomiting	• Give antihistamines as ordered. • Monitor vital signs and continue to assess. • Give epinephrine and steroids as ordered.
Bacterial contamination • Organisms that survive the cold, such as *Pseudomonas* and *Staphylococcus*	Chills, fever, vomiting, abdominal cramping, diarrhea, shock, signs of renal failure	• Give antibiotics, steroids, and epinephrine as prescribed. • Maintain strict blood storage control. • Change administration set and filter every 4 hours or every 2 units. • Infuse each unit of blood over 2 to 4 hours; stop the infusion if it lasts more than 4 hours. • Maintain sterile technique.
Febrile • Bacterial lipopolysaccharides • antileukocyte recipient antibodies directed against donor WBCs	Fever up to 104 ° F. (40 ° C), chills, headache, facial flushing, palpitations, cough, chest tightness, increased pulse rate, flank pain	• Administer antipyretics and antihistamines as ordered. • If the patient needs further transfusions, use frozen RBCs and a leukocyte filter, and give acetaminophen as ordered.
Hemolytic • ABO or Rh incompatibility • Intra-donor incompatibility • Improper cross-matching • Improperly stored blood	Chest pain, dyspnea, facial flushing, fever, chills, hypotension, flank pain, hemoglobinuria, oliguria, bloody oozing at infusion site, burning along the vein receiving blood, shock, signs of renal failure	• Monitor vital signs, including pulse oximetry. • Manage shock with I.V .fluids, oxygen, epinephrine, and vasopressors as ordered. • Obtain post-transfusion reaction blood sample and urine sample for analysis. • Observe for signs of hemorrhage from disseminated intravascular coagulation.
Plasma protein incompatibility • Immunoglobulin A (IgA) incompatibility	Abdominal pain, diarrhea, dyspnea, chills, fever, flushing, hypotension	• Administer oxygen, fluids, epinephrine, and steroids as ordered.

(continued)

Guide to transfusion reactions (continued)

EXOGENOUS

What causes it	What to look for	What to do
Bleeding tendencies • Low platelet count in stored blood, causing thrombocytopenia	Abnormal bleeding and oozing from cuts or breaks in the skin or the gums, abnormal bruising and petechiae	• Give platelets, fresh frozen plasma, or cryoprecipitate as ordered. • Monitor platelet count.
Circulatory overload • Possibly from infusing whole blood too rapidly	Increased plasma volume, back pain, chest pain or tightness, chills, fever, dyspnea, flushed feeling, headache, hypertension, increased central venous pressure, distended neck veins	• Monitor vital signs. • Use packed RBCs instead of whole blood. • Give diuretics as ordered.
Hypocalcemia • Citrate toxicity, which occurs when citrate-treated blood is infused too rapidly and binds with calcium, causing a calcium deficiency	Arrhythmias, hypotension, muscle cramps, nausea, vomiting, seizures, tingling in fingers	• Slow or stop the transfusion if ordered. Expect a more severe reaction in hypothermic patients or patients with elevated potassium levels. • Give calcium gluconate I.V. slowly if ordered.
Hypothermia • Rapid infusion of large amounts of cold blood, which decreases body temperature	Chills, shaking, hypotension, arrhythmias (especially bradycardia), cardiac arrest if core temperature falls below 86° F (30° C.)	• Stop the transfusion. • Warm the patient. • Obtain an electrocardiogram (ECG). • Warm the blood if the transfusion is resumed.
Potassium intoxication • An abnormally high level of potassium in stored plasma caused by hemolysis of RBCs	Diarrhea, intestinal colic, flaccidity, muscle twitching, oliguria, signs of renal failure, bradycardia, ECG changes with tall, peaked T waves, cardiac arrest	• Obtain an ECG. • Give Kayexalate as ordered. • Give glucose 50% and insulin, bicarbonate, or calcium as ordered to force potassium into cells.

Giving a transfusion

Administering a blood transfusion of any kind requires cooperation and vigilance on the part of a number of personnel, from the blood bank technologist to the nurse at the bedside to the support personnel throughout the facility. Follow these steps when caring for a patient having a blood transfusion.

Before starting

Prior to starting a blood transfusion, you'll want to take these actions.

• Be sure the patient or next of kin has signed an informed consent form. Explain the procedure to the patient. Many people are still afraid of receiving a blood transfusion due to the fear of contracting HIV. Educate the patient as indicated about the extremely low risk of infection due to highly effective screening procedures.

• Review your facility's policy for administering blood.

• Assess your patient, documenting vital signs and other pertinent information. Notify the doctor if the patient has a fever of 100° F (37.8° C) or higher prior to the transfusion.

• Keep in mind your patient's other treatment needs. If he is receiving an I.V. medication that can't be mixed with blood products, for instance, another I.V. line may need to be inserted.

• Check the orders for the type of transfusion to be given. (See *How to avoid transfusion errors,* page 302.)

• Triple-check the identity of your patient to ensure that the right patient receives the right transfusion at the right time.

• Ask the patient if he has ever had a transfusion reaction and if so, under what conditions the transfusion was given, and how it was resolved.

During the transfusion

While the transfusion is in progress, take these actions:

• Maintain sterile technique when setting up and transfusing blood and its components.

• Blood products should be infused through at least an 18 or 20G I.V. catheter. Never use a smaller gauge catheter or needle.

• Obtain normal saline solution, gloves, a gown, and a face shield in addition to the Y-type administration set (with filter).

• Transfuse blood using a Y-type I.V. set, and infuse the blood over 2 to 4 hours.

• When you start the transfusion, remain with the patient and observe him carefully for the first 15 minutes. (See *Teaching about blood transfusions.*) Most acute adverse reactions occur within that time period, though delayed reactions can occur up to 2 weeks later. Recheck vital signs 15 minutes after hanging the blood, and again every hour.

• A pressure bag or a specialized infusion pump may be used to administer blood more rapidly.

Flushing and filters

• Use the normal saline solution as a flush solution before and after infusing blood products. You may need to flush the I.V. line during the transfusion if the blood is dripping too slowly. Do not use a dextrose solution, which can cause hemolysis, or lactated Ringer's solution, which contains calcium and can clog the tubing.

• Filters work best when completely filled with blood. Special filters are available to trap leukocytes (leukocyte-depleting filters) or tiny clots and debris that can get through standard filters (micro-aggregate filters).

• In transfusing whole blood, reduce the risk of a reaction by adding a microfilter to trap platelets.

Getting blood ready

• Obtain blood from the lab *when you're ready to hang it.* Check the bag for leaks, discoloration, bubbles, and clots. Return questionable products to the blood bank.

• Do not use a nursing-unit refrigerator to store blood because the temperature may be inaccurate and the blood could be damaged. Blood that isn't refrigerated for 4 hours or more is at high risk for bacterial contamination.

• If the order calls for blood to be warmed prior to administration, use a blood-warming device and special tubing. The temperature should be maintained between 89.6° and 98.6° F (32° and 37° C). Blood-warming devices are useful when transfusing large quantities of blood.

How to avoid transfusion errors

Proper identification of your patient and the blood product to be given is essential. Following your facility's policy:

• Match the patient's name, medical record number, ABO and Rh status, and blood bank identification numbers with the label on the blood bag.

• Check the expiration date.

• Have another nurse verify the information.

• Sign the blood slip, filling in the required data. The blood slip will prove useful in the event of an adverse reaction.

• Double-check the doctor's order to make sure you're transfusing the correct product.

• Be sure that the type and cross-match were done within 48 hours, an FDA requirement for transfusions.

Giving platelets

- Transfuse platelets over 15 minutes. Premedicate with antipyretics or antihistamines as ordered if patient history includes a platelet transfusion reaction.
- Avoid giving platelets when a patient is febrile.
- Check the platelet count 1 hour after the transfusion ends.

Giving albumin and other fluids

- Do not mix albumin with other solutions.
- A solution of 5% albumin is equivalent to 12.5 g or 250 ml. A 25% solution is equivalent to 25 g or 50 ml.
- Be aware that albumin may be given as a volume expander until cross-matching for a whole blood transfusion is completed.
- Albumin should not be used for severe anemia and should be given cautiously in cardiac and pulmonary patients. When used for a patient with a cardiac or pulmonary disorder, heart failure may occur.
- Factor VIII's half-life is 8 to 10 hours, which means that repeated transfusions at those intervals should be given to maintain normal Factor VIII levels.
- If a patient will receive WBCs, premedicate him with diphenhydramine hydrochloride (Benadryl), if prescribed, and give antipyretics for fever. Agitate the blood container to prevent cells from settling and unintentional delivery of a bolus infusion. WBC transfusions may be given along with antibiotics to treat infection but should not be given with amphotericin B.

> **Parting points**
>
> ## Teaching about blood transfusions
>
> Be sure to cover these topics with your patient and evaluate his learning:
> - need for transfusion
> - reason for informed consent, if required
> - risks
> - length of time required
> - related procedures, such as vital sign checks and follow-up blood tests
> - adverse reactions and when to report them
> - activity restrictions during the transfusion.

After the transfusion

After the transfusion finishes, you'll want to take these actions.
- Stop the transfusion immediately if you see signs of an adverse reaction. Continue to assess the patient as you remove the blood and tubing, and hang an infusion of normal saline solution to keep the vein open.
- Observe for signs of circulatory overload, especially in the elderly. Carefully monitor the rate of infusion and the I.V. site.
- Obtain laboratory tests as ordered to determine the effectiveness of the treatment. The hemoglobin of an adult

patient receiving one unit of packed RBCs should increase by 1 g/dl. The hematocrit should increase by 3%. You should see a rise in platelets of 5,000 to 10,000/mm³ with each unit of platelets infused and an improvement in prothrombin time and partial thromboplastin time after giving clotting factors.

• Document your administration of a blood product according to facility policy. (See *Documenting transfusions*.)

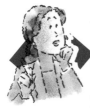

Quick quiz

1. If a hematologically stable patient receives one unit of RBCs, you can expect an increase in:
    A. hematocrit by 3% and hemoglobin by 1 g/dl.
    B. hematocrit by 5% and hemoglobin by 2 g/dl.
    C. platelet count by 5,000/mm³.

Answer: A. The hematocrit should rise by 3% and the hemoglobin by 1 g/dl.

2. The most common blood type in the United States is:
    A. type A.
    B. type B.
    C. type O.

Answer: C. Type O blood is the most common blood type in the United States.

3. Whole blood is rarely used unless the patient has lost more than:
    A. 10% of the total blood volume.
    B. 25% of the total blood volume.
    C. 50% of the total blood volume.

Answer: B. Twenty-five percent is generally considered the cutoff for using whole blood.

4. An Rh-negative mother would be most likely to have a serious hemolytic reaction when:
    A. she is first exposed to Rh-positive blood.
    B. she delivers her first child.
    C. she has a second exposure to Rh-positive blood.

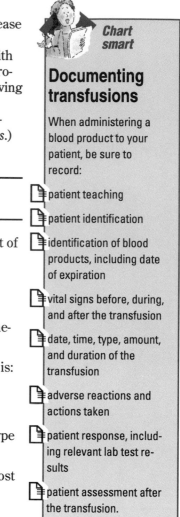

Chart smart

Documenting transfusions

When administering a blood product to your patient, be sure to record:

- patient teaching
- patient identification
- identification of blood products, including date of expiration
- vital signs before, during, and after the transfusion
- date, time, type, amount, and duration of the transfusion
- adverse reactions and actions taken
- patient response, including relevant lab test results
- patient assessment after the transfusion.

Answer: C. A mother initiates antibody formation after the first exposure. By the second exposure, the antibodies already present react and cause a hemolytic reaction to the infused Rh-positive blood.

5. To expand plasma volume or to replace clotting factors, you would expect to give:
    A. albumin.
    B. fresh frozen plasma.
    C. whole blood.

Answer: B. Fresh frozen plasma would be the product-of-choice for those conditions and others.

6. Ten minutes after you start an infusion of packed RBCs, your patient complains of chills, chest and back pain, and nausea. His face is flushed, and he is anxious. His blood pressure is 90/60 mm Hg; temperature, 101.5° F (38.6° C); heart rate, 120 beats/minute; and respirations, 24/minute. Your assessment indicates that the patient is experiencing:
    A. an HLA antibody-antigen reaction.
    B. a hemolytic reaction.
    C. circulatory overload.

Answer: B. The signs and symptoms indicate a hemolytic reaction.

7. To prevent an antibody-antigen reaction, a patient with type B blood should receive:
    A. type A or O blood only.
    B. type B or O blood only.
    C. type AB or O blood only.

Answer: B. A person with type B blood should receive only type B or O blood. Type A or AB blood would most likely cause a reaction.

8. Removal of most leukocytes in a unit of packed cells helps to prevent:
    A. an HLA antibody-antigen reaction.
    B. a febrile, nonhemolytic reaction.
    C. a plasma protein incompatibility reaction.

Answer: B. About 70% of the leukocytes in packed cells have been removed, which reduces the risk of febrile, nonhemolytic reactions.

Scoring

★★★ If you answered all eight items correctly, you've done a great job! Can you say *transfusion expert?* We knew you could!

★★ If you answered five to seven correctly, super! You're a platelet-giving powerhouse.

★ If you answered fewer than five correctly, no prob. You're simply plasma-rrrific!

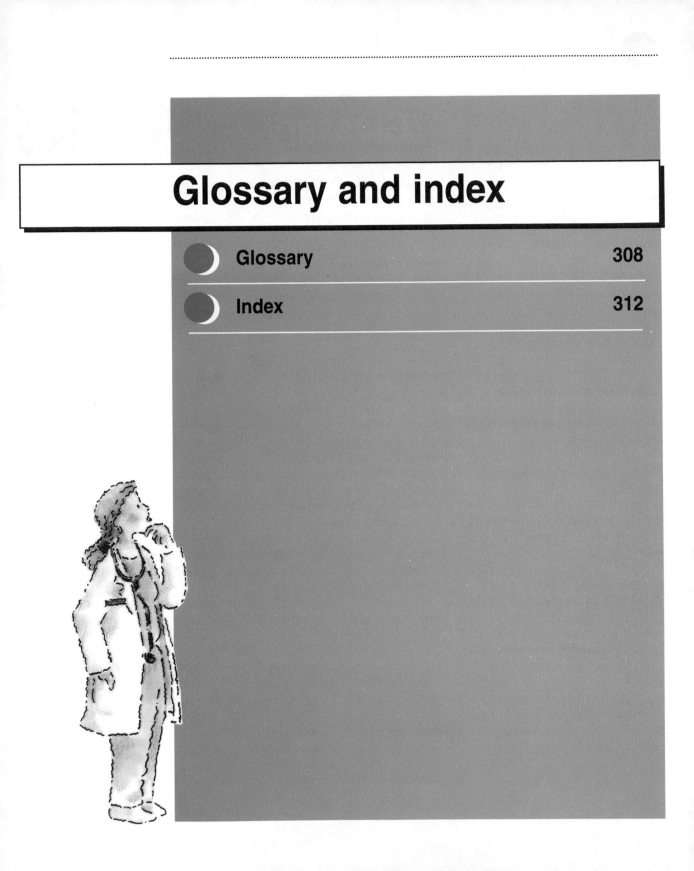

Glossary and index

Glossary

absorption: taking up of a substance by cells or tissues

acid: substance that donates hydrogen ions

acid-base balance: mechanisms by which the body's acids and bases are kept in balance

acidosis: condition resulting from the accumulation of acid or the loss of base

adenosine triphosphate: vital phosphorus-containing compound that represents stored energy in the cells; needed to carry out the body's functions

air embolism: air bubble in the vascular system

aldosterone: adrenocortical hormone that regulates sodium, potassium, and fluid balance

alkalosis: condition resulting from the accumulation of base or the loss of acid

anion: negatively charged ion, of which proteins and chloride, bicarbonate, and phosphorus are among the body's most plentiful

anion gap: measurement of the difference between the amount of sodium and the amount of bicarbonate and chloride in the blood

antibody: substance produced by the body that reacts with an antigen and causes outward signs or symptoms of that reaction

antidiuretic hormone: hormone made by the hypothalamus and released by the pituitary gland that decreases the production of urine by increasing the reabsorption of water by the renal tubules

antigen: substance that causes the body to form antibodies against it

anuria: absence of urine formation, or less than 100 ml of urine in 24 hours

arterial blood gas (ABG) analysis: measurement of arterial pH, partial pressures of oxygen and carbon dioxide, and other levels used to evaluate acid-base balance and pulmonary function

autologous transfusion (autotransfusion): reinfusion of the patient's own blood or blood components

base: substance that accepts hydrogen ions

buffer: substance that, when combined with acids or bases, minimizes changes in pH

calcification: deposit of calcium phosphate in soft tissues that can occur with prolonged high serum phosphorus levels and can lead to organ dysfunction

calcium: positively charged ion involved in the structure and function of bones, impulse transmission, blood-clotting process, and the normal function of heart and skeletal muscle

carboxyhemoglobin: molecule of carbon monoxide and hemoglobin that prevents the normal transfer of oxygen and carbon dioxide, a condition that can cause asphyxiation or death

cation: positively charged ion, of which sodium, potassium, calcium, magnesium, and hydrogen are the body's most abundant

cation-exchange resin: medication used to lower serum potassium levels by exchanging sodium ions for potassium ions in the GI tract

cerebral edema: increase in the brain's fluid content; may result from correcting hypernatremia too rapidly

chemoreceptor: special cell that senses the presence of specific chemicals in the bloodstream

chloride: most abundant anion in extracellular fluid; maintains serum osmolality and fluid, electrolyte, and acid-base balance

Chvostek's sign: abnormal spasm of facial muscles that may indicate hypocalcemia or tetany; tested by lightly tapping the facial nerve (upper cheek, below the zygomatic bone)

colloid: large molecule, such as albumin, that normally doesn't cross the capillary membrane

colloid osmotic pressure: pressure exerted by colloids in the vasculature

compensation: process by which one system (renal or respiratory) attempts to correct an acid-base disturbance in the other system

crystalloid: solute, such as sodium or glucose, which crosses the capillary membrane in solution

deep tendon reflex: involuntary muscle contraction in response to a sudden stretch that can be elicited by a hammer or finger tap on a tendon at its insertion

dehydration: condition in which the loss of water from cells causes them to shrink

2,3-diphosphoglycerate (2,3-DPG): compound in red blood cells that contains phosphorus and facilitates the transfer of oxygen from hemoglobin to the tissues

diuretics: class of medications acting at various points along the nephron to increase urine output, resulting in the loss of water and electrolytes

electrolyte: solute that separates in a solvent into electrically charged particles called ions

extravasation: leakage of intravascular fluid into surrounding tissue; can be caused by such medications as chemotherapeutics, dopamine, and calcium solutions that produce blistering and, eventually, tissue necrosis

Factor VIII (cryoprecipitate): antihemophilic factor recovered from fresh frozen plasma; instrumental in blood clotting

glomerular filtration rate: rate at which the glomerulae in the kidneys filter blood; normally occurs at a rate of 125 ml/minute

granulocytopenia: fewer than normal number of granular leukocytes in the blood

hydrostatic pressure: pressure exerted by fluid in the blood vessels

hypercalcemia: excess of calcium in extracellular fluid; when the total serum calcium level is above 10.1 mg/dl or the ionized calcium level is above 5.1 mg/dl

hypercapnia: increase in partial pressure of carbon dioxide in arterial blood greater than 45 mm Hg

hyperchloremia: excess of chloride in the extracellular fluid; occurs when the serum chloride level is above 106 mEq/L

hyperchloremic metabolic acidosis: condition resulting from a deficit in bicarbonate ions and an increase in chloride ions, which causes a decrease in pH

hyperkalemia: excess potassium in the extracellular fluid; occurs when the serum potassium level is greater than 5 mEq/L

hypermagnesemia: excess magnesium in the extracellular fluid; occurs when the serum magnesium level is above 2.5 mEq/L

hypernatremia: excess sodium in the extracellular fluid; occurs when the serum sodium level is above 145 mEq/L

hyperphosphatemia: excess phosphorus in the extracellular fluid; occurs when the serum phosphorus level is above 2.6 mEq/L

hypervolemia: excess of fluid and solutes in extracellular fluid; can be caused by increased fluid intake, fluid shifts in the body, or renal failure

hypocalcemia: deficit of calcium in extracellular fluid; occurs when the total calcium level is below 8.9 mg/dl or the ionized calcium level is below 4.5 mg/dl

hypocapnia: decrease in the partial pressure of carbon dioxide in arterial blood (less than 35 mm Hg)

hypochloremia: deficit of chloride in extracellular fluid; occurs when the serum chloride level is below 96 mEq/L

hypochloremic metabolic alkalosis: condition caused by a deficit in chloride and a subsequent increase in bicarbonate that ultimately causes an increase in pH

hypokalemia: deficit in potassium in extracellular fluid; occurs when the serum potassium level is below 3.5 mEq/L

hypomagnesemia: deficit in magnesium in extracellular fluid; occurs when the serum magnesium level is below 1.5 mEq/L

hyponatremia: deficit of sodium in extracellular fluid; occurs when the serum sodium level is below 135 mEq/L

hypophosphatemia: deficit of phosphorus in extracellular fluid; occurs when the serum phosphorus level is below 1.8 mEq/L

hypotonic: solution that has fewer solutes than another solution

hypovolemia: condition marked by the loss of fluid and solutes from extracellular fluid that, if left untreated, can progress to hypovolemic shock

hypovolemic shock: potentially life-threatening condition in which a decreased blood volume leads to low cardiac output and poor tissue perfusion

hypoxemia: deficiency of oxygen in arterial blood (lower than 80 mm Hg)

hypoxia: deficiency of oxygen in the tissues

infiltration: leakage of fluid from a blood vessel into surrounding tissue

interstitial fluid: fluid surrounding cells that, with plasma, makes up extracellular fluid

isotonic solution: solution that has the same concentration of solutes as another solution

magnesium: cation (positively charged ion) found primarily in intracellular fluid that promotes efficient energy use, aids protein synthesis, regulates nerve and muscle impulses, and promotes cardiovascular function

metabolic acidosis: condition in which excess acid or reduced bicarbonate in the blood drops the arterial blood pH below 7.35

metabolic alkalosis: condition in which excess bicarbonate or reduced acid in the blood increases the arterial blood pH above 7.45

oliguria: low urine output; less than 400 ml/24 hours

orthostatic or postural hypotension: drop in blood pressure and increase in heart rate that occurs when the body changes position and that can be caused by a loss of circulating blood volume

osmolality: concentration of a solution; expressed in milliosmols per kilogram of solution

osmolarity: concentration of a solution; expressed in milliosmols per liter of solution

osmotic pressure: pressure exerted by a solute in solution on a semipermeable membrane

osmoreceptors: special sensing cells in the hypothalamus that respond to changes in the osmolality of blood

osteodystrophy: defective bone development; can occur in the face of prolonged elevated serum phosphorus levels

osteomalacia: softening of bone tissues due to demineralization; often accompanies chronic hypocalcemia

paralytic ileus: obstruction of the bowel due to paralysis of the bowel wall

paresthesia: numbness, tingling, or other abnormal sensations occurring with no apparent cause; possible symptom of electrolyte imbalance

peripherally inserted central catheter (PICC): catheter inserted through a vein above the antecubital area that causes fewer and less severe adverse effects than a traditional central venous catheter and can be left in place for several months

petechiae: minute hemorrhagic spots in the skin

pH: measurement of the percentage of hydrogen ions in a solution; the normal arterial pH is 7.35 to 7.45

phosphorus: anion, or negatively charged ion, located primarily in intracellular fluid and involved in maintaining bone and cell structure, maintaining storage of energy in cells, and aiding oxygen delivery to the tissues

pneumothorax: presence of air or gas in the pleural cavity

potassium: major intracellular cation involved in skeletal muscle contraction, fluid distribution, osmotic pressure, and acid-base balance, and maintaining the heartbeat

pulmonary edema: abnormal fluid accumulation in the lungs; a life-threatening condition

pyelonephritis: inflammation of the renal parenchyma, calyces, and pelvis

reabsorption: taking in, or absorbing, a substance again

renin-angiotensin system: renal mechanism in which renin and angiotensin regulate blood pressure and water and sodium levels

resorption: loss of a substance through physiologic or pathologic means, such as loss of calcium from bone

respiratory acidosis: acid-base disturbance caused by a failure of the lungs to eliminate sufficient carbon dioxide; the partial pressure of arterial carbon dioxide is above 45 mm Hg and the pH is below 7.35

respiratory alkalosis: acid-base imbalance that occurs when the lungs eliminate more carbon dioxide than normal; the partial pressure of arterial carbon dioxide is below 35 mm Hg and the pH is above 7.45

respiratory failure: condition that occurs when the lungs can't sufficiently maintain arterial oxygenation or eliminate carbon dioxide

rhabdomyolysis: disorder in which skeletal muscle is destroyed; causes intracellular contents to spill into extracellular fluid

silastic: silicone rubber, the preferred material for sterile catheters intended for long-term total parenteral nutrition because it's more flexible, durable, and biocompatible than plastic

sodium: major cation of extracellular fluid involved in regulating extracellular fluid volume, transmitting nerve impulses, and maintaining acid-base balance

solute: molecules or ions dissolved in a solution

solvent: fluid in which a solute is dissolved

speed shock: dangerous condition that occurs when I.V. solutions or medications are given too rapidly; characterized by almost immediate facial flushing, irregular pulse, severe headache, decreased blood pressure, loss of consciousness, and cardiac arrest

tetany: condition caused by abnormal calcium metabolism and characterized by painful muscle spasms, cramps, and sharp flexion of the wrist and ankle joints

third-space fluid shift: movement of fluid out of the intravascular space into another body space, such as the abdominal cavity

Trousseau's sign: carpal (wrist) spasm elicited by applying a blood pressure cuff to the upper arm and inflating it to a pressure 20 mm Hg above the patient's systolic blood pressure; indicates the presence of hypocalcemia

uremia: excess of urea and other nitrogenous wastes in the blood

uremic frost: powdery deposits of urea and uric acid salts on the skin, especially the face; caused by the excretion of nitrogenous compounds into sweat

von Willebrand's disease: syndrome characterized in part by a tendency to bleed and a prolonged bleeding time

water intoxication: condition in which excess water in the cells results in cellular swelling

Index